COGNITION AND ACTION IN SKILLED BEHAVIOUR

ADVANCES IN PSYCHOLOGY

55

Editors:

G. STELMACH

P. A. VROON

NORTH-HOLLAND
AMSTERDAM · NEW YORK · OXFORD · TOKYO

COGNITION AND ACTION IN SKILLED BEHAVIOUR

Edited by

Ann M. COLLEY

and

John R. BEECH

Department of Psychology
University of Leicester
Leicester LE1 7RH
U.K.

1988
NORTH-HOLLAND
AMSTERDAM · NEW YORK · OXFORD · TOKYO

ISBN: 0 444 70493 0

Publishers:
ELSEVIER SCIENCE PUBLISHERS B.V.
P.O. Box 1991
1000 BZ Amsterdam
The Netherlands

Sole distributors for the U.S.A. and Cananda:
ELSEVIER SCIENCE PUBLISHING COMPANY, INC.
52 Vanderbilt Avenue
New York, N.Y. 10017
U.S.A.

LIBRARY OF CONGRESS
Library of Congress Cataloging-in-Publication Data

Cognition and action in skilled behaviour / edited by Ann M. Colley and John R. Beech.
p. cm. -- (Advances in psychology ; 55)
Based on selected papers from the First International Conference on Skilled Behaviour, held Apr. 1987 at Sussex University, sponsored by the Cognitive Section of the British Psychological Society and by the Dept. of Psychology of the University of Leicester.
Includes bibliographies and indexes.
ISBN 0-444-70493-0 (Netherlands)
1. Motor ability--Congresses. 2. Cognition--Congresses.
I. Colley, Ann M. II. Beech, John R. III. International Conference on Skilled Behaviour (1st : 1987 : Sussex University) IV. British Psychological Society. Cognitive Section. V. University of Leicester. Dept. of Psychology. VI. Series: Advances in psychology (Amsterdam, Netherlands) ; 55.
BF295.C63 1988
152.3--dc19 88-22775
CIP

PRINTED IN THE NETHERLANDS

PREFACE

In April 1987, the First International Conference on Skilled Behaviour took place at Sussex University. This conference was co-sponsored by the Cognitive Section of the British Psychological Society and by our own university department. It grew from a conviction that recent advances in different areas of skills research had not been presented and discussed in a major U.K. conference. The papers presented at the conference covered aspects of motor skills, cognitive skills, social skills and clinical skills. This volume contains chapters based upon selected papers on motor and cognitive skills.

The distribution of papers submitted to this conference by area, served to support an observation that we had previously made in surveying the skills literature; that "skills" is very often taken to be synonymous with perceptual-motor skills. Although the general applicability of a skills framework has been long acknowledged (see for example Fitts & Posner, 1967), researchers have been slow to look at performance in purely cognitive tasks such as memory and problem-solving from this viewpoint. Many skills have both motor and cognitive components. The relative importance and complexity of these varies with the skill in question. In recent years, considerable advances have been made in our understanding of movement skills. What is clear from this volume, and from many other publications, is that mainstream research into the acquisition and control of skilled movement has taken on board the terminology and major ideas from action systems theory. These have not necessarily been adopted in their strongest form, but their influence is discernible in many of the chapters here. In parallel with these developments in the movement skills area, have been recent theoretical advances in the central areas of memory and learning in cognitive psychology. These have had far-reaching implications for our understanding of a wide range of skills, from purely cognitive tasks to those which have a substantial motor component.

As might be expected from a conference with rather a general theme, the chapters in the book represent a number of different approaches to the study of skilled action. Three of the four sections of the book are collections of individual presentations and are grouped thematically. The remaining section is based upon a lively, but good-humoured, symposium on "The action systems / motor systems controversy" which was organised by Onno Meijer and Piet van Wieringen.

The chapters in the first two sections are concerned with the theoretical issues of programming and coordination, and the learning and performance of skilled movements, respectively. This latter section contains papers with some practical implications for everyday skills. Issues raised in the third section on action systems and motor systems approaches to motor control are basic to much of the research reviewed in this volume. There have been several recent debates on the role of cognitive processes in motor control, and the usefulness of the "psychomotor" approach (see, for example, the commentaries on Zanone and Hauert's (1987) arguments for a cognitive approach to motor control). This section summarises the various theoretical positions in this debate, and also contains chapters based on individual papers which present relevant empirical findings. The fourth section contains chapters on cognitive processes in skilled performance.

We gratefully acknowledge the assistance and support of the following individuals who have helped to make this volume possible. First we must thank John Whiting, who encouraged us to publish these proceedings, and who gave us help and advice throughout the preparations for the conference and for the book. His department has contributed substantially to both the conference and this book. Sue Lloyd made an excellent job of typing the camera-ready copy for this book, amid delays and minor calamities (not all book-related). Dr. K. Michielson and the staff at North-Holland have been both efficient and patient.

We would also like to thank colleagues who have given up their time to referee one or more of the chapters in this book:

Phillip Bairstow
Alan Beggs
Eric Brodie
Roy Davis
Ken Flowers
David Frohlich
Kerry Greer
David Hale
Nigel Harvey
Laurence Hartley
Dennis Holding
Ian Howarth
Marc Jeannerod
Beth Kerr
Tony Lambert
Judith Laszlo
David Lee
David Legge
Bob Logie
Carol McGuinness
Ruud Meulenbroek
Neil Morris
Helen Ross
Henry Shaffer
Martin Sheridan
Mary Smyth
Will Spijkers
David Sugden
John Wann
William Warren Jr.
John Whiting

References

Fitts, P.M. & Posner, M.I. (1967). Human performance. Belmont, C.A.: Brooks/Cole.

Zanone, P. & Hauert, C. (1987). For a cognitive conception of motor processes: A provocative standpoint. European Bulletin of Cognitive Psychology, 7, 109-129.

Leicester, U.K.
December 1987

Ann M. Colley
John R. Beech

CONTENTS

LIST OF CONTRIBUTORS

JOHN ANNETT - Department of Psychology, University of Warwick, Coventry, CV4 7AL, U.K.
ALAN BADDELEY - MRC Applied Psychology Unit, 15 Chaucer Road, Cambridge, CB2 2EF, U.K.
PHILLIP BAIRSTOW - Department of Developmental Paediatrics, Institute of Child Health, The Wolfson Centre, Mecklenburgh Square, London, WC1N 2AP.
JON BARTRIP - Department of Developmental Paediatrics, Institute of Child Health, The Wolfson Centre, Mecklenburgh Square, London, WC1N 2AP, U.K.
JOHN R. BEECH - Department of Psychology, University of Leicester, Leicester, LE1 7RH, U.K.
P.J. BEEK - Department of Psychology, Faculty of Human Movement Sciences, The Free University, Postbus 7161, 1007 Amsterdam, The Netherlands.
W.D.A. BEGGS - Blind Mobility Research Unit, Department of Psychology, University of Nottingham, Nottingham, NG7 2RD, U.K.
M. BUEKERS - Institute for Physical Education, Katholieke Universiteit Leuven, Tervuursevest 101, B-3030 Leuven (Heverlee), Belgium.
CLAUDIA CARELLO - Center for the Ecological Study of Perception and Action, Department of Psychology, University of Connecticut, Box U-20, 406 Cross Campus Road, Storrs, Connecticut 06268, U.S.A.
ROBERT W. CHRISTINA - Motor Behavior Laboratory, The Pennsylvania State University, University Park, Pennsylvania 16802, U.S.A.
ANN M. COLLEY - Department of Psychology, University of Leicester, Leicester, LE1 7RH, U.K.
EMANUEL DONCHIN - Department of Psychology, University of Illinois, Urbana, Illinois 61801, U.S.A.
C.M. FABER - Department of Psychology, Faculty of Human Movement Sciences, The Free University, Postbus 7161, 1007 MC Amsterdam, The Netherlands.
K.A. FLOWERS - Department of Psychology, University of Hull, Hull, HU6 7RX, U.K.
DAVID M. FROHLICH - Alvey DHSS Demonstrator Project, Department of Sociology, University of Surrey, Guildford, GU2 5XH U.K.
K.J. GILHOOLY - Department of Psychology, University of Aberdeen, King's College, Old Aberdeen, AB9 2UB, U.K.
A.J.K. GREEN - Department of Psychology, University of Aberdeen, King's College, Old Aberdeen, AB9 2UB, U.K.
YVES GUIARD - C.N.R.S., L.N.F., 31 chemin Joseph Aiguier, B.P.71,

13402 Marseille Cedex 9, France.
NIGEL HARVEY – Department of Psychology, University College London, Gower Street, London, WC1E 6BT, U.K.
C.I. HOWARTH – Department of Psychology, University of Nottingham, Nottingham, NG7 2RD, U.K.
BARRY G. HUGHES – Motor Behavior Laboratory, University of Wisconsin, Madison, Wisconsin 53706, U.S.A.
WOUTER HULSTIJN – Department of Experimental Psychology, University of Nijmegen, Postbus 9104, 4500 Nijmegen, The Netherlands.
DYLAN M. JONES – Department of Applied Psychology, U.W.I.S.T., Llwyn-y-Grant, Penylan, Cardiff, CF3 7UX, U.K.
JUDITH I. LASZLO – Department of Psychology, University of Western Australia, Nedlands, Western Australia 6009.
J.L. LEAVITT – Faculty of Human Kinetics, University of Windsor, Windsor, Ontario, Canada, N9B 3P4.
ELIZABETH LIMONS – Motor Behavior Laboratory, The Pennsylvania State University, University Park, Pennsylvania 16802, U.S.A.
ROBERT LOGIE – Department of Psychology, University of Aberdeen, King's College, Old Aberdeen, AB9 2UB, U.K.
C.L. MACKENZIE – Department of Kinesiology, University of Waterloo, Waterloo, Ontario, Canada, N2L 3G1.
CLARE MADDEN – Department of Applied Psychology, U.W.I.S.T., Llwyn-y-Grant, Penylan, Cardiff, CF3 7UX, U.K.
AMIR MANE – Department of Psychology, University of Illinois, Urbana, Illinois 61801, U.S.A.
RONALD G. MARTENIUK – Department of Kinesiology, University of Waterloo, Waterloo, Ontario, Canada, N2L 3G1.
P. MEUGENS – Department of Physical Education, Katholieke Universiteit Leuven, Tervuursevest 101, B-3030 Leuven (Heverlee), Belgium.
RUUD G.J. MEULENBROEK – Department of Experimental Psychology, University of Nijmegen, Postbus 9104, 6500 Nijmegen, The Netherlands.
CHRISTOPHER MILES – Department of Applied Psychology, U.W.I.S.T., Llwyn-y-Grant, Penylan, Cardiff, CF3 7UX, U.K.
J. PAUWELS – Department of Physical Education, Katholieke Universiteit Leuven, Tervuursevest 101, B-3030 Leuven (Heverlee), Belgium.
JIM G. PHILLIPS – Motor Behavior Laboratory, University of Wisconsin, Madison, Wisconsin 53706, U.S.A.
URSULA T. ROLFE – St. Louis University Medical Center, 221 North Grand Blvd., St. Louis, Missouri 63103, U.S.A.
G.J.P. SAVELSBERGH – Department of Psychology, Faculty of Human Movement Sciences, The Free University, Postbus 7161, 1007 MC Amsterdam, The Netherlands.
JOHN B. SHEA – Motor Behavior Laboratory, The Pennsylvania State University, University Park, Pennsylvania 16802, U.S.A.
RUSSELL SHEPTAK – Department of Psychology, University of Illinois, Urbana, Illinois 61801, U.S.A.
MARTIN R. SHERIDAN – Department of Psychology, University of Hull, Hull, HU6 7RX, U.K.
BEN SIDAWAY – Motor Behavior Laboratory, The Pennsylvania State University, University Park, Pennsylvania 16802, U.S.A.

S.P. SWINNEN - I.L.O. Group Medical Sciences, Katholieke Universiteit Leuven, Tervuursevest 101, B-3030 Leuven (Heverlee), Belgium.

M.T. TURVEY - Center for the Ecological Study of Perception and Action, Department of Psychology, University of Connecticut, Box U-20, 406 Cross Campus Road, Storrs, Connecticut 06268, U.S.A.

GERARD P. VAN GALEN - Department of Experimental Psychology, University of Nijmegen, Postbus 9014, 6500 Nijmegen, The Netherlands.

P.C.W. VAN WIERINGEN - Department of Psychology, Faculty of Human Movement Sciences, The Free University, Postbus 7161, 1007 MC Amsterdam, The Netherlands.

C.B. WALTER - Department of Physical Education, University of Illinois, P.O. Box 4348, Chicago, Illinois 60680, U.S.A.

H.T.A. WHITING - Department of Psychology, Faculty of Human Movement Sciences, The Free University, Postbus 7161, 1007 MC Amsterdam, The Netherlands.

Cognition and Action in Skilled Behaviour
A.M. Colley and J.R. Beech (Editors)

GROUNDS FOR RECONCILIATION : SOME PRELIMINARY THOUGHTS ON COGNITION AND ACTION

Ann M. Colley and John R. Beech
University of Leicester

One of the major issues to emerge from recent perspectives on the nature of attention, memory and motor control, concerns the way in which cognitive processes interact with the motor system to produce planned coordinated action. How do intentions and strategies result in well-executed movement? Tasks vary in the amount of cognitive processing they require, and, within tasks, the stage of skill acquisition will affect the nature of the processing that is undertaken. Adams (1987) has recently pointed out that theories of action have given little consideration to how perception and action are linked, and that we have little systematic knowledge of the relationship between language and action. The amount of control that can be exerted on lower-level motor processes by higher level cognitive processes should be of central concern in any account of the acquisition of skilled movement.

This issue has been taken up by the action systems theorists. Their view, which has resulted from the influence of Bernstein (1967), and the ecological approach of Turvey, Kugler and collaborators (e.g. Kugler, Kelso, & Turvey, 1982; Turvey, 1977; Turvey & Carello, 1986; Turvey & Kugler, 1984; Turvey, Shaw, & Mace, 1978), is that the acquisition of skilled movement occurs when movement structures are constrained to behave in a manner appropriate for the attainment of a particular goal. More specifically, ensembles of motor units (muscles, joints, etc.) are constrained to act as functional units or coordinative structures, thereby reducing the degrees of freedom which apply to the control of a given task, and providing the basic organisation of movement. Reflexes, or functional configurations thereof, may provide the basis for coordinative structures (Turvey, 1977). Global constraints, or organisational invariants, specify the characteristics of different types of movements. Local constraints tune a movement to its environment and are defined by the interaction between the actor and the environment. In the initial stages, acquiring a movement skill consists of discovering the appropriate organisational invariant.

The system of global and local constraints proposed by ecological theorists carries with it the implication that control of movement is distributed at a number of levels in the nervous system and is heterarchical in nature. Hierarchical control, espoused by many early theorists (e.g. Fitts, 1964; Miller, Galanter, & Pribram, 1960), uses the notion that executive control at the highest level is responsible for a global specification of how a movement, or sequence of movements will be executed. Lower levels of the hierarchy provide more detailed specifications for the enactment of the movement. However, it is apparent from neurophysiological and anatomical evidence that the relationship between higher and lower centres is more flexible than this (see Turvey, 1977, pp.224-225 for a fuller explication of this point), and that local information about the environment and the state of the limbs may modify instructions from higher centres. Because lower level coordinative structures can function autonomously in response to the environment, higher centres need not play any role in necessary small-scale adjustments and may therefore remain in ignorance of them. This sets limits on the role of higher centres in the control of movement. Turvey (1977) argues that the Action Plan which directs movement at a high level, identifies the coordinative structures necessary for a particular movement, and how these will be functionally related in the execution of the movement. The relationship specified by the Action Plan may be modified when local information from lower centres becomes available, so that a movement can be tuned by its environment. The influence of the action systems approach is discernible in the research described in many of the chapters in this volume.

One problem for any researcher concerned with learning rather than purely performance, is how constraints are selected in the first place. Saltzman and Kelso (1983) describe the early stages of motor skill learning as being characterised by a tendency to reduce the complexity of the movement by keeping much of the body stiff. Initially constraints are applied to provide a rough approximation to the necessary movement. Practice, and therefore experience, of the reactive forces which operate when the actor makes a given movement in a given environment, allows the constraints initially applied to be selectively relaxed. Therefore the dynamics of the movement are gradually discovered. This explanation points toward examining the kinematic and biomechanical properties of movements which operate over a learning period, in order to understand the mechanisms of learning. By careful description of the changes which occur, we should be able to go some way toward a description of the manner in which the constraints are applied and tuned for a particular skill. This approach does not, however, address the problem of how constraints are initially selected when a new task is encountered. Cognitive processes play a substantial role in the initial stages of learning most movement skills. Selection of the appropriate task components is mediated by symbolic representation; by coaching, instruction or imitation. Cognitive processes must be able to specify global constraints, albeit in a rather crude manner. How they do this is, as yet, far from clear.

Early studies of skill focussed on examining changes in the way in which we attend to and process perceptual information and choose appropriate responses based on this information during skill acquisition. Action system theorists have argued against a conception of information as separate from response:

> ...ecological realism denies a dualism of information (that controls and coordinates) and dynamics (that is controlled and coordinated). Fundamentally, ecological

> realism views information as arising in the dynamics of the animal-environment system, unique and specific to those dynamics and to the system's dimensions.
> (Kugler, Kelso, & Turvey, 1982, p.48.)

In the Gibsonian tradition they proposed a direct linkage between perceptual cues and the actions they "afford". In learning skilled movement, this linkage must be established. Although a direct triggering of action from perceptual cues such as tau (time to contact with an approaching surface; Lee, 1980) may provide a plausible explanation of performance of movements such as locomotion, stair-climbing and ball catching (see also Turvey & Carello, this volume), in many human skills decisional processes are necessary at all grades of performance from novice to expert. Of course, as Turvey and Carello point out, the performer must be able to perceive that the environment permits a particular action, and this argues for the existence of what Turvey and Carello describe as "smart perceptual instruments".

Epstein (1986) distinguishes "realist" (action systems) from "standard" (motor systems) views of perception and action, and does not feel that the two are incompatible. The standard viewpoint emphasises central programming of movement and error correction during execution using feedback. Epstein argues that hybrids of the two approaches provide good options to either extreme position. A rather general "hybrid" view of the role of cognition in motor control, is that there is a number of skills in which the direct linkage of perception with action underlies performance. Further processing is involved when the task or stage of learning requires it. Much of the literature on the acquisition of "perceptual-motor" skills in the 1950s and 1960s was based on tasks with an obvious cognitive component. It is therefore not surprising that the models produced at this time represented the organisation of the components of skill as a hierarchy, with a decision-making executive at the top, which structured the components of a task required to achieve a particular goal. Further down the hierarchy, smaller and smaller components, or subroutines, contained the detail of performance. At the bottom of the hierarchy were well-learned "habits" or reflexes. The model presented by Glencross (1978) illustrates this form of theorising. He distinguished four levels of "plans" which represent the cognitive structure of skills. At the top, or Directive Plan Level, the goal and desired outcome of the activity is represented. The second level contains General Plans which deal with strategic factors, and the rules and limitations of the task. The third level contains Motor Plans for spatially and temporally organised movement patterns, and at the lowest level Motor Programmes which are "response units of action". Responses are constructed from basic units into programmes and response patterns under the guidance of the directive and strategic plans, which act in an executive manner. One major difference between models such as that of Glencross, and the view-point advanced by Turvey and colleagues, concerns the amount of control exerted by "executive" levels and the interpretation of a response unit of action, which in the ecological view would be an autonomous coordinative structure. Neither viewpoint tells us very much about strategic factors or intentions in performance, although both of these are represented as plan levels by Glencross.

A distinction which can be drawn in Glencross's model, and which is common to many similar descriptions of skilled behaviour, differentiates between higher levels of control which allow goals and intentions to access the control mechanisms necessary to accomplish them, and lower levels of control which tune the performance of skill to its environment. The ecological theorists have avoided the issue of intentionality:

> ... (We respectfully ignore the problem of how an intention is determined and in addition we give due recognition to the likelihood that some of the structures responsible for determining an intention may also be responsible for its translation into an action plan and for the plan's subsequent differentiation.) Therefore, an intention is an 'event' for the action system in the way that, say, a scene is an event for the visual, perceptual system.
>
> (Turvey, 1977, p.222.)

This suggests that even the ecological theorists would support some distinction between higher level cognitive processes and those processes directly responsible for movement control. Other theorists have drawn a similar distinction more directly. Mackay (1983) distinguishes between the conceptual system which contains "cognitive units for controlling movements" and the muscle movement system which sets parameters for the execution of the task. Roy (1983) in his consideration of apraxic syndromes makes a similar distinction.

There does seem to be some utility in distinguishing between cognitive and motor processes. However, although we can justify such a distinction, it is important to give some consideration to how the cognitive system, which we assume uses representations based upon propositions or imagery, passes control to motor centres, which have to issue commands to specify the activity necessary for the muscular forces which constitute action.

Cognitive processes in action

Annett (1985) points to the possible role of imagery as the "bridge" between action and language. Words can evoke images, which in turn can summon actions. Part of the support for this notion comes from the effectiveness of using descriptions which produce imagery to convey information about posture in the early stages of coaching a skill. Annett gives the example of a squash coach who instructs novices to receive service by adopting the stance of Red Indians waving tomahawks. Further support comes from the reported spontaneous usage of imagery by subjects attempting to describe how they perform certain actions, for example, tying a bow. These examples certainly suggest that imagery has an important role in accessing action routines.

Where in the cognitive system is it necessary to place this bridge? Our access to the cognitive system is mediated symbolically, but the mode of communication of the cognitive system and the motor system is the same. The locus of the bridge must be at peripheral stages of access to the cognitive system, where we are encoding material, rehearsing it in working memory or retrieving it from storage.

One possible account of the role of imagery is that it allows access to action routines via the working memory system by providing a description of the necessary actions. In the Baddeley and Hitch (1974) working memory model there are (at least) two subsystems, the articulatory loop for verbal material and the visuo-spatial sketchpad. Imagery may be a particularly effective way of accessing stored action routines using the visuo-spatial subsystem for certain tasks which are most readily conceptualised spatially. In this sense it forms a bridge between language and action. This is not to say, however, that action routines might not be accessed more directly using language. As Logie, Baddeley, Mane, Donchin and Sheptak (this volume) point out, the role of working memory in skill acquisition, particularly in the early stages, has yet to be systematically explored.

Working memory is a major component of Anderson's (1982) ACT* system, which also has a declarative memory or database for the storage of factual information and a procedural memory for the storage of information about how to perform tasks and actions. Procedural information is contained in productions which represent individual steps in a task, and are condition-action units which initiate an action if their condition is fulfilled. Conditions can be matched with the output of other productions or with information active in working memory.

Allport (1980) also puts forward the view that cognitive processing mechanisms and action are directly coupled in a version of a production systems framework. Although production systems models have been used with increasing frequency to explain and simulate the learning and performance of purely cognitive tasks, they have made relatively little impact on models of cognitive-motor tasks. Allport discusses the starting points for understanding action control. The first concerns different levels of control, with higher levels providing an abstract specification of a course of action, and lower levels controlling constraints applied to limbs to enact a given task. The second concerns the necessity for stored "action patterns", which need not be separate from the processing mechanisms themselves, and function as content-specific control mechanisms for a particular class of actions. Allport suggests that these content-specific mechanisms are accessed via production-like mechanisms. To return to the role of imagery in skilled action, the production-like mechanisms may be accessed via one of the working memory subsystems, and the visuo-spatial subsystem may provide the most effective means of access for complex motor tasks.

Accessing motor control centres from cognitive mechanisms, then, can be accomplished directly via the neural equivalent of condition-action rules. Note that there is still a distinction to be made, between the function of higher and lower levels of control. The role of higher level processes is to specify a course of action and the role of lower level processes is to enact it. There still remains the possibility that the enactment of movement can be triggered directly via perceptual cues in the case of skills such as locomotion which need be modified only by environmental considerations without recourse to strategic factors. We appear to be in a position of advocating (at least) two routes to the movement system: a direct route from perceptual affordances and a route via the cognitive system. The second "mediated" route can presumably be used under conditions of controlled or automatic processing by the cognitive system (Schneider & Shiffrin, 1977). In many sports skills, for example, decisions made at high speed by expert performers may be automatic. We should add the caution here, that the concept and definition of automaticity is still the subject of some debate (see Phillips & Hughes, this volume). In the initial stages of learning some skills such as balancing or interceptive components of ball skills, mediated processing may allow the learner to make an approximation to the correct movement. During the course of practice, the learner is exposed to the dynamic properties of the movement and to the perceptual cues which afford the movement, thus allowing the direct route to develop.

Intentions and movement

The problem of how intentions and goals are represented has been discussed by a number of investigators (e.g. Allport, 1980; Mackay, 1983). Pew (1984) summarises this problem:

> Perhaps the highest level of motor control, namely, the level at which the motor activity to be performed is selected, is the least well understood. Most of our representations gloss over this process by one of two dodges. Either we deny the admissibility of such questions because they cannot be addressed without retreat into mentalism (Gallistel, 1980) or else we draw a box and label it 'Executive Routines', letting that substitute for an explanation.
>
> (p.20)

Again we have to examine carefully the content of the problem we have set ourselves. How does an intention, which initiates action, differ from the goals and subgoals realised at other levels of control? Each level can be described as having a goal, which is set by the shift of control from another level. At the highest levels, there are two possible ways in which a goal can be set: directly by an external cue or internally from information active in working memory as a result of some previous decision-making or problem-solving activity.

Hierarchical theories of intentions and their enactment, such as that of Mackay (1983), allow for the successive differentiation of an intention through a number of different processing levels. This view may well be oversimplified in the light of recent neuropsychological evidence. Marcel (in press) describes some preliminary findings from some research that he has undertaken on neurological patients with movement disorders. This research has examined the effects on performance of movements of the status of the intention which generates them. When the apraxic patients were asked to make a voluntary movement, such as copying letter-like shapes or picking up an object, some patients could not make the movement while others showed considerable impairment of movement. When the same voluntary movements formed part of a self-initiated sequence (e.g. lifting a glass to drink, or writing to dictation) some patients showed much better execution of the movements. This finding has been noted many times by clinicians and researchers (e.g. Roy, 1983).

Marcel's novel finding concerned the performance of the same movements by patients as part of everyday routines, which was even better. The only distinguishing feature of the situations in which the best performance was evident was the context of the action, which was as part of a socially or culturally significant intention. Marcel found, for example, that lifting and grasping were performed better when the patient was serving tea, than when lifting a glass to drink, and that writing a diary was performed better than writing to dictation. These findings point to a very significant role for context and the status of intentions in movement control. Even sequences of movements which rely on direct perception of lawful environmental events, such as locomotion, are not performed in isolation. They form just one part of the enactment of a more complex intention, for instance, walking to the pub for a drink with some friends.

There is more to movement than meets the eye

The ecological theorists emphasise the importance of the environmental context in the control of movement. There are good examples in the literature of the way in which the "affordances" (Gibson, 1979) of different objects in the environment relate to goal-directed action, for example, riser height and stair climbing (Warren, 1984). What remains to be explained is how the intention to climb a flight of stairs at a particular point in time initiates the movement. There is also the problem that properties of the staircase will affect the way in which it is climbed. For example, stairs which are constructed of concrete will be climbed more rapidly and less tentatively than stairs made of rickety and rotten wood, even if both have the same riser height. Thus prior knowledge of the different properties of concrete and rotten wood will affect the stepping movements of the climber. An empirical demonstration of this point is provided by Marteniuk, MacKenzie, Jeannerod, Athenes and Dugas (1937) and described by Marteniuk, MacKenzie and Leavitt (this volume). Marteniuk et al. (1987) demonstrated the prior knowledge of the properties of objects (the fragility of a light bulb and a tennis ball respectively) affected movements of reaching and grasping. In a second experiment they demonstrated that the movements of the wrist in picking up a wooden disk differed according to whether the disk had to be placed in a tight-fitting well or thrown into a cardboard box. They concluded that this finding is evidence of the influence of high level planning processes on the control of movement.

Strategic factors also play an important role in determining the course of some movements. The environment in which a movement occurs must be considered, both as the physical context in which a movement is performed, and in broader terms. In many skills, the performer must choose between a number of similar types of response the most appropriate of which can only be determined by making decisions based on perceptual cues. This is true of many sport skills. The skilled batsman in cricket not only has to intercept the ball with the bat, but must rapidly select the appropriate stroke to accomplish the interception and convey the ball to a part of the field where it cannot be quickly fielded. The essence of a truly skilful movement is its flexibility and adaptability.

Conclusion

It is nearly impossible to write anything in this area without displeasing someone, however the first point to be made is that action theorists have neglected planning processes in movement, and motor theorists have neglected to take account of the neurological substrate of motor control and the lawful properties of the perceptual environment. Sheridan, van Wieringen and Marteniuk, MacKenzie and Leavitt (all this volume) present compelling arguments for the substantial influence of high level processes on movement control, and they together with other authors advocate a "mixed" approach.

The influence of cognitive processes is most readily seen in the performance of the "family" of skills in which it is necessary to translate symbolic material into a response sequence, such as writing, typing, speech and musical performance (Shaffer, 1976; see Colley, 1988, for a review). There is also clear evidence that cognitive processes play a role in determining movements which do not obviously have a cognitive component. As we have seen, Marteniuk et al. (1987) have demonstrated that high level processes affect grasping and reaching movements. Another example is the study by Kerr, Condon and McDonald (1985) which demonstrated that performance on the Brooks (1967) spatial matrix task, generally regarded as a working memory task, was impaired when subjects were required to adopt a difficult standing position. This indicates that regulation of posture and concurrent cognitive spatial processing share common mechanisms, implicating a role for high-level mechanisms in postural control. One objective for future research should be to extend the results of these studies using different types of movements with different planning demands. Theoretical accounts of the role of high level processes in the execution of different types of movement can then be founded on a reasonably extensive database.

Action theorists do not deny the role of higher processes in motor control, although they might seek to define "cognition" in a rather different way to traditional motor systems accounts:

> If cognition is defined as it should be in my opinion — as the appreciation of the affordances of the environment, an appreciation that is based on direct perception but can go beyond it through symbolic and other processes, then there is no doubt that action is organized in part by cognition.
>
> (Reed, 1987, p.186.)

A major problem remains in embodying such a definition in a testable theory. Reed (1987) goes on to criticize the "inadequate theory of perception" used by information processing theorists which takes no account of direct perception, and their separation of planning from movement, which he interprets as requiring a "rigid dualism of mind separated from body". The first criticism has some justification, as recent research attests (e.g. Lee, 1980; Warren, 1984; Warren, Young, & Lee, 1986). Further research should discover more lawful properties of the perceptual environment and their role in the direct control of action. This would contribute to the development of an "adequate" theory of perception.

As for the second criticism, the separation of planning and execution processes of movement is a result of our current state of knowledge, and the metaphors used to guide research and describe the findings. We doubt that this separation is really founded on the notion of dualism with its "dis-integration" of cognition and action. In recent years computational models have guided the modelling of cognitive processes, while physical models have provided good descriptions of the mechanisms of motor control. It is impossible to integrate the two in any satisfactory way, nevertheless the two approaches do share common aims. Many cognitive psychologists (e.g. Allport, 1980; Anderson, 1982; McClelland & Rumelhart, 1985; Rumelhart & Norman, 1981) have removed the executive from models of learning and memory, just as Turvey (1977) has toppled the homunculus from his cortical keyboard. The computational approaches in cognitive psychology and the physical models used to describe movement control are both seeking to provide <u>simple</u> descriptions. For the time being may both prosper! The action systems approach has led to the questioning of many of the assumptions which have traditionally been made in research on skilled movement with some benefit for the development of the area. After all, as Persse McGarrigle asked in a rather different context: "What do you <u>do</u> if everybody agrees with you?" (Lodge, 1985, p.319.)

References

Adams, J.A. (1987). Historical review and appraisal of research on the learning, retention and transfer of human motor skills. <u>Psychological Bulletin</u>, <u>101</u>, 41-74.

Allport, D.A. (1980). Patterns and actions: Cognitive mechanisms are content-specific. In G. Claxton (Ed.), <u>Cognitive psychology: New directions</u>. London: Routledge & Kegan Paul.

Anderson, J.R. (1982). Acquisition of cognitive skill. <u>Psychological Review</u>, <u>89</u>, 369-406.

Annett, J. (1985). Motor learning: A review. In H. Heuer, U. Kleinbeck & K-H. Schmidt, (Eds.), <u>Motor behavior: Programming, control and acquisition</u>. Berlin, Heidelberg: Springer-Verlag.

Baddeley, A.D., & Hitch, G.J. (1974). Working memory. In G. Bower (Ed.), <u>Recent advances in learning and motivation</u>, <u>Vol. 8</u>. New York: Academic Press.

Bernstein, N. (1967). <u>The coordination and regulation of movements</u>. London: Pergamon.

Brooks, L.R. (1967). The suppression of visualization by reading. <u>Quarterly Journal of Experimental Psychology</u>, <u>19</u>, 289-299.

Colley, A.M. (1988). Cognitive motor skills. In D.H. Holding (Ed.), <u>Human Skills</u> (2nd ed.). Chichester: Wiley.

Epstein, W. (1986). Contrasting conceptions of perception and action. <u>Acta Psychologica</u>, <u>63</u>, 103-115.

Fitts, P.M. (1964). Perceptual-motor skill learning. In A.W. Melton (Ed.), <u>Categories of human learning</u>. New York: Academic Press.

Gallistel, C.R. (1980). <u>The organisation of action: A new synthesis</u>.

Hillsdale, N.J.: Erlbaum.
Gibson, J.J. (1969). The ecological approach to visual perception. Boston: Houghton Mifflin.
Glencross, D.J. (1978). Cognitive structure and the acquisition of skill. In D.J. Glencross (Ed.), Psychology and sport. Sydney: McGraw-Hill.
Kerr, B., Condon, S.M., & McDonald, L.A. (1985). Cognitive spatial processing and the regulation of posture. Journal of Experimental Psychology: Human Perception and Performance, 11, 617-622.
Kugler, P.N., Kelso, J.A.S., & Turvey, M.T. (1982). On the control and coordination of naturally developing systems. In J.A.S. Kelso & J.E. Clark (Eds.), The development of movement control and coordination. New York: Wiley.
Lee, D.N. (1980). Visuo-motor coordination in space-time. In G.E. Stelmach & J. Requin (Eds.), Tutorials in motor behavior. Amsterdam: North-Holland.
Lodge, D. (1985). Small world: An academic romance. Harmondsworth : Penguin.
Mackay, D.G. (1983). A theory of the representation and enactment of intentions. In R.A. Magill (Ed.), Memory and control of action. Amsterdam: North-Holland.
Marcel, A.J. (in press). Phenomenal experience and functionalism. In A. Marcel & E. Bisiach (Eds.), Consciousness in contemporary science. Oxford: Oxford University Press.
Marteniuk, R.G., MacKenzie, C.L., Jeannerod, M., Athenes, S., & Dugas, C. (1987). Constraints on human arm movement trajectories. Canadian Journal of Psychology, 41, 365-378.
McClelland, J.L. & Rumelhart, D.E. (1985). Distributed memory and the representation of general and specific information. Journal of Experimental Psychology: General, 114, 159-188.
Miller, G.A., Galanter, E., & Pribram, K. (1960). Plans and the structure of behavior. New York: Holt, Rinehart & Winston.
Pew, R.W. (1984). A distributed processing view of human motor control. In W. Prinz & A.F. Sanders (Eds.), Cognition and motor processes. Berlin, Heidelberg: Springer-Verlag.
Reed, E.S. (1987). The ecology of agency. European Bulletin of Cognitive Psychology, 7, 186-189.
Roy, E.A. (1983). Neuropsychology of apraxia. In R.A. Magill (Ed.), Memory and control of action. Amsterdam: North-Holland.
Rumelhart, D.E. & Norman, D.A. (1981). Analogical processes in learning. In J.R. Anderson (Ed.), Cognitive skills and their acquisition. Hillsdale, N.J.: Erlbaum.
Saltzman, E. & Kelso, J.A.S. (1983). Toward a dynamical account of motor memory and control. In R.A. Magill (Ed.), Memory and control of action. Amsterdam: North-Holland.
Schneider, W. & Shiffrin, R.M. (1977). Controlled and automatic human information processing: I. Detection, search and attention. Psychological Review, 84, 1-66.
Shaffer, L.H. (1976). Intention and performance. Psychological Review, 83, 375-393.
Turvey, M.T. (1977). Preliminaries to a theory of action with reference to vision. In R. Shaw & J. Bransford (Eds.), Perceiving, acting and knowing: Toward an ecological psychology. Hillsdale, N.J.: Erlbaum.
Turvey, M.T. & Carello, C. (1986). The ecological approach to

perceiving-acting: A pictorial essay. Acta Psychologica, 63, 133-155.

Turvey, M.T. & Kugler, P.N. (1984). An ecological approach to perception and action. In H.T.A. Whiting (Ed.), Human motor actions: Bernstein reassessed. Amsterdam: North-Holland.

Turvey, M.T., Shaw, R.E., & Mace, W. (1978). Issues in a theory of action: Degrees of freedom, coordinative structures and coalitions. In J. Requin (Ed.), Attention and performance VII, Hillsdale, N.J.: Erlbaum.

Warren, W.H. (1984). Perceiving affordances: Visual guidance of stair climbing. Journal of Experimental Psychology: Human Perception and Performance, 10, 683-703.

Warren, W.H., Young, D.S., & Lee, D.N. (1986). Visual control of step length during running over irregular terrain. Journal of Experimental Psychology: Human Perception and Performance, 12, 259-266.

Welford, A.T. (1976). Skilled performance: Perceptual and motor skills. Glenview, Ill.: Scott Foresman.

Part I

PROGRAMMING AND COORDINATION

Cognition and Action in Skilled Behaviour
A.M. Colley and J.R. Beech (Editors)

ARE MODELS OF THE FUTURE USED TO ANTICIPATE TARGETS IN TRACKING TASKS?

Nigel Harvey
University College London

Anticipation of targets in tracking tasks was investigated in a study in which signals stepped between windows arranged horizontally on a screen. Subjects tracked them by using a linear slide to move a cursor. The signals were generated by a second-order autoregressive algorithm with coefficients set so as to produce a non-deterministically periodic sequence. Each signal lasted one second and there was a second interval between them. Subjects were instructed to place the cursor over the signals as soon as, and for as long as, possible but to use the interstimulus interval to anticipate the position of the next signal. They each tracked a total of 10 blocks of 100 signals. Half way through and at the end of the experiment they were asked to enter a series of 100 signal positions such that their simulated signal sequences would be of the same type as those which they had been tracking. Over the session, subjects learned to produce beneficial anticipations of future signals. Also, the similarity between the simulated sequences and the tracked sequences was greater at the end of the experiment than half way through it. However, simulation performance was not correlated with prior anticipation performance. Possible mechanisms subserving anticipation are discussed.

In this chapter, I shall be concerned with subjects' ability to predict the future position of a target on the basis of its previous positions. This ability, sometimes known as perceptual anticipation (Poulton, 1957), was discussed in a review written by Schmidt (1968). In his conclusion, Schmidt commented that "the general lack of interesting theoretical ideas is certainly one reason for the relative lack of research in the area" (p.643).

In fact, at about the same time that Schmidt (1968) was writing, work by Soviet psychologists (Anokhin, 1969; Bernstein, 1967) was appearing in the West and supplying some of the missing theory. They argued that we incorporate anticipation into our model of the world and use forecasts in motor control. Bernstein's work on this topic has been considered to be the most important of his many and varied contributions to the study of movement (Requin, Semjen, & Bonnet, 1984). Curiously, though, it has been subject to little, if any, experimental investigation. The work to be reported here represents an initial attempt to remedy this situation.

What role did Bernstein think that anticipation has in motor control? To answer this question I must briefly outline his general theoretical stance. He argued that movement coordination is achieved by use of mechanisms that control muscles as global units. These mechanism impose certain constraints on the muscles prior to the delivery of commands for the movement itself. He argued that the global unit encodes, as a manipulable whole, the complete time course of a particular class of movement (e.g. walking). "There exist in the central nervous system formulae or engrams (that) contain in some form of brain trace the whole process of the movement in its entire course in time." (Bernstein, 1935; see Bernstein, 1984a, pp.97-98.) He argued that variants within a particular class of movement (e.g. walking uphill versus walking downhill) are specified or tuned by altering the values of certain parameters in the motor formula responsible for the whole movement class. The parameter values that are inserted into this formula depend on, a) the required outcome of the movement, b) feedback received during the movement, and c) anticipation of the future (Bernstein, 1957; see Bernstein, 1984b). Determination of movement by the first two of these factors has been the subject of intensive experimentation in recent years. Importance of the third factor has been demonstrated (e.g. Pew, 1974) but Bernstein's model of its operation has yet to be tested.

What psychological processes did Bernstein propose to subserve anticipation? He argued that:

> In the brain there exist two unitary opposed categories or forms of modelling the perceptual world: the model of the past-present, or what has happened and is happening, and the model of the future. The latter proceeds directly from the former and is organized in it. These are necessarily distinct from each other, chiefly because the first type of model is single-valued and categorical, while the latter can only operate by means of extrapolation to some or other degree of confidence or probability.
>
> (Bernstein, 1961; see Bernstein, 1984c, p.455)

In other words, Bernstein proposed that anticipation is based on a stochastic model of the future that is extracted from experience with the past. Here I shall be concerned with two questions that arise from this proposal. First, does more experience result in better anticipation? Second, is anticipation based on a model of the future?

Does anticipation improve with more experience of the target track?

In step-tracking tasks, signals jump from one position on a screen to another. Subjects are required to move a slide, joystick or other manipulandum to ensure that a cursor on the screen remains in contact with the signals for as much time as possible. With a minor modification these tasks can be used to examine perceptual anticipation. An interstimulus interval (ISI) is placed between the offset of a signal and the onset of its successor. Subjects are instructed to move the slide during each of these intervals so as to bring the cursor to the position where they anticipate that the next signal will occur. The extent to which the anticipation moves the cursor closer to the signal can be measured and, hence, any improvement in anticipation over an experimental session can be determined.

The sort of technique just outlined was first used by Poulton (1952). He argued that subjects could learn to make use of predictability that had been built into signal sequences. Later, however, Trumbo, Noble and their colleagues reported a series of studies that have been taken to indicate that people are very poor at learning to exploit signal predictability. For instance, Trumbo, Noble, Cross, and Ulrich (1965) found that subjects could learn to predict tracks that were made up of a fixed repeating sequence of twelve signal positions but that when every alternate signal in the sequence was fixed and the remainder were random, subjects were no better at learning to predict the signals than when all of them were in random positions.

I suggest that this result may have occurred not because subjects were poor at predicting per se but because they had to support a much greater load in working memory with the alternating fixed-random sequence track than with the totally fixed track. In the latter case, Trumbo et al. (1965) presented subjects with the fixed repeating sequences 4, 1, 11, 10, 4, 7, 1, 15, 5, 4, 5, 10. (Positions are coded from the left with the leftmost location designated 1.) Now assume that this sequence has been stored in long-term memory (LTM) and that the current signal is at location 5. It would only be necessary for the subjects to remember that the previous signal was in position 15 in order to predict that the next one will be in position 4. In the alternating fixed-random condition, the stimulus sequence could be represented as 4, R, 11, R, 4, R, 1, R, 5, R, 5, R. (R signifies a randomly chosen signal position.) Assuming again that this sequence has been stored in LTM and that the current stimulus is 5, it would now be necessary for the subject to remember that the previous signal but one was in position 1 in order to predict that the next signal but one will be in location 5. Thus both past signals and predictions would have to be retained for longer in working memory than when the sequence is fixed. Furthermore, and in contrast to the fixed sequence condition, these working memory traces of past signals and predictions would both be subject to interference from intervening signals and movements.

In the experiment to be reported here, no fixed sequences had to be stored in LTM and the working memory load necessary for successful prediction was kept low. Signals stepped between windows arranged horizontally on a screen and subjects tracked them by using a linear slide to move a cursor across the screen. The sequence of signals was generated by a second-order autoregressive algorithm. For this purpose, the window in the centre of the screen was designated zero, windows increasingly to the right of this position were given increasingly positive numbers and windows increasingly to the left of it were given increasingly negative ones. The position of the next signal (X_t) in a sequence of steps was then derived from the positions of its two immediate predecessors (X_{t-1}; X_{t-2}) according to the rule

$$X_t = 0.707X_{t-1} - 0.5X_{t-2} + e_t$$

where e_t was a normally distributed random error with a mean of zero and a standard deviation of 2.6. Signals lasted for one second and there was a one second ISI between them. Subjects were told to use the ISI to anticipate each signal before its appearance.

Although none of the signals produced by the algorithms are determined, it would be possible for subjects to learn to produce beneficial anticipation to them by various means, none of which would involve a heavy working memory or LTM load. These possible means of anticipation are discussed in the next section.

Is successful anticipation based on a model of the future?

If successful anticipation does occur, what psychological processes could be responsible for it? Bernstein argued that they would involve use of an internalised probabilistic model of the future acquired from experience with the past. Such a model would provide a non-deterministic specification of the temporal pattern that is present in the signal sequence. For instance, an internal representation of an autoregressive algorithm similar to the one used to generate the signal sequence would constitute such a model.

Of course, beneficial anticipations can be made without such a model. It is not necessary to have specified the temporal pattern in a sequence of signals up to the present in order to make successful predictions abouı future signals in that sequence. There are certain general algorithms that act as useful heuristics for predicting future signals on the basis of those that have appeared in the past. These heuristics do not involve the extraction of temporal patterns from past signals. Instead, they depend for their success on certain general principles that concern the way that the future relates to the past. For instance, the future is usually more like the recent past than like the distant past. Anticipation using these prediction heuristics is quite distinct from anticipation based on a knowledge of the temporal patterns in the signal sequence.

Prediction heuristics all involve some sort of smoothing or averaging of past signal values. The simplest heuristic would involve averaging all previous values of the signal and using the average as the prediction for the next signal in the sequence. For a signal sequence generated by the autoregressive algorithm given above, adoption of this strategy would lead, after experience of a number of signals, to the central position (i.e. zero) always being the prediction for the next signal. This strategy need not impose a heavy memory load on the subject because the mean could be determined recursivelv. (After n signals, the new estimate of the mean (M_n) is given by the previous estimate (M_{n-1}) plus a modification determined by the value of the current signal (X_n) – i.e. $M_n = M_{n-1} + (X_n - M_{n-1})/n$.) While this heuristic would provide subjects with some success in predicting signals, it would not allow them to improve their anticipation performance after the mean had settled on its asymptotic central value.

A rather more sophisticated prediction heuristic would not use the average of all past signal positions but, instead, employ a moving average of the last n signal positions. Of course, if n were very large, this strategy would not be distinguishable from the previous one. If, on the other hand, n were set equal to one, then no active prediction movements would be made by the subject. The prediction for the next signal position would always be the previous signal position, where the cursor rests. In fact, the best value of n to use for prediction depends on the characteristics of the signal sequence. Consequently, if anticipation performance improves with experience of a signal sequence, this may be because subjects are able to learn a more effective value of n for predicting that sequence. Again, as long as the moving average is determined recursively, this strategy need not involve a heavy memory load.

A still more sophisticated prediction heuristic would involve not just a simple moving average but use a weighted average with weights exponentially decreasing backwards in time. Thus the immediately preceding signal would be more important than the last signal but one for determining the prediction for the next signal. Similarly, the last signal but one would make a more important contribution to this prediction than the signal before that - and so on. The steepness of the decrease in the values of the weights that are attached to signals further and further back in time depends on the coefficients of the exponential decay function governing the values of these weights. The optimum value of this coefficient depends on characteristics of the signal sequence. Thus, if anticipation performance improves with experience of the signal sequence, this may be because subjects are able to modify the exponential coefficient they are using so as to produce better predictions. Like other prediction heuristics, exponential smoothing may be carried out recursively. Memory load would be minimal. The forecast for the next signal would just be a modification of the previous forecast that had been made to predict the current signal. The modification would depend only on the current signal and the value of the exponential coefficient. However, with exponential smoothing as a prediction heuristic, there may be advantages in not using recursive estimation. Trace decay theories of memory (e.g. Wickelgren, 1970) have typically assumed that the memory for a stimulus decays exponentially over time. Thus, rather than prediction imposing a load on memory, the characteristics of memory decay would themselves underlie prediction.

Instead of using the sort of prediction heuristics that I have just outlined, subjects may learn something about the temporal pattern in the signal sequence. This pattern would be characterised either in terms of time domain parameters or in terms of frequency domain parameters. The autoregressive algorithm used to generate the signal sequence in the experiment is an example of a time domain representation of a signal sequence. An internal representation of a rule such as this could be acquired without imposition of a heavy memory load by recursive estimation of the autoregressive coefficients (Young, 1984). With more experience of the signal sequence, the internal representation of the pattern in it would become increasingly veridical. This internal representation could be considered as a mental model of the history of the sequence. However, given that the temporal pattern in the sequence is to be maintained, it also provides a mental model of the future of the sequence (Bernstein, 1984c). Possession of such a model would allow subjects to use recent signal positions to predict future ones. Therefore, experience with the signal sequence that allows recursive refinement of the coefficients in the model should also allow subjects to produce better anticipations of future signal positions.

The coefficients of the autoregressive algorithm used to generate the signal sequences were chosen so as to produce a non-deterministically periodic sequence. Figure 1 shows the spectral density function of one of the sequences produced by this algorithm. It is clear from this that the band of frequencies in the signal falls mainly between 0.1 and 0.2 cycles per event interval. (As signals appeared every two seconds, this is equivalent to 0.05 - 0.1 Hz). It may be that subjects internalise information about the temporal pattern in the signal sequence by representing it in terms of frequency characteristics such as this rather than in terms of the time domain parameters discussed above. In fact, there have been a number of recent suggestions that both movements (Gallistel, 1980; Pribram, Sharafat, & Beekman, 1984) and temporal changes in the environment (Kruse, Stadler, Vogt, & Wehner, 1983) are represented in the brain in frequency analysed form. Both Pew (1974) and Stadler and Wehner (1985) feel that anticipation in tracking tasks is based on a frequency domain characterisation of the temporal pattern in the target. Like the equivalent time domain description, such a characterisation can be regarded as a model of both the past and the future of the signal sequence.

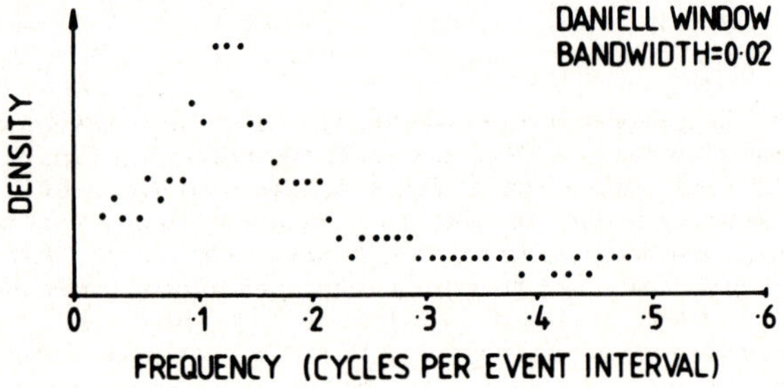

Figure 1. Spectral density function of a sequence produced by the signal generating algorithm.

Experiment

The experiment addressed two issues. First, does more experience with a signal sequence result in better anticipation performance? To examine this, I asked subjects to use the ISIs in a step-tracking task to predict the positions of the signals that would appear next in the sequence. I looked for an improvement in this ability over the experimental sessions.

Second, if subjects can anticipate signals, how do they do so? In particular, does a model of the future subserve performance? This question was tackled by asking subjects to enter a sequence of signal positions such that their simulated sequences would be of the same type as those which they had been tracking. They did this half way through the experiment and at the end of it. If subjects have learned to anticipate signals by developing an internal model that specifies the temporal pattern in the sequences, then they could use this model to generate a series of signals having that pattern. If this is what they do, then their generation performance should be correlated with their immediately preceding anticipation performance.

Use of prediction heuristics to anticipate signals will not lead to acquisition of the knowledge that is needed to generate signal sequences. The total sample, moving or weighted average of a sequence of signals does not preserve information about the temporal pattern in that sequence. Thus there is no reason to suppose that subjects using prediction heuristics to anticipate signals will be able to generate sequences similar to those they have experienced during the anticipation and tracking phase of the experiment.

Subjects using prediction heuristics to anticipate signals may still develop internal models of the temporal patterns in the signal sequences and may use these models to perform the generation task. However, this would mean that quite separate processes subserve the two types of task. There would be no reason to expect generation performance to be correlated with the anticipation performance immediately preceding it.

Method

The experiment employed a step-tracking paradigm. Subjects tracked the signals but also used the ISI between each signal to anticipate the position of the next one. Each subject anticipated and tracked a total of ten sequences of 100 signals. After the fifth and tenth sequence, they each generated their own series of 100 signals to simulate the type of sequences that they had been tracking.

Tracking ability was measured by hit rate and by the time taken to reach the target. Ability to anticipate was measured by the percentage reduction in the absolute distance between cursor and target that the prediction produced and by the percentage of predictions that moved the cursor away from the target. Subjects' assessments of their own tracking and anticipation performance were also recorded to examine how subjective monitoring of performance in the current task compares with that in other tasks (Berry & Broadbent, 1984; Broadbent, FitzGerald, & Broadbent, 1986; Harvey, Garwood, & Palencia, 1987; Phillips, 1987; Schmidt & White, 1972). Finally, time series analysis was performed on the sequences generated by subjects and the autoregressive coefficients obtained were compared with those used by the experimenter to produce the tracked sequences.

Apparatus and stimuli

Stimuli were generated by computer and presented on a fast phosphor colour monitor. A series of 19 outline (i.e. hollow) white squares was arranged horizontally across the screen at eye level throughout the presentation of each sequence of 100 signals. Each of these windows subtended horizontal and vertical visual angles of 0.4° and was separated from its neighbour by 0.6°. Signal presentation was accomplished by filling in one of these squares so that its area was a uniform white. Each signal in a sequence lasted for one second and was separated from its successor by an interstimulus interval (ISI) of one second.

The order of presentation of the signals was governed by the second-order autoregressive algorithm given above. This was done as follows. The value X_t at time t = 0 was set to zero. This value was not transformed into a screen position and did not result in stimulus presentation. The value X_t at time t = 1 was then determined from the algorithm. This value was just e_t because X_{t-1} equalled zero and X_{t-2} did not exist. Again, this value was not transformed into a screen position and did not result in stimulus presentation. The value of X_t at time t = 2 was then determined from the algorithm. This value and the 99 succeeding values of X_t were transformed into screen positions and did result in presentation of stimuli. This transformation simply involved rounding X_t to the nearest whole number. A stimulus was then presented in the window corresponding to this number. For this purpose, the central window was designated zero, windows increasingly to the right of this position corresponded to increasingly positive numbers up to +9 and windows increasingly to left of it corresponded to increasingly negative numbers down to -9. None of the realisations of the algorithm that were used in the experiment contained values outside the range ± 9.

Subjects responded by moving a low friction linear slide. This slide controlled the position of a cursor on the screen. The cursor was a vertical line centred on an imaginary horizontal axis joining the centres of the square windows. The slide moved the cursor along the axis. When the slide was in its central position, the cursor vertically bisected the central window. When the slide was in its leftmost position, the cursor was 0.6° to the left of the left side of the leftmost window. Similarly, when the slide was placed in its rightmost position, the cursor was 0.6° to the right of the right side of the rightmost window. The cursor itself subtended 0.8° of vertical visual angle. Thus when it was placed across a window, it protruded from the top and bottom of the window by 0.2°. The slide had a movement range of 47 cm. and this corresponded to a cursor movement of 22.4 cm. - a gain factor of 0.48.

Subjects tracking a sequence of signals heard a tone during the time that their cursor was placed over a target signal. The same tone sounded when subjects entered stimuli during the sequence generation phases of the experiment.

Subjects used the keyboard of the computer to enter subjective estimates of their performance at the end of each tracking sequence. They also used the keyboard when generating their own stimulus sequences.

Subjects

12 subjects aged between 18 and 35 years each served for one session of approximately 60 minutes' duration. All subjects were right-handed. Each of them received a payment of £1.00 for their participation in the experiment.

Experimental design

Each of the 12 subjects tracked ten sequences of 100 signals. Each of the 120 target sequences used in the experiment was a separately generated realization of the second-order autoregressive algorithm specified above. After the fifth and tenth target sequences, subjects entered their own sequences of 100 signals to simulate those that they had been tracking.

Procedure

Subjects were run individually in a quiet artificially lit room. Each one sat 60 cm. in front of the screen and controlled the linear slide with the right (dominant) hand. At the start of the experiment, the following instructions appeared on the screen:

> This is a tracking task. A sequence of signals will appear in different horizontal positions on this screen. You move the slide. It controls the position of the cursor on the screen. Your aim is to place the cursor over the signals as soon as possible after they appear. The sequence of signals is not totally random. To some extent you can predict them. When you hit a signal, you will hear a tone. Stay on the signal till it vanishes then move the cursor to where you think the next signal will occur. Press a key to start.

After each sequence of signals had been tracked, two questions appeared on the screen and subjects answered them by typing numbers on the computer keyboard. The first question was, "What per cent of signals do you think you missed?" The second one was, "What per cent of the occasions on which you tried to anticipate the target resulted in you moving further away from it rather than closer to it?" After answering these questions, subjects pressed a key when they were ready to continue with the experiment.

After the fifth and tenth signals sequences, the following message appeared on the screen:

> Next, move the cursor from one window to another to produce a sequence of signals that is just like those you have tracked. Once the cursor is over a window, press a key to make the signal appear there. Then move on to your next window and repeat.

Subjects then entered a sequence of 100 signals. When they placed the cursor over a chosen signal window and pressed a key, they saw a signal appear in that window and heard a one-second tone to confirm that the computer had registered that signal position.

The position of the linear slide was sampled every 10 ms. and this was used to provide data concerning the tracking and anticipation of experimenter-generated target sequences and to record the location of the signals in the subject-generated sequences. These data were stored to disc during a five-minute break half way through the experiment and, again, at the end of the experiment.

Results

Possible changes over the experimental session in subjects' ability to track and anticipate signals and to estimate their own performance levels were examined using analyses of variance. Time series analysis was used to investigate the signal sequences generated by subjects.

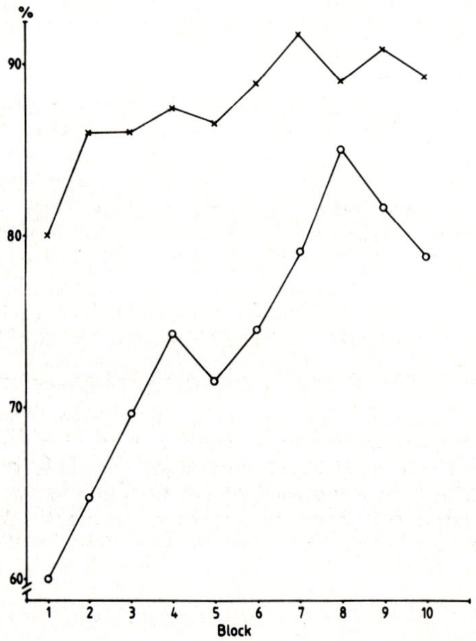

Figure 2. Mean hit rates (X—X) and mean subjective estimates of hit rates (0—0) for the ten blocks of signals.

Tracking performance

Figure 2 shows a significant increase in signal hit rate over the experimental session ($F(9,99) = 6.87$; $p < 0.001$). There was no evidence that this was associated with a reduction in the time taken to reach the target. This time remained fairly constant over blocks with a mean of 577 ms. and a standard deviation of 8.7 ms.

Anticipation performance

An active anticipation was observed when there was a difference in cursor position of at least 0.025° of visual angle between the start and end of the ISI. As the top row of Table 1 shows, practice produced an increase in the percentage of ISIs containing active anticipations ($\underline{F}(9,99) = 2.8$; $\underline{p} < 0.01$) - though this effect appears to have been restricted to the first three blocks of the experimental session.

Table 1

Mean % ISIs containing anticipation movements, together with the mean % of these that were in the wrong direction and the mean % of them estimated by subjects to be in the wrong direction.

	Block of signals									
	1	2	3	4	5	6	7	8	9	10
% ISIs with anticipation movements	71	74	80	79	78	81	78	83	81	78
% anticipations in wrong direction	28	31	35	33	31	34	32	35	32	32
% anticipations estimated to be in wrong direction	46	43	43	37	42	40	36	32	31	32

The absolute distances between the cursor and the target at the start and at the end of each ISI were averaged over all the ISIs in a block. To obtain the anticipation score for a block, the second of these values was subtracted from the first and the difference between them was expressed as a percentage of the first. Figure 3 shows

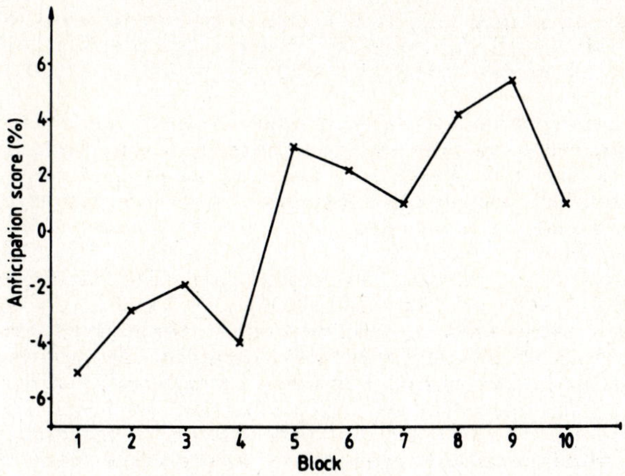

Figure 3. Mean anticipation score over the ten blocks of signals.

a significant increase in this score over the experimental session ($F(9,99) = 3.06$; $p < 0.01$). This improvement in anticipation performance did not appear to be due to better prediction of the direction of target movement. This is because there was no evidence that the percentage of active anticipations that moved the cursor away from the target decreased over the session. As the second row of Table 1 shows, this percentage remained quite constant over blocks with a mean of 32% and a standard deviation of 2%. Thus when subjects learn to anticipate signals, they appear to be learning something about how far to move in a given direction rather than about which direction to move in.

Subjective estimates of performance

Figure 2 shows a significant increase over blocks in subjects' own estimates of their tracking performance ($F(9,99) = 5.1$; $p < 0.001$). The impression that this increase is steeper than the one observed for actual tracking performance was confirmed with a two-way analysis of variance. This showed not only significant main effects of actual versus estimated hit rate ($F(1,11) = 22.1$; $p < 0.001$) and block ($F(9,99) = 7.6$; $p < 0.001$) but also a significant interaction between these factors ($F(9,99) = 2.3$; $p < 0.025$). Thus, although subjects remained underconfident in their tracking performances, their degree of underconfidence declined over the session.

Subjects' confidence may have increased either because they were monitoring their improving performance or else just because they expected to get better with practice. To investigate this issue, the z'-transformed within-subject correlations between actual and estimated hit rates were examined. These were found to have a mean value of 0.63 and to be significantly greater than zero ($t_{11} = 3.96$; $p < 0.01$). Thus it appears that the increase in confidence was related to the improvement in performance.

As the third row of Table 1 shows, there was a slight decrease in subjects' own estimates of the percentage of their predictions that moved the cursor away from the target ($F(9,99) = 2.1$; $p < 0.05$). By the end of the session, subjects' underconfidence in their ability to predict the direction of the target seems to have vanished. This impression was supported by the results of two-way analysis of variance in which the only effect found to be significant was the interaction between block and actual versus estimated performance at predicting direction of target movement ($F(9,99) = 3.1$; $p < 0.01$).

The group means of actual and estimated performance in predicting direction of target movement appear to have been similar because of subjects' ability to monitor their own anticipation performance. Z'-transformed within-subject correlations between these two variables across blocks had a mean of 0.29, a value significantly greater than zero ($T_{11} = 1.81$; $p < 0.05$).

Generation performance

Each series of positions generated by subjects was transformed into a sequence of numbers. As before, this was done by designating the central screen position to be zero. Positions increasingly to the right of it were then assigned increasingly positive numbers and positions increasingly to the left of it were given increasingly negative ones. Time series analysis was then performed on each of the 24 resulting sequences. This was done by fitting autoregressive moving average (ARMA) models via Pandit and Wu's (1983) stepwise modelling strategy. This uses an F-test to determine whether a higher order model produces a significantly better fit than a lower order one. (Additionally, t-tests showed that all the parameters in the models selected with this procedure were significantly different from zero.)

Table 2 provides a classification of the best fitting models. This shows that after the first half of the experiment, a third of the subjects generated sequences of the same form (AR2) as the track-generating algorithm. However, after the second half of the experiment, over half the subjects were generating sequences of the correct form. Figure 4 shows two typical sequences generated by subjects, together with their best fitting (AR2) models.

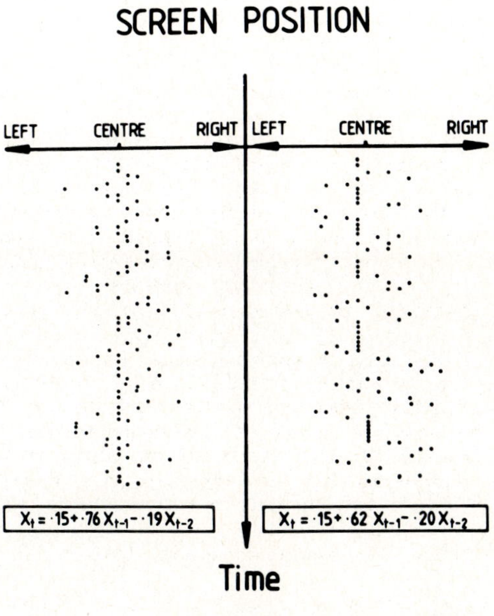

Figure 4. Two typical sequences of signals generated by subjects, together with their best fitting AR2 models.

To examine the numerical similarity between the autoregressive coefficients in the track-generating algorithm and those in the sequences generated by subjects, all subject-generated sequences were fitted to AR2 models. The means of the resulting AR1 and AR2 coefficients are shown in Table 3, together with the target coefficients that were entered into the track-generating algorithm. The mean AR1 coefficient was significantly different from the target value after the first half of the experiment ($\underline{t}_{11}$ = 3.44; $\underline{p} < 0.01$) but no longer significantly different from it after the second half ($\underline{t}_{11}$ = -0.23; ns). The mean AR2 coefficient was significantly different from its target value after both the first half ($\underline{t}_{11}$ = 7.16; $\underline{p} < 0.01$) and the second half ($\underline{t}_{11}$ = 5.28; $\underline{p} < 0.01$) of the experiment - although, as Table 3 shows, it was clearly numerically closer to the target in the latter case.

Table 2

Classification of the ARMA models obtained after time series analysis of the signal sequences generated by the 12 subjects. Successful generation of the form of the previously anticipated sequences is indicated by production of AR2 models.

Sequence Generated	Type of model		
	AR1	AR2	ARMA 2, 1
After first half of experiment	6	4	2
After second half of experiment	4	7	1

Table 3

Values of autoregressive coefficients in signal sequences generated by the experimenter, together with the mean value of those obtained after fitting AR2 models to the sequences generated by subjects.

Sequence	Autoregressive coefficient	
	AR1	AR2
Experimenter-generated target	0.7071	- 0.5000
Subject-generated after first half of experiment	0.5441	- 0.1235
Subject-generated after second half of experiment	0.6840	- 0.2001

Subjects learnt both to anticipate and to generate sequences. Was generation performance related to anticipation performance? To examine this issue, the generated sequences from both halves of the experiment were fitted to the target AR2 form. Then absolute deviations in the parameters (AR1, AR2, mean, error variance) of generated sequences from those used in the experimenter's algorithm were extracted to form indices of generation performance. If the same model of the temporal pattern in the sequences that is used for generation is also used for anticipation, then it should be possible to predict a given subject's anticipation score for a given half of the experiment from these indices of generation performance. However, stepwise mutliple regression showed that none of the four indices of generation performance could predict anticipation score. In fact, together they were unable to account for any of the variance in the anticipation scores (Adjusted $\underline{r}^2 = 0.0\%$).

Discussion

The experiment showed that subjects are able to learn to anticipate signals that appear in non-deterministic sequences. The contrast with Trumbo et al.'s (1965) results may have occurred because successful anticipation in their experiments required subjects to support a much greater memory load than was necessary for successful anticipation in the present case. Their subjects' poor performance may have arisen from an inability to store or retain the information required for prediction rather than from an inability to use stored information to produce good predictions.

Subjects were also able to simulate sequences similar to those that they had tracked and performance in this generation task appeared to be better at the end of the experiment than half-way through it. This means that subjects must have acquired some information about the temporal pattern in the signals. They must have developed a model of the future of the sequences they had been tracking and then used it in the simulation phases of the experiment. However, this model does not appear to have been used for anticipating targets in the sequences from which it was extracted. Anticipation performance was not based on the temporal pattern information, the model of the future, that subserved generation performance.

So how was anticipation accomplished? There appear to be two possibilities. First, it could have been based on a different type of model of the future from the one used in the generation task. For instance, the model used for anticipation may have expressed the temporal pattern in the signal sequence in terms of time domain parameters whereas the model used for the generation task may have expressed that same pattern in terms of its frequency domain parameters. Thus, two separate but equivalent models would have been independently extracted from the tracked sequences and used for different purposes - anticipation and generation. On the other hand, subjects may have used prediction heuristics to anticipate signals. More experimental work is needed to distinguish between these two alternatives.

Finally, it is interesting to compare subjects' monitoring of their own performance in the current task with that found in other tasks. In dynamic systems control (Berry & Broadbent, 1984; Broadbent et al., 1986) and in some cases of motor control (Harvey et al., 1987), subjects seem poor at monitoring their own performance. However, in other motor control tasks (e.g. Schmidt & White, 1972) and in judgmental forecasting (Phillips, 1987) they are much better at estimating their own performance. The present task appears to have been of the latter type. Subjects' estimated and actual performance were correlated and their initial underconfidence was reduced over the session. The extent to which subjects can monitor their own performance probably depends on the availability of relevant feedback and on the ease with which that feedback can be used. However, clarification of this issue requires further experimentation.

References

Anokhin, P.K. (1969). Cybernetics and the integrative activity of the brain. In M. Cole & I. Maltzman (Eds.), A handbook of contemporary Soviet psychology. New York: Basic Books.

Bernstein, N.A. (1967). The coordination and regulation of movement. London: Pergamon Press.

Bernstein, N.A. (1984a). The problem of the interrelation of co-ordination and localization. In H.T.A. Whiting (Ed.), Human motor actions: Bernstein reassessed. Amsterdam: North-Holland. (Originally published, 1935.)

Bernstein, N.A. (1984b). Some emergent problems of the regulation of motor acts. In H.T.A. Whiting (Ed.), Human motor actions: Bernstein reassessed. Amsterdam: North-Holland. (Originally published, 1957.)

Bernstein, N.A. (1984c). Trends and problems in the study of investigation of physiology of activity. In H.T.A. Whiting (Ed.), Human motor actions: Bernstein reassessed. Amsterdam: North-Holland. (Originally published, 1961.)

Berry, D.C., & Broadbent, D.E. (1984). On the relationship between task performance and verbal knowledge. Quarterly Journal of Experimental Psychology, 36A, 209-231.

Broadbent, D.E., FitzGerald, P., & Broadbent, M.H.P. (1986). Implicit and explicit knowledge in the control of complex systems. British Journal of Psychology, 77, 33-50.

Gallistel, C.R. (1980). The organization of action: A new synthesis. Hillsdale, New Jersey: Erlbaum.

Harvey, N., Garwood, J., & Palencia, M. (1987). Vocal matching of pitch intervals: Learning and transfer effects. Psychology of Music, 15, 90-106.

Kruse, P., Stadler, M., Vogt, S., & Wehner, T. (1983). Raum-zeitliche integration wahrgenormmener bewegung durch frequenzanalyse. Gestalt Theory, 5, 83-113.

Pandit, S.M., & Wu, S.M. (1983). Time series and system analysis with applications. New York: Wiley.

Pew, R.W. (1974). Human perceptual-motor performance. In B.H. Kantowitz (Ed.), Human information processing: Tutorials in performance and cognition. Hillsdale, New Jersey: Erlbaum.

Phillips, L.D. (1987). On the adequacy of judgmental forecasts. In G. Wright, & P. Ayton (Eds.), Judgmental forecasting. Chichester: Wiley.

Poulton, E.C. (1952). On the basis of perceptual anticipation in tracking. British Journal of Psychology, 43, 295-302.

Poulton, E.C. (1957). On prediction in skilled movements. Psychological Bulletin, 54, 467-478.

Pribram, K.H., Sharafat, A., & Beekman, G.J. (1984). Frequency encoding in motor systems. In H.T.A. Whiting (Ed.), Human motor actions: Bernstein reassessed. Amsterdam: North-Holland.

Requin, J., Semjen, A., & Bonnet, M. (1984). Bernstein's purposeful brain. In H.T.A. Whiting (Ed.), Human motor actions: Bernstein reassessed. Amsterdam: North-Holland.

Schmidt, R.A. (1968). Anticipation and timing in human performance. Psychological Bulletin, 70, 631-646.

Schmidt, R.A., & White, J.L. (1972). Evidence for an error detection mechanism in motor skills. Journal of Motor Behavior, 4, 147-153.

Stadler, M., & Wehner, T. (1985). Anticipation as a basic principle in goal directed action. In M. Frese, & J. Sabini (Eds.), Goal directed behavior: The concept of action in psychology. Hillsdale, New Jersey: Erlbaum.

Trumbo, D., Noble, M., Cross, K., & Ulrich, L. (1965). Task predictability in the organization, acquisition, and retention of tracking skill. Journal of Experimental Psychology, 70, 252-263.

Wickelgren, W.A. (1970). Multitrace strength theory. In D.A. Norman (Ed.), Models of human memory. New York: Academic Press.

Young, P. (1984). Recursive estimation and time-series analysis: An introduction. Berlin: Springer-Verlag.

Cognition and Action in Skilled Behaviour
A.M. Colley and J.R. Beech (Editors)

HAND MOVEMENT TO MOVING TARGETS : PLANNING AND ADJUSTMENTS OF SPEED AND DIRECTION

Phillip J. Bairstow
Institute of Child Health, University of London

Adult subjects were used in a study of the way in which the hand approaches and intercepts a moving target. The speed and trajectory of the target was varied. Hand movement was analysed in terms of: initial speed and direction; ongoing modifications to the speed and the path of movement. Results showed that initial speed was scaled specifically for the target's speed and trajectory, while initial direction was scaled only roughly. During the movement, there was usually only one adjustment to the speed of the hand, but frequent adjustments to the path of the hand. Braking of the hand was crucial for intercepting the target accurately. Control over the speed of movement was independent of control over the path of movement. There was evidence for direct and rapid links between input systems and output systems.

This paper reports the first attempt to examine systematically in adults the way in which the hand approaches and intercepts targets which move on different trajectories and with different speeds. There has been little work published previously on this topic (e.g. Alderson, Sully & Sully, 1974) in contrast to a number of recent detailed analyses of hand movement to stationary targets (e.g. Atkeson & Hollerbach, 1985; Flash & Hogan, 1985). Moving targets place different demands on a subject than stationary targets, and the nature of the hand's response could be expected to depend on the target's motion.

The task to be described requires subjects to intercept targets moving on a television monitor. Subjects move on the surface of the screen; they aim directly at the target with their hand, and are free to adjust their speed and direction of movement. The task, therefore, has spatial and temporal characteristics, and data on the speed and direction of hand movement will be reported. The task is essentially different from coincident timing or anticipatory timing tasks, which have targets moving through fixed and predictable paths of motion, and are constrained spatially in requiring subjects to make a unidimensional manual response with a demand for accurate timing only. In one group of these studies, subjects were required to press a button to coincide with the arrival of a target at a fixed point (Belisle, 1963; McGown, Dobbins, & Rarick, 1973; Slater-Hammel, 1960). In another group of studies, subjects viewed a screen which had a vertically moving target, and a horizontally moving cursor. The subject controlled the motion of the cursor by moving a handle along a slide (Ball & Glencross, 1985; Dorfmann, 1977) or turning a knob (Gerhard, 1959), and the task was to intercept the target with the cursor. There was only one possible point of interception, hence the tasks had a low spatial demand. Timing data from such spatially constrained tasks are not relevant to the present situation in which it is possible to substitute precise timing with a combination of aiming and timing. Indeed, it will be shown that when given the freedom, subjects do adjust the direction in which they move as they approach a moving target.

Experimental data to be described, shows that visual and kinaesthetic input is converted by the central nervous system into motor output, more rapidly than tradition reaction time data would seem to allow. Data shows also that the direction of movement of the hand is controlled independently from the speed of movement. Indeed, there may be a ranking in the order of control; contrary to what one might think intuitively, the speed of movement may be specified by the perceptuo-motor system, earlier in the response than the direction of movement.

Method

Subjects

The subjects were 12 adult volunteers, varying in age from 22 to 55 years (mean age 31 years 4 months). All wrote with their right hand, and had normal or corrected-to-normal vision.

Apparatus and task

The task required subjects to intercept targets moving on a television monitor. The monitor's screen was 61 cm, high line rate, and had a frame frequency of 58.19 Hz. It was mounted to slope upwards and away from the subject at 18 degrees from the horizontal. Subjects held a pen-like cursor in the right hand and moved to intercept the targets by sliding the cursor on the surface of the screen. The cursor was a sparking device of a Series 6 GRAF/PEN sonic digitizer, and the microphone sensors were mounted along the left and far side of the monitor. The apparatus used to regulate the moving targets, record the motion of the hand and calculate whether the target was intercepted, was an LSI 11/23 microcomputer with 64 K bytes RAM, and a SUPERVISOR 214 SB12 stand-alone monochrome graphics display system.

At the commencement of a trial, a cross (1cm x 1cm) was displayed at the near right hand corner of the television screen. The subject held the pen of the digitizer in the right hand with a pencil grip, and positioned the pen over the cross. This was the subject's "home position" at the commencement of every trial. The subject was instructed to look toward the far edge of the screen. A square target (1cm x 1cm) appeared and moved toward the near edge in a straight line with a constant speed. The subject's tasks were to slide the pen on the surface of the screen and intercept the approaching target before it disappeared off the near edge. The trial ended either with the subject intercepting the target at which point it halted and changed into an exploding pattern (this was a source of motivation and knowledge of the accuracy of performance), or if not intercepted, the target passed off the near edge of the screen. Subjects were seated but were otherwise unrestrained in their posture or movements. Subjects were instructed to be accurate (i.e. to intercept the targets). They were free to choose how fast they moved and to intercept the target anywhere along its path. They could intercept the target by slowing down and stopping, or by crossing over and following through at speed.

The display of successive target positions, and the measurement of hand position was synchronized to the monitor frame pulse. The targets appeared to move continuously and smoothly. The position of the hand was sampled every 17.2 ms (similar to recent studies of reaching to stationary targets; Fisk & Goodale, 1985; Soechting, 1984).

Design and procedure

Subjects had five blocks of 12 trials. The speed of the target varied between trial blocks. Within a trial block, the speed was constant, while the target's trajectory varied (there were six trajectories). The target appeared at one of three locations at the far edge of the screen, and from each location either moved parallel to the Y-axis of the screen or at an angle (see Figure 1). Hence,

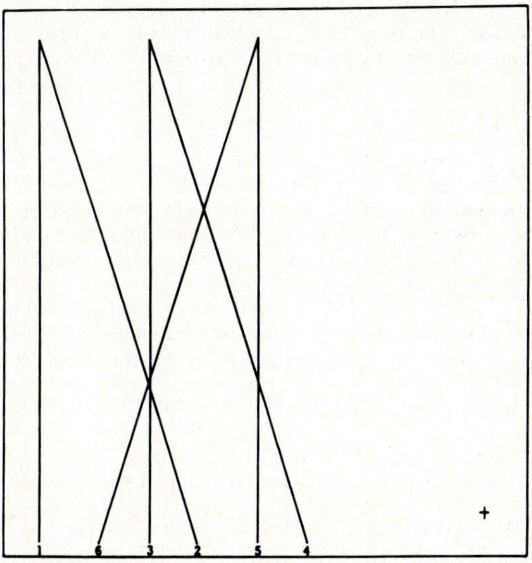

Figure 1 A hard copy of the six trajectories. The subject's home position is shown at the bottom right hand corner.

an essentially new response had to be generated for each trial because the subject could not predict the target's trajectory before it was seen. The 12 trials were made up of two random orders of the six trajectories. Subjects were unaware of the repetition of trials. The second six trials of each block were analysed.

Testing began with the target speed at 375 mm/s, to familiarize the subject with the task requirements, and to imply a need to respond quickly (albeit subjects were not instructed to move rapidly). For the remaining five blocks, the target speed was 125, 200, 275, 375 and 500 mm/s. Subjects were forewarned before each trial block that the target speed would be higher. This design allowed for an examination of the way in which performance changed with an ordered increase in the temporal demands of the task. Trials from three blocks were analysed in detail (target speed 125, 375, 500 mm/s). For each dependent variable, an analysis of variance was performed for a two-factor experiment, (six trajectories and three speeds) with repeated measures on both factors (Ferguson, 1981).

Data analysis

The raw data was a record of pixel locations for both the target and the hand-held cursor (see Figure 2). These were converted to mm. The analysis was performed partially automatically, and partially by employing an interactive computer graphics mode of analysis. The following seven measures were calculated.

Movement initiation time
This was the time between the appearance of the target and the first significant movement of the cursor. The criterion for the latter was that the cursor moved by more than one millimetre in a frame, and over the next four frames the movement amplitude was sequentially larger (i.e. the cursor was accelerating). This removed occasional starting artifacts due to jitter or tremor at the home position.

Three measures were made relevant to the speed of motion of the cursor. The tangential velocity of the cursor was calculated by measuring the distance moved in each 17.2 ms television frame (velocity = distance / .01718s). The velocity profile was plotted on the television screen for each trial. (See Figure 3.)

Initial acceleration of the cursor
This was calculated over four television frames following the first significant movement. A line was fitted to the plot of tangential velocity against time, and the slope of the line is the measure of initial acceleration. (See Figure 3.)

Movement duration
This was the time interval between the first significant movement of the cursor, and the cursor's closed approach to the target.

Speed units
This was a measure of how often the hand accelerated and decelerated. In the case of the velocity profile shown in Figure 3, the hand accelerated once then decelerated once, and this was counted as two speed units.

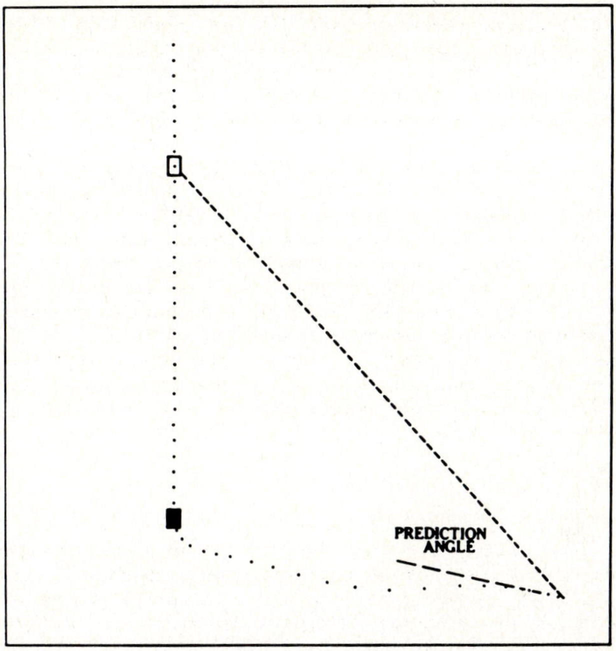

Figure 2 A hard copy of a replay of a single trial, showing pixel locations in each TV frame for both the target on trajectory 3, and the hand-held cursor. The unfilled square is the location of the target when the subject made the first significant movement; the filled square is the location of the target when the subject made the closest approach. The long-dashed line is the initiai direction of movement of the cursor. The short-dashed line is the theoretical line of direct approach to the target. In this trial the subject aimed initially well ahead of the target (positive prediction angle).
N.B. The aspect ratios of the monitor and the line-printer are different, hence the target in the hard copy is oblong, whereas the target on the monitor was square.

Three measures relevant to the direction of motion of the hand were made as follows (see Figure 2):

Initial direction of movement
This was calculated over the first three frames following movement initiation. The angle between the location of the cursor when the first significant movement occurred, and the location of the cursor three frames later was measured relative to the Y-axis of the screen

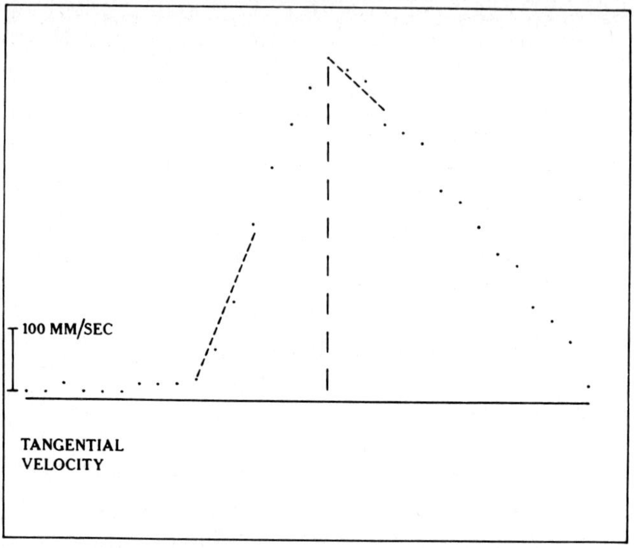

Figure 3 A piot of tangential velocity of the cursor in each TV frame from the trial shown in Figure 2. The line fitted to the first four measures of tangential velocity is shown (the slope of the line was used to calculate the initial acceleration). The peak velocity is marked. The line fitted to the four measures of velocity after the peak, for the calculation of deceleration, is also shown. 100 mm/s tangential velocity is indicated by the bar on the left.

(0° was a downward motion in the Y direction, 180° was an upward motion, with graded angles in between). Measuring the angle over three frames avoided quantization measurement errors that would arise from single pixel increments in cursor motion.

Prediction angle
This was calculated from the frame in which the first significant movement occurred. It was a measure of how far ahead or behind the target the subject aimed initially; it was the included angle between the initial direction of movement of the cursor (the initial angle) and the line of direct approach to the target. This is analogous to Von Hofsten's (1980) β angle. When subjects aimed their hand behind the target, the prediction angle was given a -ve sign, when aimed ahead, the angle was +ve.

Direction units
This was a measure of how often the curvature in the path of hand movement changed, as the hand approached the target. Firstly, a measure of curvature was made by performing a lineation of the movement path between each point sampled, and calculating the angular deviation from a straight line between adjacent segments.

When the deviation was clockwise the angle was positive, when anti-clockwise it was negative. The cumulative angle change was plotted on the television screen (see Figure 7). When the hand was moving in a straight path, the slope of function was zero, when in a clockwise arc the slope was positive, when in an anti-clockwise arc the slope was negative. The number of changes in slope was counted and this was a measure of the number of direction units. It will be noted that a straight path of movement, or a constant curvature in the path of movement were counted as "units" of direction. In the trial shown in the left of Figure 7 there are three direction units (anti-clockwise—anti-clockwise—clockwise); on the right there is one clockwise direction unit.

Results and Discussion

Movement initiation time

The time between the appearance of the target and the onset of acceleration of the cursor was, on average, 220 ms. This value is similar to traditional visual reaction time data.

Initiation time to targets on distant trajectories did not differ from initiation time to close targets. This is contrary to data on reaching to stationary targets (see Sidaway, Christina & Shea, this volume; and Kerr, 1983, for conflicting data). Chronometric data on aiming to stationary targets has been used in discussions of processes involved in motor control. It has been argued that aiming at distant targets involves greater constraint on the neuromotor system than aiming at close targets. The response to a distant target is, therefore, more difficult to organize - it needs to be more accurate - and this is an explanation for the extra time that is sometimes needed to translate input into motor output.

The lack of variation in movement initiation time in the present task is of limited interest when the target moved slowly, because there was no speed requirement, and any kind of initiation time/movement speed trade-off would be possible. However, when the target moved rapidly, there was an implicit demand on the subject to move as quickly as possible. The continued failure to find an increase in initiation time with increase in the distance of the target, suggests that there may be a difference in how the neuromotor system translates input from a stationary target, and input from a moving target, into motor output. There is a need for further systematic study of reaching to non-previewed, rapidly moving targets, of varying distance and size, to establish the relevance of Fitts' index of difficulty, to initiation time.

While initiation time did not vary with the target's trajectory, data on the initial 52 ms of movement shows that subjects had prepared, during the initiation interval, a response that was specific for the target.

Initial acceleration

Acceleration of the hand in the initial 52 ms had been scaled for the target's trajectory ($\underline{F}(5,55)=5.02$, $\underline{p}<.01$). Targets that were close were approached with lower acceleration than those far away (this is consistent with data on reaching to stationary targets: Accornero, Barardelli, Argenta, & Manfredi, 1984; Benecke, Meinck, & Conrad, 1985; Flash & Hogan, 1985). Targets that moved obliquely towards or away from the subject's home position were approached with lesser and greater acceleration (respectively) than targets moving vertically from the same starting position. Initial acceleration was also greater for fast targets than slow targets ($\underline{F}(2,22)=23.40, \underline{p}<.01$). In other words, acceleration at the onset of movement was scaled for all characteristics of the target — its origin, angle of motion, and speed (see Figure 4).

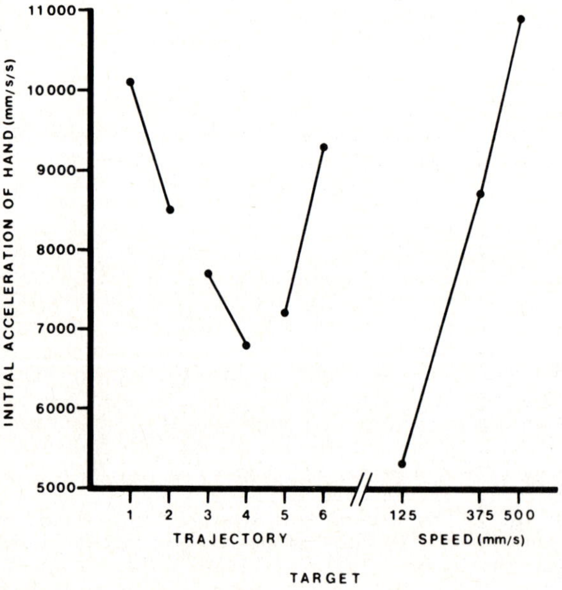

Figure 4. Mean initial acceleration of the hand for the six target trajectories (see Figure 1), and three speeds.

The acceleration of the limb depends on the resultant force of active (muscle contraction) and passive (e.g. viscoelastic resistance) factors, both aiding and hindering limb motion. Quite clearly subjects could plan finely the force of muscle contraction (and hence acceleration), prior to movement onset. Planning for target speed was assisted by the speed being potentially predictable. Target trajectory, however, was not predictable, and the planning of force was possible only after the target appeared and during the 220 ms movement initiation time.

Initial direction

Direction of movement over the initial 52 ms showed that the hand was aimed ahead of the target - not to where the target was seen (see Figure 2). However, the direction of hand movement did not vary with the target's trajectory; subjects aimed indiscriminately to the left regardless of the location of the target. Subjects aimed lower on the screen for fast targets than slow targets ($F(2,22)=12.15$, $p<.01$), but they did not aim further ahead of faster targets (i.e. the prediction angle did not vary with target speed).

These results show that in contrast to acceleration, the initial direction of movement was not scaled finely for different targets - direction was not adjusted for different trajectories, and only adjusted crudely for different speeds. The direction of movement is determined primarily by the balance of activity in the muscle groups controlling movement of the limb. This balance of activity was not finely planned prior to movement onset.

Movement duration

As Figure 5 suggests, the time between the onset of acceleration and interception of the target varied with the target's trajectory ($F(5,55)=4.19$, $p<.01$) and the speed ($F(2,22)=26.29$, $p<.01$).

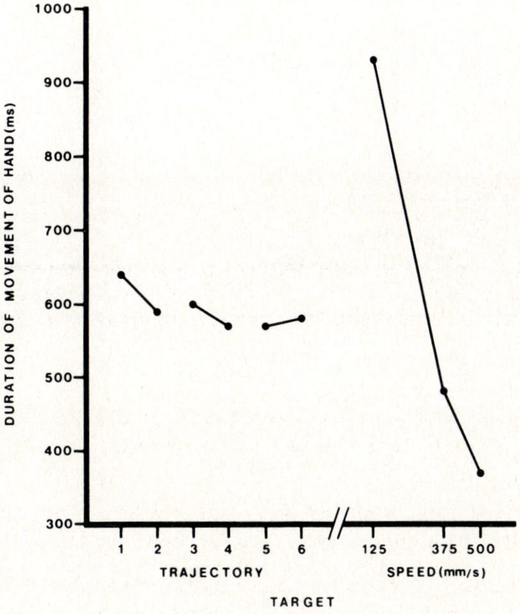

Figure 5. Mean duration of movement of the hand, for the six target trajectories (see Figure 1), and three speeds.

During this interval there were adjustments to both the speed and direction of the hand, even when the duration was as short as 365 ms.

Adjustments to movement speed

The tangential velocity of the hand was changing throughout the response. In the absence of EMG recordings, it is possible only to infer likely adjustments in muscular activity underlying the observable changes in velocity. Initial acceleration was generated by the force of muscular contraction in agonist muscles, with a constant force generating a constant acceleration. The sudden onset of deceleration was generated by muscular activity in antagonist muscles, because the subjects were moving on the surface of a screen of low friction, and in a horizontal plane essentially. A change between acceleration and deceleration was taken as the clearest possible sign, and also a conservative sign, that the neuromotor system had specified an adjustment to speed through an adjustment in activity in antagonistic muscles.

Most commonly there was only one major adjustment to speed (see Figures 3 and 6a). After the initial acceleration, the hand reached a peak in tangential velocity and then there was a longer braking phase, though the hand was still moving when it intercepted the target.

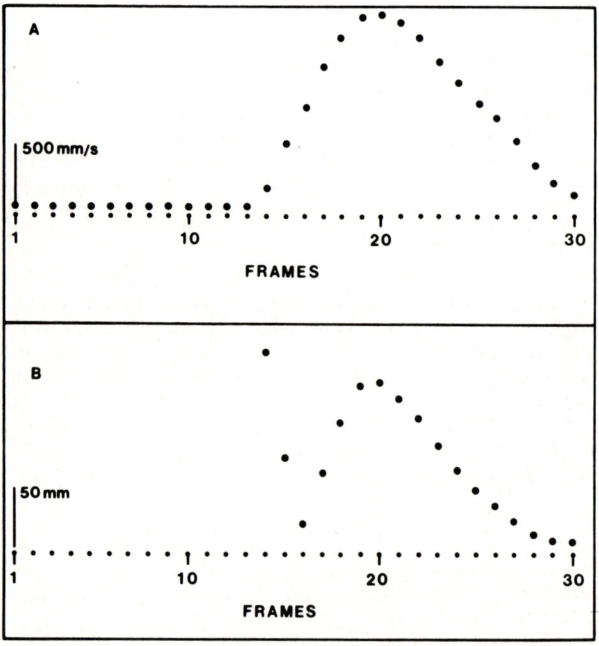

Figure 6. (a) Tangential velocity of the handheld cursor in each TV frame (58.19 Hz) on a typical trial; 500 mm/s is indicated by the bar on the left. b) From the same trial, the distance between the extrapolated location of the target and extrapolated location of the cursor in each TV frame (see text); 50 mm is indicated by the bar on the left. The target appeared in Frame 1.

It is interesting that, even though the initial acceleration of the hand was scaled for different targets, the braking phase was vital for bringing the hand to the target. This can be shown in the following way: the movement of the target and the movement of the hand in each television frame was extrapolated over the number of frames remaining before interception of the target. The distance between the extrapolated target and extrapolated cursor location was calculated; the smaller the distance, the more appropriate was the subject's speed and direction of movement in a particular frame, for reaching the eventual interception point on time. The plot in Figure 6b shows that early in the response the subject was accurately "on target" (frame 16 distance = 2 cm). But the subject was in an acceleration phase (Figure 6a), behaving in an apparently inappropriate way, leading to a peak in error (frame 20 distance = 15 cm) which coincided with a peak in velocity of the hand. The second steady decrease in distance between extrapolated target and cursor leading to interception of the target, coincided with deceleration of the hand. If the subject had continued moving at the peak velocity, the target would have been missed by a large margin. Clearly, the breaking phase after the peak in velocity was crucial for bringing the hand to the target accurately.

It is well known that braking is a feature of reaching to stationary targets (e.g. Fisk & Goodale, 1985; Soechting, 1984). The present data shows that the braking phase of reaching is important in situations where the environment - a moving target - is not dictating implicitly a terminal deceleration, and when the subject has the option of intercepting and passing over the target at speed. Indeed, it is rare to see trials in which subjects adopt spontaneously the strategy of intercepting the targets while still accelerating.

Adjustments to the path of the hand

It was common for the hand to move through a curvilinear path; that is, the direction of the hand was changing continually. Movement of the hand along a path of constant curvature can be caused by motion around a single joint (e.g. the elbow). Movement of the hand along a straight path can occur only if a number of joints are synergistically involved in the response. Changes in the curvature of the path of the hand was taken as the clearest possible outward sign that the neuromotor system had specified an adjustment to the path of the hand through an adjustment in the balance of activity in muscle groupings determining limb movement. In contract to the single adjustment to speed, there were multiple adjustments to the path of movement. The number of adjustments did not vary with the target's trajectory, but decreased as the target speed was increased (7,5,4 adjustments; $F(2,22)=36.45$, $p<.01$). The initial crude setting of movement direction for a particular target is compensated for during the movement by multiple adjustments to the path.

Independent control over the direction and speed of hand movement

There is evidence, both in initiation and in ongoing control, that the direction of movement of the hand is controlled independently from the speed of movement. As shown above, the initial acceleration is scaled for the origin, direction of motion, and speed of a target,

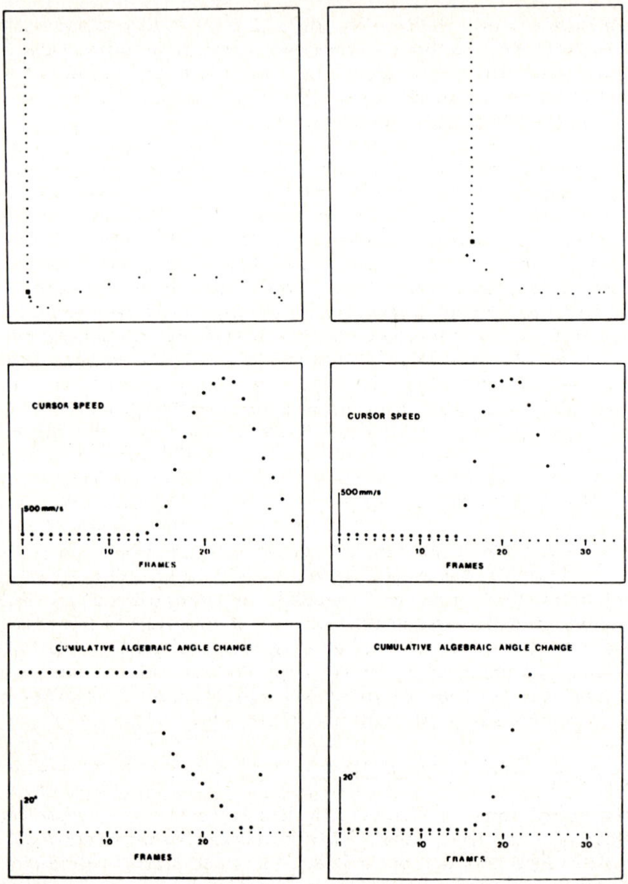

Figure 7. Data from two trials are shown. In the top part of the figure are hard copies of the trials, showing pixel locations for the target and the hand in each TV frame. In the bottom part of the figure are plots of the tangential velocity of the handheld cursor and curvature in the path of the hand in each TV frame (58.19 Hz); 500 mm/s tangential velocity, and 20° cumulative algebraic angle change is indicated by the bars on the left. The target appeared in Frame 1. In both trials there was one adjustment to the speed of the hand - acceleration to a peak, followed by deceleration (two "speed units"). In the trial on the left there were three "direction units" (two anticlockwise units, followed by a clockwise unit). In the trial on the right there was one "direction unit" (a smooth clockwise motion of the hand). In both trials it can be seen that adjustment in speed and adjustment in the path of the hand did not occur at the same time.

while initial direction of movement is scaled only crudely for target speed. During the movement there is usually only one adjustment to speed, but multiple adjustments to the path of movement. Indeed, as Figure 7 shows, speed and direction adjustments can occur at different times during the movement; this is seen quite commonly.

Acceleration depends on the force of contraction in a group of muscles; the path of movement depends on the balance of activity in that group of muscles. Present results suggest that a balance of activity and an overall level of activity need not be specified together. Perhaps it is not surprising that one can continue a movement on a certain path but make it slower. This can be a matter of scaling down activity in an already active group of muscles. However, if antagonist muscles have to be activated, then there is a control problem if these now active muscles should not upset the path of movement - they have the potential to throw the hand off course, yet one commonly sees smooth deceleration, and no adjustment to the path. The recorded motion of the hand is a complex function of the total EMG activity in a group of antagonistic muscles. It is interesting to see a recent study which suggests that the late burst of agonist activity in a goal directed movement moderates the antagonist braking forces and redirects the movement back to the target (Wierzbicka, Wiegner, & Shahani, 1986).

There seems to be another complex control problem involved in maintaining a constant acceleration, and making adjustments to the path of movement — that is, changing the balance of activity in the group of muscles but maintaining an overall level of activity. I do not believe we yet have an explanation for how the motor system solves these sorts of control problems.

Another point to make here is that the speed of hand movement seems to be specified earlier in the response than the direction of movement. This leads one to think about how sensory input may be used to control the aiming response. First, visual input from the target's origin, angle, and speed of motion is used by the central nervous system to prepare and specify a level of activation of muscles, although the initial balance of activity is specified only crudely. Then input, possibly visual and kinaesthetic, from the now moving hand, plus the visual input from the target, is used to control the hand as it makes its approach to the target. The frequent adjustments of the path of movement indicate that direction is best specified "en route". Perhaps the balance of activity in muscle groupings can only be finely adjusted by input from the moving hand, while visual input from the target alone is adequate for specifying the force of contraction at the onset of movement.

Fast conversion of sensory input into motor output

Data on the initiation and ongoing control of movement shows that input is converted by the central nervous system into motor output more rapidly than traditional reaction time data would allow. Movement initiation time was 220 ms on average. Although this interval is similar to traditional visual reaction time, it seems short considering the major differences between the present task and the usual simple and choice reaction time tasks. Subjects were not given a preview of the target, were not warned about it, and did not know which way it would move. And while there is more to aiming at a moving target than a stationary target, subjects managed within 220 ms to finely adjust the force of muscle contraction for the origin, path, and speed of the particular target. Given that there are a number of activities going on during initiation time - like the activation of neuromuscular components - the actual planning and scaling of force for a particular target must take even less time than 220 ms.

Movement duration was 365 ms on average, when the target moved rapidly. During this time, four adjustments to the movement path were commonly seen. Each adjustment therefore took place once every 91 ms on average. These short intervals which were needed to prepare and adjust a response to a moving target lead one to think that there must be direct and rapid links between input systems and output systems. This notion can be found in a number of recent publications dealing with reaching to stationary targets (e.g. Beaubaton & Hay, 1986; Pelisson, Prablanc, & Goodale, 1986; Prablanc, Pelisson, & Goodale, 1986).

It is certain that subjects were unaware of the control processes they manifestly have at their command. They did not make explicit judgements or conscious decisions. When subjects had trials played back immediately to them, their comments were illuminating. Invariably they expressed surprise at how far down the screen the target moved, before they themselves began moving. To them it seemed as if they moved as soon as the target appeared, and they were unaware of needing to spend as much as 40 per cent of the time available observing the target and initiating a response. They were also unaware of making adjustments, most notably when the target moved rapidly; they thought that they intercepted the targets at maximum speed, and were unaware of braking; they thought that they made a direct approach, and were unaware of changing the path of the hand. The control of the hand that is evident in these types of data must be the domain of rather "low" functional levels of the central nervous system.

The results of a study being conducted presently with normal and "clumsy" children (see Laszlo, Bairstow, Bartrip, & Rolfe, this volume) suggest that it may be possible to measure with the present task, the functioning of different levels of the perceptuo-motor system. When clumsy children, in particular, are started off with slow target speeds, they do not perform very well. When the speed is increased, performance deteriorates initially as one might expect. But if the target speed is increased still further, some children seem to switch to a different mode of control, and start moving very rapidly and accurately. How sensory input is rapidly and effectively converted by the central nervous system into motor output in this way has yet to be explained.

Acknowledgements

The research was supported by a grant from the Medical Research Council. Paul Laszlo wrote the software to control the task. My thanks go to Jon Bartrip and Kathleen Leadbetter for help in the preparation of the manuscript.

References

Accornero, N., Barardelli, A., Argenta, M., & Manfredi, M. (1985). Two joint ballistic arm movements. Neuroscience Letters, 46, 91-95.

Alderson, N., Sully, D.J., & Sully, H.G. (1974). An operational analysis of a one-handed catching task using high speed photography. Journal of Motor Behavior, 6, 217-226.

Atkeson, C.G., & Hollerbach, J.M. (1985). Kinematic features of unrestrained vertical arm movements. Journal of Neuroscience, 5, 2318-2330.

Ball, C.T., & Glencross, D. (1985). Developmental differences in a coincident timing task under speed and time constraints. Human Movement Science, 4, 1-15.

Beaubaton, D., & Hay, L. (1986). Contribution of visual information to feedforward and feedback processes in rapid pointing movements. Human Movement Science, 5, 19-34.

Belisle, J.J. (1963). Accuracy, Reliability and refractoriness in a coincidence—anticipation task. Research Quarterly, 34, 271-281.

Benecke, R., Meinck, H.M., & Conrad, B. (1985). Rapid goal-directed elbow flexion movements: limitations of the speed control system due to neural constraints. Experimental Brain Research, 59, 470-477.

Dorfmann, P.W. (1977). Timing and anticipation: A developmental perspective. Journal of Motor Behavior, 9, 67-79.

Ferguson, G.A. (1981). Statistical analysis in Psychology and Education. London: McGraw-Hill.

Fisk, J.D., & Goodale, M.A. (1985). The organization of eye and limb movements during unrestrained reaching to targets in contralateral and ipsilateral visual space. Experimental Brain Research, 60, 159-178.

Flash, T., & Hogan, N. (1985). The coordination of arm movements: an experimentally confirmed mathematical model. Journal of Neuroscience, 5, 1688-1703.

Gerhard, D.J. (1959). The judgement of velocity and prediction of motion. Ergonomics, 2, 287-304.

Kerr, B. (1983). Preplanning for aimed movements: disruption from a preliminary task. Journal of Experimental Psychology: Human Perception and Performance, 9, 596-606.

Laszlo, J.I., Bairstow, P.J., Bartrip, J., & Rolfe, U. Clumsiness or perceptuo-motor dysfunction? In A.M. Colley, & J.R. Beech (Eds.), Cognition and action in skilled behaviour. Amsterdam: North Holland (in press).

McGown, C.M., Dobbins, D.A., & Rarick, G.L. (1973). Intra-individual variability of normal and educable mentally retarded children on a coincidence timing task. Journal of Motor Behavior, 5, 193-198.

Pelisson, D., Prablanc, C., Goodale, M.A., & Jeannerod, M. (1986). Visual control of reaching movements without vision of the limb. II. Evidence for fast unconscious processes correcting the trajectory of the hand. Experimental Brain Research, 62, 303-311.

Prablanc, C., Pelisson, D., & Goodale, M.A. (1986). Visual control of reaching movements without vision of the limb. I. Role of retinal feedback of target position in guiding the limb. Experimental Brain Research, 62, 293-302.

Sidaway, B., Christina, R.W., & Shea, B. An information theory interpretation of the response complexity effect on programming time. In A.M. Colley, & J.R. Beech (Eds.), Cognition and action in skilled behaviour. Amsterdam: North Holland (in press).

Slater-Hammel, A.T. (1960). Reliability, accuracy and refractoriness of a transit reaction. Research Quarterly, 31, 217-228.

Soechting, J.F. (1984). Effect of target size on spatial and temporal characteristics of a pointing movement in man. Experimental Brain Research, 54, 121-132.

Von Hofsten, C. (1980). Predictive reaching for moving objects by human infants. Journal of Experimental Child Psychology, 30, 369-382.

Wierzbicka, M.M., Wiegner, A.W., & Shahani, B.T. (1986). Role of agonist and antagonist muscles in fast arm movements in man. Experimental Brain Research, 63, 331-340.

Cognition and Action in Skilled Behaviour
A.M. Colley and J.R. Beech (Editors)

UNPACED AIMING – A CONTROL THEORY EXPLANATION

W.D.A. Beggs and C.I. Howarth
University of Nottingham

Most experiments in the field of motor control use one of two paradigms, paced or self-paced aiming. Measures of performance, either of accuracy or of time respectively, are then used to generate models. Most of these models are of limited generality. In an experiment in the self-paced tradition, both response accuracy and movement time were recorded. In addition, measures of hand trajectories towards the strip targets were obtained. The intermittent correction hypothesis of Howarth and Beggs predicts a linear relationship between the width of the dispersion of hits and the point at which the last correction to a closed-loop movement is made; this prediction was confirmed. By including the hypothesis that subjects make strategic changes to the way that they move their hand towards the target, this model can account for aiming accuracy in both paced and self-paced tasks. In addition, it offers a new way of understanding Fitts Law.

Two main theoretical perspectives on the control of movement dominated the literature of the last thirty years; models based on Information Theory (e.g. Fitts, 1954; Welford, 1968) and models based on Control Theory, specifically the iterative correction hypothesis (e.g. Crossman & Goodeve, 1963, 1983; Keele, 1968; Howarth, Beggs, & Bowden, 1971). In the last few years, new approaches, deriving from neuro-physiological and biomechanical considerations have made their appearance (Meyer, Smith, & Wright, 1982; Schmidt, Zelaznik, Hawkins, Frank, & Quinn, 1979). The emergence of this change in emphasis is at least partly because of the limitations in the scope of the earlier work.

One of the major weaknesses in all approaches is their inability to account for data which is more easily described by an alternative model. For example, the Impulse Variability models are at the moment limited to accounting for ballistic errors made in the same direction as the movement itself, while the Iterative Correction model proposed by Howarth et al. (1971) is unable to account for the accuracy of movements which are self-paced, only those where the subject has to move in time to a metronome. This failure of any one approach to give a general account of movement accuracy and speed is at least one reason why there is such a plethora of models.

One of the most widely known systematic analyses of the relationship between movement time, movement distance and the required accuracy of responses was due to Fitts (1954). His theory, based on the concept of the noisy channel, predicted a function where MT is the

$$MT = a \log 2A/W + b \qquad (1)$$

movement time, A is the amplitude of movement, W the width of the target, and a and b are constants. This relationship remains a reasonable description of data from a wide range of tasks (Fitts, 1954; Fitts & Peterson, 1964; Knight & Dagnall, 1967; Langolf, Chaffin, & Foulkes, 1976) and is generally able to predict performance speed when accuracy is constrained.

There have been several attempts to erect models of movement control which would predict Fitts Law; the first of these came from workers in the Information Theory tradition (Fitts, 1954; Fitts & Peterson, 1964; Welford, 1968). Later, the Iterative Correction camp produced their own attempts (Crossman & Goodeve, 1963, 1983; Keele, 1968; Langolf, Chaffin, & Foulke, 1976). Recently, Keele (1981) reviewed these theoretical perspectives and concluded that they contained unrealistic assumptions. For example, they do not predict the apparently continuous relationship of terminal error and movement time. Meyer, Smith, and Wright (1982) have tried to account for Fitts Law by an extension of Impulse Variability theory, but like earlier workers, their modelling also relies on a number of as yet imperfectly tested assumptions. Clearly, it would be a considerable step forward if the generality or the limitations of a given approach were more accurately known.

At least one attempt has been made to investigate the boundary conditions for the Information Theory model and one of the Iterative Correction models. Kerr and Langolf (1977) showed, using an experimental set-up very like that described by Howarth et al. (1971), that the accuracy of movements made with a dart-throwing action without releasing the stylus were well described by Fitts Law. A very similar task reported by Howarth et al. produced data which was well described by their model, but could not be accounted for by Fitts Law. Unlike Howarth et al., however, Kerr and Langolf used self-paced movements, and it looked as if the description of aiming advanced by Howarth et al. was altogether too specific, and concerned only with paced movements, while Fitts Law and its explanations were concerned with self-paced movements.

Howarth et al. proposed a probabilistic model of aiming. In this, the width of the distribution of terminal errors is seen as a function of two fundamental parameters; σ_θ , the angular accuracy of aiming, and d_c, the distance from impact at which a final correction to a movement is implemented. A crucial factor in this model was the corrective reaction time, which they had earlier estimated as 290ms (Beggs & Howarth, 1970). The model predicted that after a correction had been made, if the remaining time to impact was less than this value, further corrections to the movement could not occur, and the hand would move ballistically from this point in time and space onto the target. Howarth and Beggs had nothing to say about paced or self-paced movements, although the data which they used to support their model came exclusively from paced aiming experiments.

Very conveniently, it was found that d_C had a relatively simple relationship to the movement time, and so it proved possible to predict the effect of movement time on terminal accuracy by the following equation

$$E_\varepsilon^2 = E_O^2 + KD^2\sigma_\theta^2 t_C / T^{2.8} \quad (2)$$

where E_ε^2 is the variable error, E_O^2 is a residual error, probably tremor, K is an arbitrary constant, D is movement distance, t_C is the corrective reaction time, σ_θ is the angular accuracy of aiming, and T is movement time (Howarth & Beggs, 1985).

Recently, several workers have suggested that visual corrective reaction time may be much less than 200 to 300 ms. However, there are a number of reasons why their data have to be treated with caution. For example, Smith and Bowen (1980) used an on-line discrete aiming task with a number of criterion movement times and conditions of feedback. They noted that mean errors at a movement time of 150 ms were significantly affected by a delay in feedback of 66 ms, and concluded that this showed that feedback must have operated faster than 150 ms. Unfortunately, they failed to discuss the curious nature of the variable errors at the same movement time. These suggest that an anomaly may have occurred, because the distribution of errors at this movement time under normal conditions was very low, and markedly failed to follow the trend of increased error distribution width with decreasing movement time. In any case, as discussed by Howarth and Beggs (1985), no theoretical account of performance based on corrections to a movement considers mean error rather than the distribution of errors; and their experiment was not designed in the first place to test for the effects of visual information on corrections to movements.

Zelaznik, Hawkins, and Kisselborough (1983) presented a series of experiments intended, rather indirectly, to measure visual corrective reaction time. However, although they measured errors aimed at a dot target in the dimensions parallel and perpendicular to the direction of movement, they failed to separate constant and variable errors. By using a root-mean-square error, the logical and theoretical differences between the width of the distribution, and its centre relative to the target are confounded. These differences, and the differing effects of movement time and other variables have been commented on before (e.g. Beggs, 1971; Howarth, 1978; Howarth & Beggs, 1985).

The theory of movement control based on intermittent corrections advanced by Howarth et al. (1971) is specifically concerned with errors measured at right angles to movement. These errors of direction (Zelaznik et al., 1983) or errors of aiming (Howarth & Beggs, 1985) are much less likely than errors of stopping to suffer distortions when constant and variable errors are combined in a single score (Beggs, 1971), simply because constant errors in this dimension are relatively small, and not much affected by movement time. In fact, Zelaznik et al.'s data for errors of aiming or direction did seem to show that t_C may lie between 180 and 260 ms. Such a value, somewhere between those found by Keele and Posner (1968) and Beggs and Howarth (1970) may fit the data for repetitive aiming rather better than the 290 ms of the latter: Howarth and

Beggs (1985) allude to this possibility. Zelaznik et al.'s data suggest that the same may be true for single-shot aiming; their contention that t_c is less than 100 ms is simply not supported by their experiments. It remains possible that corrections with a latency of this magnitude are the ripple effect identified by Crossman and Goodeve (1963, 1983), implicating a peripheral kinaesthetically-mediated corrective loop.

Carlton (1981) used a single shot aiming paradigm, and reported that at about 290 ms into the movement, a discontinuity in the trajectory of the hand was observed. This was in spite of the subject being unable to see most of his movement. However, he then suggested that corrective reaction time must be markedly lower than earlier estimates because the subjects could only see the last very short portion of their hand movements. Unfortunately, his assumption that vision of the hand as it comes into view from under an occluding shield is the only source of information about its position, is unwarranted, and relating the time at which this event occurs to the later presence of a correction to the movement is not an acceptable method of estimating t_c. Like Stubbs (1976), we have assumed that when the target is fixated, visual hand position information is not used for control. Rather, kinaesthetic or proprioceptive information about the hand, and visual target position information, may be used to generate an intersensory error signal. In this explanation, the sight of the hand, either on the target or in motion, is used to keep the visual and kinaesthetic spatial information in synchrony (e.g. Howarth, 1978; Howarth & Beggs, 1985).

It is interesting to note that the corrections found by Carlton appear to have a periodicity of precisely that which we earlier reported (Beggs & Howarth, 1970), suggesting that after 290 ms, a correction is made to an ongoing movement. Carlton's work makes it clear that we should have explicated our ideas rather more carefully, although we have recently somewhat extended and clarified them (Howarth & Beggs, 1985). If the corrective reaction time is, say, 290 ms, then clearly it is impossible for two corrections to be made inside this time to impact, if one is made precisely 290 ms away from the target. The point in the trajectory where the hand is 290 ms from impact is thus crucial; we have called this d_c, and identified discontinuities in performance associated with it (Beggs & Howarth, 1970). However, this point of inflection describes the worst case. If a correction is made here or later, no further corrections are possible, and the hand finishes the movement ballistically. If a correction is made earlier in the movement, another may then be fitted in before the hand reaches the target - possibly very close to the target. Thus, although for theoretical and practical convenience d_c is measured from impact, the subject may be able to fit corrections in at any part of the movement, assuming that the latency period after starting the movement is exceeded. Carlton's result, that a correction can be observed at around 290 ms after the start of the movement, is consistent with our intermittent correction hypothesis. It is, however, interesting to speculate that corrections need not be synchronised to the start of the movement; in fact, our data (Beggs & Howarth, 1970) preclude this. Perhaps they are "elicited" by the "affordance" of the target? In fact, these data suggested that some corrections can occur inside d_c; the small positive slope of the curves between impact and d_c suggest that the hand was not in fact always moving ballistically. Second, these data suggest that in slower movements, t_c is less than 290 ms, although we did not comment on this. Jagacinsky, Repperger, Moran, Ward, and Glass (1980) showed that a number of successive corrections to movements can be identified kinematically. Reading the data from their Figure 3, it seems that the first took about 320 ms, the second 240, the third 200, and a fourth about 175 ms. Clearly, the number of corrections that can be made to a movement will be determined by the movement time. Although Keele (1981) has called our theory a single correction model, in fact we have never claimed that only a single correction is made. Rather, we have focussed on the importance for terminal accuracy of the final correction to a movement (e.g. Howarth & Beggs, 1985). It is a weakness in our approach that we assume that each one is accomplished with the same latency, but for medium speed movements, this is largely true. These findings do not seriously challenge the conclusion that t_c lies somewhere between 200 and 300 ms. Although we have measured it in a paced aiming situation (Beggs & Howarth, 1970), we will again use our own value for this parameter, mainly because it was measured on the equipment used for this experiment. It may be that t_c varies somewhat in different situations.

The exponent in the above equation is an empirically determined one, which described the decelerative portion of the approach trajectory of the hand towards the target. In paced aiming experiments where naive subjects were used, this exponent remained remarkably stable, and independent of movement speed (Beggs & Howarth, 1972a; Beggs, Graham, Monk, Shaw, & Howarth, 1972; Howarth et al., 1971). On the other hand, a number of experiments have shown that there is more than one way of approaching a target. Annett, Goldby, and Kay (1958) showed that the approach trajectory of the hand had a very different shape to that reported by Howarth et al. (1971) or by Beggs and Howarth (1972a). Instead of a relatively uniform deceleration described by an exponent of about 1.5, Annett et al. found that subjects decelerated sharply near the target, and hovered close to it before their final approach; such a trajectory would have a much higher value for the exponent. The task used by Annett et al. was self-paced, which means that the subjects would be asked to achieve high accuracy at the expense of time, instead of the accurate timing demanded by metronome pacing.

More recently, a task-related change in the approach trajectory of the hand, or torsional wrist movements was demonstrated by Langolf et al. (1976) and Jagacinski et al. (1980), who both examined the microstructure of the movement involved in different sorts of aiming tasks. The effect of practice, too, can change how a subject performs a task, in a quite subtle way. Beggs and Howarth (1972b) showed that a subject adjusted the approach trajectory with practice, so that accuracy was improved. The critical change was that the distance d_c was reduced, resulting in smaller terminal error distributions which were still linearily related to the values of d_c at different movement times. It seems that subjects are well aware of their own capabilities at an intuitive level, and adopt or change their strategies appropriately, depending on the particular aiming task they are asked to do. This work suggests the possibility that the Howarth and Beggs model may be able to account for accuracy in self-paced aiming, as well as paced aiming, simply by considering any strategic changes in hand approach trajectories which may occur. This paper reports an experiment which investigates this possibility.

Method

In the paced aiming experiment reported by Howarth et al. (1971), the approach trajectory of the hand towards the target was measured by recording the time to impact of the hand at different distances to impact, using an infra-red beam which was interrupted by the moving hand. From these data, a set of averaged approach curves was constructed, which allowed the values of d. to be calculated for each movement time. This method differs from the technically more advanced kinematic methods used by subsequent workers, and produces a "probable" approach trajectory. Nevertheless, these data are adequate for our probabilistic model, although individual corrections can only be inferred, not directly observed. The equipment used in that experiment was again employed in this experiment, but in this case, the task was self-paced.

However, the description "self-paced" is perhaps a misnomer. The movement time on this task was constrained, not by a metronome, but by requiring the subjects to move at such a speed that their attempts to hit a strip target did not fall outside it. Changes in movement times were thus caused by the combination of instructions to the subjects and changes in the physical size of the target strip. This is a familiar paradigm, but in this experiment, the actual position of hits was recorded, both within and around the strip.

This experiment tested the hypothesis that the width of the distribution of hits on each target in a self-paced aiming task would also be linearly related to d. In addition, any changes in trajectory shape due either to the change from metronome pacing to target width pacing, or to differences in strategy with different target widths would become apparent. Finally, from data on movement times and target widths, the ability of Fitts Law to describe these data could be assessed. Following the work of Kerr and Langolf (1977), it was expected that there would be a good fit to this function.

Apparatus

The equipment used in this experiment was a hybrid of two pieces of apparatus that have been described in detail before (Beggs, Wilkinson, & Howarth, 1975; Howarth et al., 1971). The subject sat on a stool and made repeated aiming movements from a home position just over the right shoulder to a target mounted on a fronto-parallel plane at eye-level. The movement distance was 50.0 cm, and the trajectory of the hand was sampled at eight intermediate distances from the target, namely 2.5, 5, 10, 15, 20, 25, 30, and 35 cm. This was achieved by arranging that a "wing" of cardboard fixed to the stylus broke a vertical beam of infra-red light, which was placed at each of these eight positions on successive trials. Breaking this beam started a timer, which was stopped when the stylus hit the target. These timing data, together with a second total movement-time figure collected at each trial produced a set of readings which described the movement of the hand towards the target.

The target was formed from printed-circuit board, with vertical copper lines 1 mm wide separated by 1 mm gaps. Each line produced a bit-code on paper tape, which could then be read and stored in a computer for later analysis. On the target board was drawn one of six "strip" targets, using a black felt-tip pen; the copper line in the centre of these targets was known. The strips were 5, 7.5, 12.5, 17.5, 25, and 50 mm in width: these were chosen to span the range of widths used by Kerr and Langolf (1977), which were from 0.25 to 2 inches. The vertical height of the target "strips" was 6 cm.

Subjects and Procedure

A total of 24 subjects were used, assigned in groups of 4 to one of the six target widths. This design was a consequence of the practical difficulties of arranging for a change in the target width during the course of the experiment. All subjects had normal or corrected to normal sight, and were right-handed undergraduates, aged between 19 and 22 years, with half of the sample being male. An equal number of males and females were assigned to each target sub-group, each of whom was told that they must make eight trials of 20 repetitive attempts to place the tip of the stylus within the target strip. They were unaware that accuracy was being measured but were told to avoid errors; that is, hits which failed to land inside the black borders of the target.

Hand trajectories were sampled by placing the infra-red beam at each of the eight positions for a trial of 20 hits. The positions were randomly selected for each subject, who thus did a total of 160 hits on a single strip target. After a sub-group of four subjects had been run, a new target was drawn on the target board, and the procedure repeated until all six widths were used.

Results

Hand movements

First, the data on hand trajectories was pooled for the four subjects in each of the six sub-groups. A plot of these pooled data showed, as in Howarth et al.'s (1971) experiment, a family of curves, with different total movement times. These data are displayed on Figure 1.

The values of d_c can be estimated by reading off from these curves the distance to impact when the hand was 290 ms away from impact. A more accurate method is to calculate an equation for each J-shaped part of these curves, up to a value of 350 ms. This equation takes the form $d = t^n$. By substituting a value of 290 ms for t, a value of d_c was arrived at for each curve. The values of the exponents, n, and the values of d_c arrived at by both methods are shown in Table 1.

Clearly, while the observed and calculated values are in very close agreement, the calculation produced a meaningless result for the widest target. This was because the hand was, in reality, still accelerating at 290 ms from impact, and this procedure assumes that

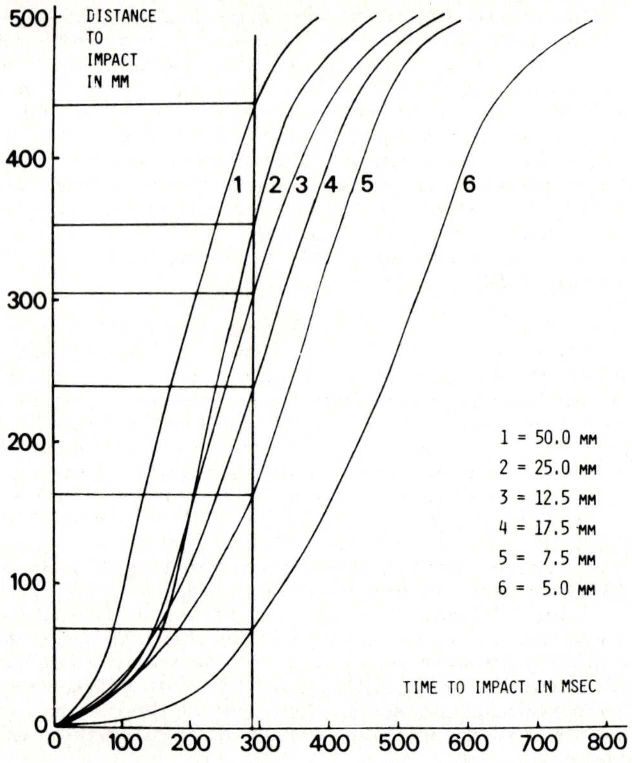

Fig. 1. The relationship between time to impact and distance to impact when aiming at strip targets.

Table 1

The exponents of the decelerative portions of the approach curves, the calculated values of d_c and the error variances. All measurements are in mm.

Strip Width (mm)	5	7.5	12.5	17.5	25	50
Exponent	2.46	1.85	2.12	1.85	1.99	1.75
Calculated d.(mm)	76.4	172.2	354.7	223.8	287.5	549.3
Observed d.(mm)	75	165	345	225	295	435
Error s.d.(mm)	2.3	3.0	4.0	4.0	4.4	6.7
Movement time (ms)	773	584	468	571	522	376

it was decelerating (see Figure 1). The by-eye estimate of d_c for this target is about 43.5 cm. However, given that the movement time for this target was within 90 ms of the estimate for corrective reaction time reported by Beggs and Howarth (1970), and that a correction at this point would be only 6.5 cm from the start of the movement, it may be that subjects tended to complete this movement without correcting it. The option to use feedback to correct movements or make them ballistically has been commented on by Zelaznik, Shapiro, and McColsky (1981). In the event that no correction was made to the movement to the widest target, it would be expected that the width of the distribution of errors would be related to the total movement distance of 50 cm, rather than d_c.

Accuracy

The analysis of the dispersion of hits on the targets will focus primarily on the variance of the distribution. In the case of targets in this orientation, constant errors are very small (Beggs, 1971) and this was confirmed in this experiment. The group mean constant errors were about 1 mm, and apparently independent of target width. They will not be discussed further. The standard deviation of the error distributions is shown in Table 1, as the group mean value for each target. The value for the smallest target, 2.3 mm, describes a dispersion in which many of the hits must have failed to land inside the strip. On the other hand, the value for the widest target, 6.7 mm, represents a distribution with 96% of the hits falling within a dispersion about 28 mm wide on a target 50 mm wide. This result further reinforces the likelihood that subjects may have had very little need to aim particularly accurately at the widest target; that is, they may not have needed to use corrections to the movement at all in order to easily ensure that their hits landed on target.

A regression equation was calculated, using the five calculated and one by-eye estimates for d_c and the corresponding values of E_ε. This equation accounted for 83.7% of the variance, and took the form

$$E_\varepsilon^2 = 0.0001888 d_c^2 + 3.15$$

This relates the width of the distribution of hits to the distance from impact where the last correction was made, by the angular accuracy of aiming. Because there is a positive intercept on the error axis, we have assumed that this represents an additional and separate source of error. Accordingly, the terminal error variance is shown, rather than the standard deviation, and the two sources of error are assumed to be additive. This technique was used by us in previous work (e.g. Beggs & Howarth, 1972a; Howarth et al., 1971).

In this case, calculation shows that the value of σ_θ, the angular accuracy of aiming was 47' of arc, and E_0^2 the irreduceable error variance, which we have attributed to tremor, was 3.15 mm². These data are displayed in Figure 2. In addition, on the assumption that no corrections were in fact made to the movements to the 50 mm target, a point representing the total distance over which the movement was uncorrected is also shown.

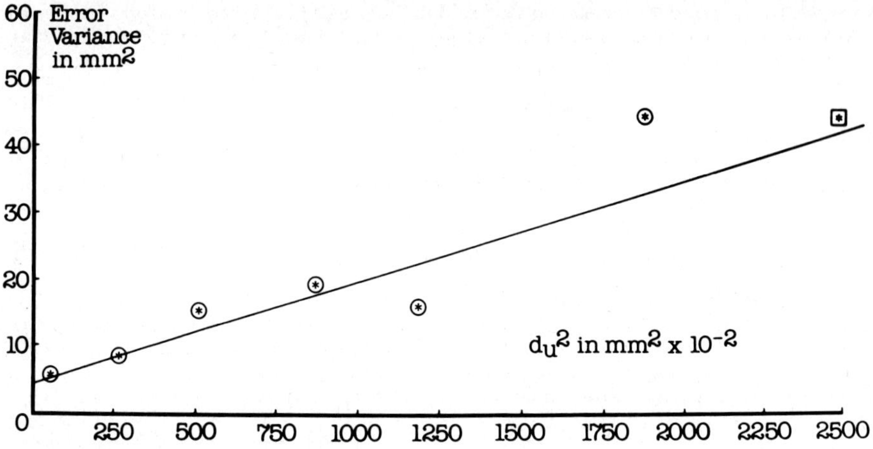

Figure 2. The relationship between the variance of the error distribution and the distance from the target where the final correction was implemented. Points shown thus ⊛ are by-eye estimates of the distance to impact when the hand was 290 ms before impact; the point shown thus ⧆ assumes that no corrections were made and that the effective distance over which the movement was uncontrolled was the same as the movement distance.

Next, a second regression equation was calculated, using the data for movement times and the value of I.D., that is, log 2A/W. This took the form

$$MT = 0.0953 \text{ I.D.} - 0.03$$

This equation accounted for 73% of the variance, and produced a value of 10.5 bits/s for the channel capacity.

Discussion

The results of this experiment confirm the Kerr and Langolf (1977) finding, that Fitts Law can describe the relationship between target width and movement time in this sort of task configuration. However, they also enable this finding to be understood in a new way, and are consistent with the Howarth and Beggs model of movement control.

First, the data support the prediction from our theory that aiming accuracy is a linear function of the maximum distance from the target where the final correction could be implemented. The slope of this function is a measure of the angular accuracy of aiming; Howarth et al. (1971) reported a value of 36' of angle for this parameter, while Beggs and Howarth (1972a) found it to be 41' of angle. In this experiment, it was about 47' of angle when all six estimates of d_c are assumed to reflect the distance over which the hand was uncorrected. The regression line fitted to these points passes somewhat above the point for the probable open-loop movement to the widest target; a line fitted through the first five points and this point accounts for 94% of the variance, and gives a value of 42' of arc for σ_θ. This line is shown on Figure 2. The combination of the error distribution lying well within the target strip, the fast movement time and the somewhat unlikely value for d_c suggest that subjects probably operated ballistically when aiming at the widest target. This raises the interesting possibility that aiming strategies, even within the same experiment, need not be constant.

Second, an intercept on the error axis as on Figure 2 has been reported before by us. Howarth et al. (1971) reported a value of 5.87mm^2 for this, with a value of 4.59mm^2 reported by Beggs and Howarth (1972a). In this experiment, this parameter was somewhat lower at 3.15mm^2 for the line fitted to the six points representing a possible strategy of corrections to all movements; this would be consistent with our "selection from tremor" hypothesis (Howarth and Beggs, 1985). However, it is more likely that strategies of aiming varied within this experiment, so that the regression line through the open loop point for the widest target produced an intercept of 4.59mm^2. Beggs, Graham, Monk, Shaw and Howarth (1972), in a multiple target aiming experiment, reported values between 0.9mm^2 and 7.8mm^2. The value found in this experiment seems, therefore, to be credible.

Explanations for this source of error differ. We have assumed that it represents irreducible physiological tremor, as did Schmidt et al. (1979). Recently, Wright and Meyer (1983) reported the same phenomenon but were unable to account for it in terms of their Impulse Variability model. It may, as they suggest, be related to some form of perceptual problem related to the subjects' difficulty in locating the target. We would, however, expect that to show up in a change in the value of the slope, that is, in the value of σ_θ.

Third, this experiment has produced clear evidence that the major difference in performance between this self-paced task and a paced aiming task is in the way that subjects approach the target. The prediction was that they would decelerate their hand more sharply, like Annett et al. (1958) and Beggs and Howarth (1972b) had found. This was demonstrated by the values of the exponents of the functions fitted to the deceleration portions of the approach trajectories. These varied from 1.75 to 2.46, with a distinct trend towards a more extreme slowing down on the narrower targets. It would seem that subjects were indeed aware of their inability to correct movements continuously, and were attempting to get as close as possible before the final correction. The result of this strategy was to minimise the error distribution on the narrower targets. It is difficult to see what other model would predict, or indeed explain this subtle change in strategy.

Finally, like the paced aiming situation reported by Howarth et al. (1971), there was a simple relationship between d_c and movement time. A regression line fitted to the five calculated values of d_c which fell on the J-portions of the approach curves and 1/T accounted for 96.9% of the variance. This enables the relationship between error and movement time to be derived, at least for those targets where corrections to the movement were likely. It is worth noting that when the exponent in the relationship between d and t remains constant across movement time, as in paced aiming, the same exponent appears in the relationship between E and T. The linear relationship observed here may be a fortuitous result of the changes in the exponent referred to above, and shown in Figure 1.

A fundamental assumption of the Howarth and Beggs model is that errors of aiming are a function of the distance through which the hand travels uncorrected, d_c, and the angular error of aiming, σ_θ. In Howarth and Beggs (1985), we showed the D, the total movement distance can simply be taken into account as follows:

$$E = aD\sigma_\theta d_c \tag{3}$$

where a is an arbitrary constant.

But for the movements in this task where corrections were made

$$d_c = b/T + c \tag{4}$$

where T was the movement time, and c another arbitrary constant. Thus, combining (3) and (4)

$$E = KD/T + J \tag{5}$$

and so

$$T = LD/E + M \tag{6}$$

where K, J, L and M are constants containing a number of terms, all of which may be estimated.

Where strip targets are sufficiently narrow as to require the subject to correct self-paced movements aimed at them, our model thus predicts that the reciprocal of the width of the error distribution, scaled by the total movement distance, will be linearly related to the movement time. In fact, a regression line fitted to our data accounted for 89.4% of the variance, and a regression line fitted to Kerr and Langolf's (1977) data, collected over a wide range of distances and widths, accounted for 90.8% of the variance.

Fitts Law assumes that in equation (6), T should be proportional to the logarithm of 2A/W (or D/E), rather than linearly as our analysis predicts. Since most of the data published over the last thirty years or so can be reasonably fitted by the logarithmic function, this seems at first sight like very strong evidence against the theory being presented here. However, the changes in strategy which are demonstrated by the changes in the exponent in the relationship between d and t form no part of any other theory which attempts to explain Fitts Law. In any case, the evidence presented in our papers since 1970, and in Woodworth (1899) argue strongly against Information Theory and other explanations of Fitts Law, and by assumption, aiming.

It may be that a way out of this impasse is to consider the nature of Fitts Law itself. The data reported here make it reasonably easy to understand why it takes the form it does. One obvious factor concerns the nature of the data usually reported in self-paced aiming. Fitts Law does not concern itself with the accuracy of aiming at all, but describes the effect on movement time of the size of the target which has to be aimed at. Although Crossman (1957) suggested that target width and the width of the error distribution within targets could be linearly related — that subjects would fit their hits neatly into each target — our data show that error width and target width are not linearly related over the entire range of target widths. Casting data in the form of Fitts Law may distort the relationship between actual error and movement time, because actual error width is unrelated to large values of target width. This has been known for nearly twenty years (Welford, 1968).

Replotting Fitts' (1954) data from his reciprocal dotting task shows that the relationship between T and mean A/W is a negatively accelerating curve; this changes to a slightly positively accelerating one when the logarithm A/W is used. The data reported by Kerr and Langolf (1977) look very similar. Both of these studies report only target width; the subjects, like ours, may not have completely filled, say, the two inch (50 mm) target with hits, with the result that A/W and D/E are not equivalent at short movement times. In effect, A/W is smaller than D/E for short movement times, and this may account for some of the nonlinearity.

This analysis suggests that it may be possible to account for one of the most robust findings in the field of movement in terms of strategic decisions by the subject to use corrections where necessary, and to optimise their effect by getting as close to the target as possible, as quickly as possible. It also predicts that the width of the error distribution is a function of movement speed (equation

(5)). This is a prediction from Impulse Variability theory, but it is difficult to see how this might be credibly extended to relatively slow movements which are subject to corrections.

There is a minor effect of movement distance to account for, which we have not discussed. The slopes of the lines relating T and A/W in Fitts' and Kerr and Langolf's data change as a function of target distance. This factor is frequently ignored. It may be that subjects adopt different strategies when the targets are at different distances; this, however, is a relatively small effect, and its explanation must await further experimental work.

Kerr and Langolf alluded to possible differences between aiming at a line target and aiming at a strip target. This experiment has shown that they were correct in their suspicion, and suggests that the reason for the difference lies purely in the subjects' strategies. There are a number of experiments which will need to be done before these ideas are confirmed. Nevertheless, the way may now be clear for a less fragmented approach to the problem of aimed movements. The Howarth and Beggs model of the control of movement has been extended from paced tasks to self-paced tasks; the concept of strategy (Howarth, 1978) has been incorporated, and subtle changes in the performance of subjects when faced with differing task demands have been identified. The proposal that apparatus and task differences fundamentally affect data, and thus models, has been made before (Beggs, 1980). This experiment is confirmation of this point of view, and suggests that a great deal of theorising in this area may have been "apparatus bound".

Acknowledgements

This research was completed while the senior author was working in the Blind Mobility Research Unit, at the University of Nottingham; this group is supported by the D.H.S.S., contract number J/R 131/60, and is directed by Professor C.I. Howarth.

References

Annett, J., Goldby, C.W., & Kay, H. (1958). The measurement of elements in an assembly task — the information output of the human motor system. Quarterly Journal of Experimental Psychology, 10, 1-11.

Beggs, W.D.A. (1971). Movement Control. Unpublished Ph.D. thesis,

University of Nottingham.

Beggs, W.D.A. (1980). The apparatus effect in experimental psychology. Paper presented at the British Psychological Society Conference, December 1980.

Beggs, W.D.A., & Howarth, C.I. (1970). Movement control in a repetitive motor task. Nature, 225, 752-753.

Beggs, W.D.A., & Howarth, C.I. (1972a). The accuracy of aiming at a target — some further evidence for intermittent control. Acta Psychologica, 36, 171-177.

Beggs, W.D.A., & Howarth, C.I. (1972b). The movement of the hand towards a target. Quarterly Journal of Experimental Psychology, 24, 448-453.

Beggs, W.D.A., Graham, J.C., Monk, T.H., Shaw, M.R.W., & Howarth, C.I. (1972). Can Hick's Law and Fitts' Law be combined? Acta Psychologica, 36, 348-357.

Beggs, W.D.A., Wilkinson, H.P., & Howarth, C.I. (1975). An on-line apparatus for hand movement research. Quarterly Journal of Experimental Psychology, 29, 220-223.

Carlton, L.G. (1981). Processing visual feedback information for movement control. Journal of Experimental Psychology: Human Perception and Performance, 7, 1019-1030.

Crossman, E.R.F.W. (1957). The speed and accuracy of simple hand movements. In E.R.F.W. Crossman & W.D. Seymour (Eds.), The nature and acquisition of industrial skills. Report to M.R.C. and D.S.I.R. Joint Committee on Individual Efficiency in Industry.

Crossman, E.R.F.W., & Goodeve, P.J. (1963). Feedback control of hand-movement and Fitts' Law. Unpublished communication to the Experimental Psychology Society, Oxford. Published in Quarterly Journal of Experimental Psychology, 1983, 35A, 251-278.

Fitts, P.M. (1954). The information capacity of the human motor system in controlling the amplitude of movement. Journal of Experimental Psychology, 47, 381-391.

Fitts, P.M., & Peterson, J.R. (1964). Information capacity of discrete motor responses. Journal of Experimental Psychology, 67, 103-112.

Howarth, C.I. (1978). Strategies in the control of movement. In G. Underwood (Ed.), Strategies of information processing. London: Academic Press.

Howarth, C.I., Beggs, W.D.A., & Bowden, J. (1971). The relationship between speed and accuracy of movement aimed at a target. Acta Psychologica, 35, 207-218.

Howarth, C.I., & Beggs, W.D.A. (1985). The control of movements by multisensory information. In Heuer, H., Kleinbeck, U., & Schmidt, K-H. (Eds.), Motor behaviour: Programming, control and acquisition. Berlin: Springer-Verlag.

Jagacinsky, R.J., Repperger, D.W., Moran, M.S., Ward, S.L., & Glass, B. (1980). Fitts' Law and the microstructure of rapid discrete movements. Journal of Experimental Psychology: Human Perception and Performance, 6, 309-320.

Keele, S.W. (1968). Movement control in skilled motor performance. Psychological Bulletin, 70, 387-403.

Keele, S.W. (1981). Behavioral analysis of movement. In V. Brooks, (Ed.) Handbook of physiology: The nervous system: Vol. 2. Motor control. Baltimore, Md: American Physiological Society.

Keele, S.W., & Posner, M.I. (1968). Processing of visual feedback

in rapid movements. Journal of Experimental Psychology, 77, 155-8.
Kerr, B.A., & Langolf, G.D. (1977). Speed of aiming movements. Quarterly Journal of Experimental Psychology, 29, 475-481.
Knight, A.A., & Dagnall, P.R. (1967). Precision in movements. Ergonomics, 10, 321-330.
Langolf, G.D., Chaffin, D.B., & Foulkes, J.A. (1976). An investigation of Fitts' Law using a wide range of movement amplitudes, Journal of Motor Behavior, 8, 113-128.
Meyer, D.E., Smith, J.E.K., & Wright, C.E. (1982). Models for the speed and accuracy of aimed movements. Psychological Review, 89, 449-482.
Schmidt, R.A., Zelaznik, H., Hawkins, B., Frank, J.S., & Quinn, J.T.Jr. (1979). Motor output variability: A theory for the accuracy of rapid motor acts. Psychological Review, 86, 415-451.
Smith, W.M., & Bowen, K.F. (1980). The effects of delayed and displaced visual feedback on motor control. Journal of Motor Behavior, 12, 91-101.
Stubbs, D.F. (1976). What the eye tells the hand. Journal of Motor Behavior, 8, 43-58.
Welford, A.T. (1968). Fundamentals of skill. London: Methuen.
Woodworth, R.S. (1899). The accuracy of voluntary movement. Psychological Review Monographs, Supplement 3, 13.
Wright, C.E., & Meyer, D.E. (1983). Conditions for linear speed-accuracy trade-off in aimed movements. Quarterly Journal of Experimental Psychology, 35A, 279-296.
Zelaznik, H.N., Shapiro, D.C., & McColsky, D. (1981). Effects of a secondary task on the accuracy of single aiming movements. Journal of Experimental Psychology: Human Perception and Performance, 7, 1007-1018.
Zelaznik, H.N., Hawkins, B., & Kisselborough, L. (1983). Rapid visual feedback processing in single-aiming movements. Journal of Motor Behavior, 15, 217-236.

Cognition and Action in Skilled Behaviour
A.M. Colley and J.R. Beech (Editors)

LEVELS OF MOTOR PROGRAMMING IN WRITING FAMILIAR AND UNFAMILIAR SYMBOLS

Wouter Hulstijn and Gerard P. van Galen
University of Nijmegen

Rapid action sequences like the successive movements in speech, handwriting and other skilled motor activities, have to be planned or programmed before their execution. One class of data supporting such a view are reaction time data, in particular the effect of movement complexity on reaction time. In handwriting experiments this effect is not easily observed however. Five studies will be presented showing that at least one variable is crucial in this type of research: the amount of practice one has with the movements, or the familiarity of the movement pattern. The first two studies tried to find evidence for either the stroke or the letter as the basic unit of motor programming. In the third experiment the writing of novel symbols was contrasted with letter combinations of the same complexity. As expected, when only the first stroke of a character had to be written, the movements were initiated much faster. Unexpectedly this only held for the novel symbols. The overlearned letters could be initiated slightly faster than their first stroke. In the fourth study the number of strokes of the writing patterns was varied from two to seven. Choice reaction time increased with number of strokes for only the symbols, and not for the more practiced letters. In the final study only capitals had to be written in either the normal way, or an unusual way by adding spaces between the individual strokes. This unpracticed way of writing considerably increased reaction time. The combined results of these studies strongly suggest that the programming of motor commands proceeds on at least two levels, one for well-practiced movement sequences and one for novel movement patterns.

The rapid execution of an action requires it to be prepared before it can be initiated. The nature of this process, in which the successive elements of the action are planned or organized in advance, is one of the major issues in the study of motor control. The term "motor program" is often used, but this term is ambiguous and a lot of terminological confusion still remains. This ambiguity is revealed clearly in comparing two often cited definitions of a motor program, both given by Keele (1968, 1981). The definition that is quoted most was given by Keele some twenty years ago. It describes a motor program as "a set of muscle commands that are structured before a movement sequence begins, and that allows the entire sequence to be carried out uninfluenced by peripheral feedback" (Keele, 1968, p.387). In the more recent definition, the 'set of muscle commands' has been replaced by the more abstract notion of a 'central representation', "... that can lead to patterned movement in the absence of feedback" (Keele, 1981, p.1400). Common to both definitions is the unimportance of feedback. Recently, a number of authors have commented on the possible role of feedback even during very fast, preprogrammed movement execution (Hulstijn, 1987; Keele, 1982; Rosenbaum, Inhoff, & Gordon, 1984; Schmidt, 1982a), but that issue will not be dealt with here. The central theme of this chapter concerns the nature of the motor program. Even in the most recent literature on motor programming (Harrington & Haaland, 1987; Ivry, 1986; Semjen & Garcia-Colera, 1986; Zelaznik & Hahn, 1985) this difference in emphasis on either the muscle command level or on the abstract level can still be found. The problem is often formulated in terms of the "unit" of programming. But it is more the level than the unit which is at issue. If handwriting is taken as a typical example of a complex skill, then the level problem can be re-phrased in the question: is writing programmed at a word level, at a letter level, at a stroke level, or, even at a lower level, at which the program specifies the onsets and forces of the muscles involved (see Hulstijn & van Galen, 1983; Teulings, Mullins, & Stelmach, 1986; van Galen & Teulings, 1983)? One obvious, but seldom recognised, solution to this problem is to dismiss the question by not selecting only one level, but instead by accepting the possibility that actions can be represented at more levels (van Galen, Smyth, & Meulenbroek, 1987; van Galen & Wing, 1984). In the traditional use of the term "program", a program has the unwanted connotation of a fixed entity, that can simply be retrieved from memory. In a multilevel view a program may instead be conceived of as the very transient result of a programming process, in which abstract representations are transformed into more specific commands at lower and lower levels. By its very nature this process does involve different levels (Hulstijn, 1987). Which of the possible levels will consume most of the programming time will be dependent on a number of factors, including the type of task, the strategy that the subject has chosen, and his or her skill in the task.

The study of this programming process is related to two other unresolved issues in programming research. The first is concerned with the extent of the program. How far ahead is the movement sequence planned or organized? Particularly in continuous skills like writing, typing, piano-playing and speech this question is very relevant. It may be answered differently for some of these skills (Hulstijn & van Galen, 1983) and the answers will probably also depend on the skill level of the subject and the strategy that he or she employs. The second issue, which is closely related to the first, is the extent to which programming and response execution can be done at the same time (see Harrington & Haaland, 1987; Hulstijn & van Galen, 1983). Is an undisturbed continuation of the movement possible during the programming of the movements that are to follow, or is movement execution delayed or even stopped when the next elements have to be planned?

As has been stated earlier, it may well be that the answers to these three questions are different, depending on the skill that is being investigated. The experiments that will be described focus on one type of skill: handwriting. Handwriting, like typing and speech, makes it possible to obtain well defined, very complex and long movement sequences simply by asking the subjects to write letters, or words, or whole sentences. But in contrast to speech and typing, handwriting is much slower. An average letter in fast typing requires about 200 ms per letter, while in fast handwriting a letter takes about 600 ms to complete. Quite recently, Semjen and Garcia-Colera (1986) convincingly demonstrated, by varying the rate of a fingertapping task, that at slow rates with 600 ms intervals, sequence planning (the authors prefer the term "planning" instead of the term "programming" which is used in the present chapter) is different from planning at fast rates. At these low rates (intervals greater than 300 ms), only the first element of the sequence is planned in advance and the rest of the sequence is planned during the execution of the first elements. Obviously there are more differences between handwriting and typewriting, and between handwriting and speech, than simply the rate of letter production. Yet it is an important factor to mention, if only to explain the contradiction of a general decline in the use of handwriting in practical communication and a very remarkable increase in the amount of research on handwriting (Kao, van Galen, & Hoosain, 1986; Plamondon, Suen, Deschenes, & Poulin, 1987; Thomassen, van Galen, & Keuss, 1983).

One experimental approach to the study of programming is to measure the time it takes to initiate a movement sequence. Following Henry and Rogers (1960), the basic assumption in these reaction time experiments is that the time needed for programming will increase with the number of units that have to be programmed. Both a simple reaction time task and a choice reaction task have been advocated as the optimal paradigm (see Hulstijn, 1987, for a short review). Each of these tasks has advantages as well as disadvantages. Therefore, both tasks should be used. The data that will be presented here have been acquired in both paradigms.

The leading question in the following experiments concerns the level problem. At what level is handwriting programmed? Originally in our research this question was formulated as the search for the basic unit in writing. Consequently, the first two studies were designed to test whether a stroke can be properly considered as the basic unit, or whether a complete letter is the best candidate. These studies have been fully reported in earlier publications, therefore only their most relevant results will be presented. In the second study, and more extensively in the third study, the main variable for the rest of this chapter is introduced: the amount of practice that one has in writing or drawing a specific grapheme. This variable turned out to have an unexpectedly large influence on reaction time. A summary of the data from this experiment has been included elsewhere (Hulstijn, 1987), but the results have not yet been published in detail. Novel graphemes which had not been thoroughly practiced were initiated much later than their control movements, i.e. the first of their strokes. Very familiar letters, on the contrary, differed only slightly from their control movements. This experiment had a limitation, however, in that the complexity of its graphemes occupied only the two extreme positions: a single stroke and the complete grapheme. Therefore, in the fourth study letters and symbols of intermediate complexity had also to be written. This experiment, which was only a pilot experiment due to the low number of subjects and trials, indeed suggested that the increase in reaction time with the number of strokes was larger for the unpracticed symbols than for the letters. Besides being a pilot, this experiment had another drawback: it only made use of a choice reaction task. Symbols probably require more time to be recognized than letters, so the reaction time effects that were found could be due solely to non-motoric factors. The final study that will be reported was designed to circumvent these problems.

In search of the basic unit

The first two studies were modelled after the well-known study of the rapid initiation of speech and typewriting by Sternberg, Monsell, Knoll and Wright (1978). In a simple reaction time paradigm Sternberg et al. demonstrated that reaction time increased linearly with the length of the utterance. Each additional word in the utterance, irrespective of whether it was a one- or a two-syllable word, added about 10 ms to the reaction time. To Sternberg et al. this and similar findings suggested that rapid movement sequences in speech are programmed not in syllables but in words, or "stress-groups". By using the same methodology it should be possible to find the programming unit in handwriting.

Study 1

Experiments performed by Mullins, Teulings and Stelmach in the Nijmegen handwriting laboratory used this experimental strategy on the level of strokes (Stelmach, Mullins, & Teulings, 1984; Teulings, Mullins, & Stelmach, 1986). If handwriting movements are programmed in units of single strokes then reaction time should increase linearly with the number of strokes. If however a pair of down-and-upward strokes are the programming elements then this should reveal itself in a more marked reaction time increase between pairs than between single strokes.

Method

In two subsequent experiments the same four subjects had to write curved "U"-like patterns in the first experiment and straight "V"-like patterns in the second experiment (see Figure 1). The number of strokes varied from 1 to 5 or 6.

Each trial followed a simple reaction, count-down procedure. It started with the presentation of the pattern on a display screen (Vector General Graphics Display, Series 3, Model 2D3) for 500 ms. This was followed by a 2500 ms. rehearsal or preparation period, and two 500 ms. periods. These were marked by short tones and ended with a high frequency tone, the go-signal. The subject was instructed to complete the writing of the pattern as fast and accurately as possible. In order to standardize the pre- and post-writing movements, the subject held his or her pen still on the X-Y tablet before writing and as soon as the last stroke was finished. The different movement patterns were presented randomly in each block of trials. One out of seven trials was a catch trial on which no go-signal was presented. The subjects were given a large amount of practice - 75 trials for each of the five or six patterns. Each of the points in Figure 1 is based on a further 75 experimental trials.

Writing was done on normal paper fixed on an X-Y tablet and with an almost normal ballpoint pen connected to a computer-controlled digitizer (Vector General Data Tablet DT1). The X- and Y-coordinates of the electronic pen position had a combined RMS error better than 0.2 mm; they were sampled with 200 Hz and lowpass filtered at 16 Hz. For each trial the tangential velocity was calculated and displayed on a screen. The reaction time was taken as the time between the start of the go-signal and the very first beginning of the pen movement in writing the first stroke.

Results and Discussion

The mean reaction times are presented in Figure 1. Instead of the expected linear increase, a U-shaped curve was found. The reaction time decreased from the one- to three-stroke patterns and then increased with further increase in the number of strokes. One can argue (see Sternberg et al., 1978, and Stelmach, Mullins, & Teulings, 1984) that the first and final elements have special characteristics requiring the increase in reaction time to be measured as a function of the number of intermediate strokes. This is particularly true for this and similar writing experiments in our laboratory, since the subjects were asked to hold their pen motionless both at the start and at the end of the writing movements. Although most subjects quickly learn to do this, it adds an extra element to the task, which, since it is not highly practiced, slightly increases reaction time. To explain the decrease in reaction time from the one- to three-stroke patterns, the additional assumption is required that only for very short sequences the programming of the final pen stop is done in the reaction time period, while for longer sequences the stop is programmed during the execution of the movement sequence, one or two strokes before the end. Although this explanation is not very parsimonious, it provides a good account of the results of the other experiments to be reported in this chapter.

If these arguments are accepted, the effect of sequence length on reaction time should be calculated from the three-stroke patterns onward. Both curves in Figure 1 do indeed show the expected increase in reaction time, but this increase was rather small, about 5 ms per stroke, and it was only significant for the lower curve. Curved patterns were initiated an average of 22 ms later, but it is not yet clear whether curved movements are more complex, causing more programming time, or whether mechanical factors should be held responsible.

It must be concluded that these data do not present very strong evidence for either accepting or refuting the hypothesis that the stroke is the unit of programming in handwriting. Alternative models should be considered. But before discussing these, we will present the results of similar reaction time experiments which attempted to discover whether the programming unit in handwriting can be found at another level: the letter level.

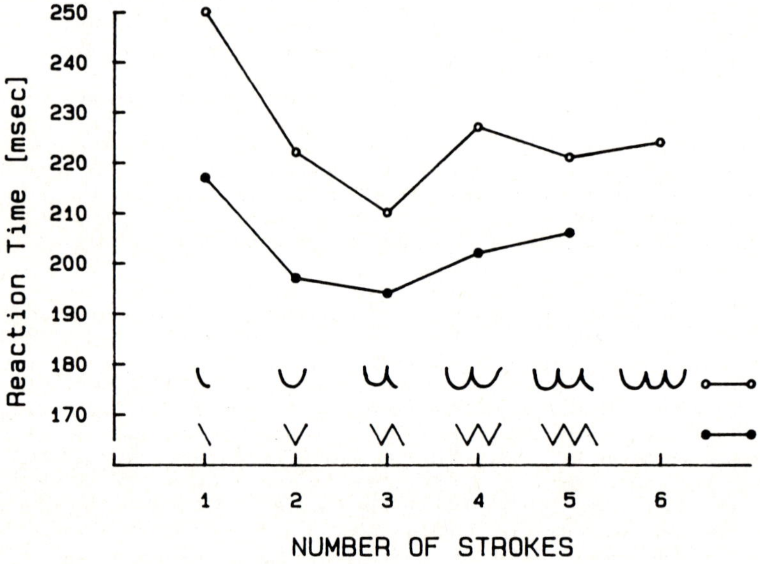

Figure 1. Reaction time as a function of the number of strokes in "V"-type patterns and "U"-type patterns.

Study 2

In three consecutive experiments the same experimental strategy that was used in Study 1 was applied, but this time the sequences consisted of letters or digits. In addition to the number of characters in the sequence, a few extra variables that were thought to influence movement complexity were manipulated. In the first of these three experiments, the number of strokes of the letters, as well as the size of the letters which had to be written, were varied. The second experiment varied the amount of practice that the subjects had received with the movement trajectories of the digits which had to be written. The third experiment varied the ease with which the letter strings could be remembered, by comparing nonsense letter strings with strings of the same letters forming a word. Full details of this study were published in Hulstijn and van Galen (1983).

Method

The three experiments were conducted several days apart with the same four subjects. In Experiment 1 the letter sequences consisted of combinations (without repetitions) of the simple letters "e", "i", "j" and "l", written in their usual size (condition "eijl-normal") or four times larger (condition "eijl-large"), and of combinations of the more complex letters "v", "o", "p" and "b" (condition "vopb-normal") written at their normal size only.

In Experiment 2 the digits "3", "4", "8" and "9" were written either in a normal way, which may be said to be overlearned, or in an unfamiliar way, by not starting at the beginning of the normal movement trajectory but at the end. The digit "8" is normally started by a Dutch subject in the middle between the two circles. In the unfamiliar condition the subject had to begin at the top.

In Experiment 3 either words or nonsense letter strings were presented. Twenty-eight different five-letter words were used, the shorter words were obtained by omitting letters, as in "blank", "bank", "ban", and "ba". The nonwords were formed by holding the initial letter at the same position and reordering the other letters, e.g. "bklna", "bkna", "bka" and "bk".

In general the same procedure, stimulus presentation and data recording were used as in Study 1. The few differences are of no importance in the present context. Subjects were trained on a separate day with at least 250 trials. These practice trials all belonged to the "eijl-normal" condition. Each experimental trial block — consisting of 112 trials — was preceded by 60 practice trials in the corresponding condition. The points in Figure 2 are based on 288 observations, or 384 observations in the third experiment.

Results and Discussion

Figure 2 presents the average reaction times of the various conditions in the three experiments.

In Experiment 1 a similar initial decrease in reaction time can be observed as was found in the stroke experiments of Study 1. However from two characters onwards, the expected linear increase was seen. The slope was 1.7 ms/letter in the "eijl"-normal condition, 6.5 ms/letter in the "eijl"-large condition and 11.7 ms/letter in the "vopb"-normal condition. This difference in slope was statistically significant.

However, before concluding that, as a result, the unit of programming in handwriting has to be located lower than the letter-level, a complicating feature of the experimental design should be considered. This complication has to do with the fact that the practice session and the three experiments were conducted on the same subjects in the same order. Within each experiment very large practice effects were found. In the first experiment the slope in reaction time, averaged over conditions, significantly decreased from 12.1 ms/letter in the first block to 3.8 ms/letter in the third block. In the second experiment the average slope decreased from 7.0 ms/digit in the first block to 1.8 ms/digit in the third block.

In the final experiment only a meagre 2.1 ms/letter was left, which even decreased to a final 1.5 ms/letter. These practice effects, occurring within each experiment, suggest that from one experiment to the next, practice may have played a role also, which may have caused the very low slopes in the final experiment. Also, the differences in slope between the three conditions in Experiment 1 can

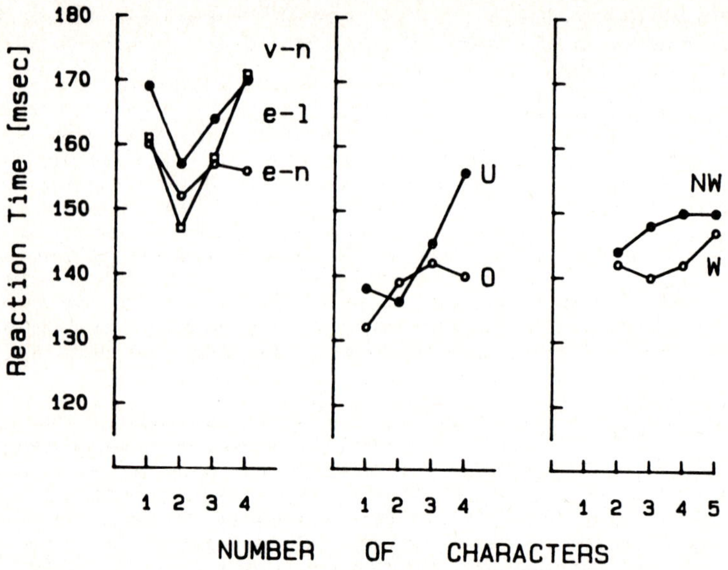

Figure 2. Reaction time as a function of sequence length. The first panel presents the data of the conditions "eijl"-normal (e-n), "eijl"-large (e-l) and "vopb"-normal (v-n). The second panel gives reaction time in the unfamiliar condition (U) and in the overlearned condition (O). The third panel presents reaction time in the nonword-condition (NW) and in the word-condition (W).

be attributed to a practice effect, due to the fact that the subjects on the training day only practiced with trials from the "eijl"-normal condition. The three conditions in Experiment 1 differ in their similarity to the training condition and the differences in slope are ordered along that dimension.

Therefore, the only conclusion that can safely been drawn is that practice had a large effect. The initial 12 ms/letter, which was similar to the slope reported by Sternberg et al (1978), levelled off with practice to only 1.5 ms/letter. A decrease in slope has also been reported by Sternberg et al. (1978), although the slopes in their experiments did not reach such a low value as was found in Experiment 3. A decreasing slope as a result of practice has often been found in a great number of slightly different studies testing Hick's law, which states that reaction time is a logarithmic function of the number of stimulus and response alternatives (see Schmidt, 1982b, for an introductory review). These studies are different in that they required only a short response and not a response varying in sequence length. Yet they suggest that in the present study the effect may be explained by more efficient memory search processes. An alternative explanation for the decrease in slope is that the subjects got more efficient in performing two activities together. If the motor programming of a unit can be done perfectly in parallel with the execution of the previous unit, then no effect of movement length will show up in reaction time and a zero slope will be predicted. This explanation is in accord with numerous observations that highly learned, automatized, movements allow a second task to be performed more easily. But accepting this explanation does mean that the unit of programming cannot be studied without addressing the related issue of the possible overlap between programming and response execution.

Apart from this, the question of what the subject actually had to program should be considered. If he or she retrieved the next letter from a short term store, and if writing this letter was done very automatically, then no movement sequence had to be planned at all. The plan, i.e. the order of the individual strokes and the correct starting point, may have simply been retrieved from a long term store. If, on the contrary, the movement sequence was not highly familiar, not practiced thousands of times, and not stored in long term memory, then the planning of the sequence might cause delays. The second of these three experiments was set up to test this.

The subjects had to write rapidly one, two, three or four digits either in the way they normally write these digits (indicated by the term "overlearned") or in an unfamiliar way: by starting at an unusual point. The middle panel of Figure 2 presents the reaction times. As can be seen, there was no difference in reaction time between the overlearned and the unfamiliar condition. The figure suggests a small difference in slope between the curves for both conditions, but this difference was far from significant. However, this lack of a difference is only true for the reaction time, i.e. for the time interval preceding the writing of the first digit. If the periods preceding the next digits are inspected, large differences emerge. The average interval between the writing of the digits in the overlearned condition was about 120 ms, but the period preceding the unfamiliar movement trajectories was, on the average, more than 110 ms longer, i.e. 230 ms.

These results suggest that programming an unfamiliar movement sequence takes considerably more time (100 ms as a rough approximation) but that this time is not reflected in the simple reaction time, probably because all this extra programming has already been done before the go-signal. It is interesting that the interdigit interval was not influenced by the number of digits in the rest of the sequence. Therefore, this effect, due to the programming of an unfamiliar movement, seems to be restricted to only the next digit ahead.

The results of Studies 1 and 2 can be summarised by concluding that the search for the basic unit in handwriting has met two obstacles. The increases in reaction time with sequence length that were found were very small — in the order of a few milliseconds — while the effects of practice (shown over blocks of trials and between unfamiliar and well learned movements) proved to be very large.

Effects of practice on reaction time

It was suggested earlier that the extra programming of an unfamiliar movement can be done before the go-signal. If this conjecture is right, then a choice reaction paradigm would be more suited to study this programming. The next study was an attempt to do this.

Study 3

A few years ago, the second author (van Galen, 1980) did an experiment in which the subjects had to draw rapidly, or "write", two graphemes, that they learned just before the start of the experiment. That experiment focussed on repetition effects: when the same pattern was written as in the previous trial, the reaction time shortened considerably. In subsequent experiments, in which letters were used instead of newly learned graphemes, this result could not be replicated however. The experiment that will be described here was the last in a series of experiments, which were all set up to investigate why these replication failures occurred. An obvious factor was the difference in practice between letters and newly learned graphemes. But the influence of a specific preparatory strategy could not be ruled out in advance. This strategy, i.e. to prepare another pattern than the one that was just presented, was used by the subjects, presumably because only two patterns had to be written. Therefore, the next study contrasted letters and newly learned graphemes, that were presented in blocks with two and with four alternatives.

The third variable that was manipulated was the extent of the movement that had to be made. The choice reaction time in starting to write the novel graphemes may be larger than the time to initiate letters, simply because of a longer stimulus recognition process. In order to test this, the same stimuli were also presented in a condition in which only the first stroke of the total stimulus pattern had to be made.

Method

The three experimental variables, i.e. practice (graphemes versus letters), number of alternatives (two versus four) and length of the movement trajectory (first stroke versus complete pattern), resulted in eight blocks of trials. These were presented to eight student subjects, in a different order, on two separate days.

The four graphemes, and the four letter combinations that were used, are presented in Figure 3. The movement of each of the four alternatives started in another direction, in order to exclude pre-programming of the first stroke. The letter combinations were considered to be at least as complex, in the number of straight and curved strokes, as the novel graphemes. In the one-stroke conditions the same stimuli were presented as in the complete-pattern conditions, the only difference being the instruction to the subjects to restrict their writing movements to the first stroke. The two alternatives in the two-choice conditions were chosen from the complete set of four alternatives. The subset was systematically varied over subjects.

All the writing patterns (graphemes and letters, single strokes as well as complete patterns) were practiced before the start of the experiment by copying them 25 times. The new patterns were learned quickly. None of the subjects made any mistake at the beginning of the experiment, although of course they were not as fluent on the graphemes as on the letters. In addition to this pre-experimental practice, each condition was practiced just before the trial block in which it was presented, for 40 or 30 (the latter for the two-alternative blocks only) trials.

The three experimental variables were held constant over a trial block; only the stimuli varied randomly over trials. There were 88 trials in blocks with four alternatives and 64 trials in the two-alternative blocks. The first four trials of each block were discarded.

Each trial started with a 500 ms low frequency warning tone, followed by a 1000 ms foreperiod, that ended with a 4000 ms display of the pattern that had to be written. Subjects were asked to initiate and finish the writing of this pattern as fast as possible. At the end of the 4000 ms recording period, their reaction time and movement time (in ms) were displayed on the screen.

The apparatus, used for stimulus presentation and pen recording, as well as the data analysis, were the same as in Study 1.

Results

The reaction time, averaged over all 84 or 60 trials per condition and averaged over all 8 subjects, is presented in Figure 3. In an analysis of variance, the main effects of each of the three independent variables turned out to be significant (graphemes versus letters: $F(1,7) = 7.32$, $p < .05$; first stroke versus all strokes: $F(1,7) = 36.19$, $p < .001$; number of alternatives: $F(1,7) = 14.52$, $p < .01$). But these main effects are less important than the interactions. It is quite clear from Figure 3 that the difference, between writing the full movement pattern and only drawing its first stroke, was very dissimilar between graphemes and letters ($F(1,7) = 14.82$, $p < .01$). The initiation of a full not-well-learned grapheme took much longer, 87 ms to be exact, than the start of its first stroke. The letters, however, were even initiated slightly (but not significantly) sooner than their first stroke. The finding that the increase in reaction time between two and four alternatives is higher for letter stimuli than for graphemes ($F(1,7) = 12.00$, $p = .01$) was unexpected. The other interactions were not significant.

Discussion

Novel graphemes were initiated after a longer reaction time than both their single stroke controls and letter combinations of equal complexity. It is tempting to explain this longer reaction time by differences in the motor programming of these movements. Choice reaction paradigms such as this usually suffer from the possibility that differences in perceptual processes cannot be fully excluded. However, the finding that, in a condition in which the same novel stimuli were presented but only the first stroke had to be drawn, reaction time was as low as in the letter conditions makes an

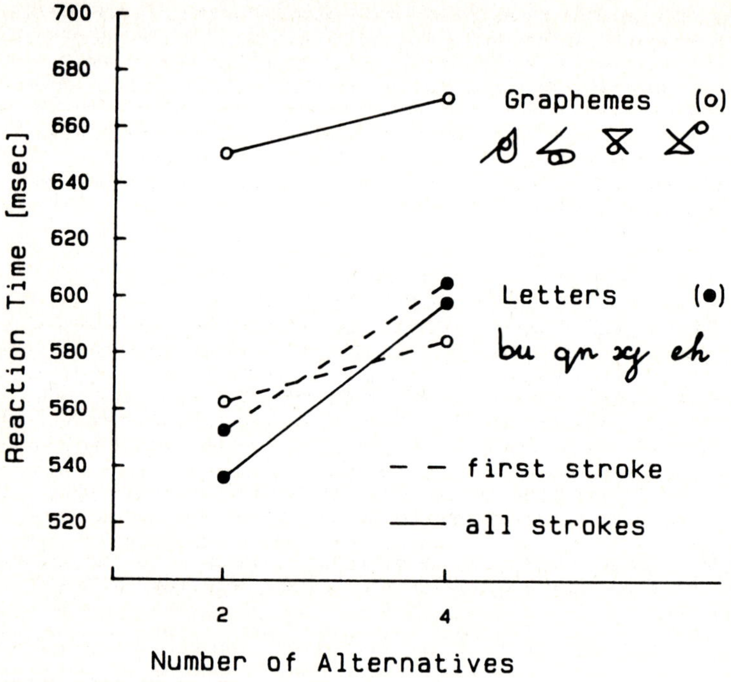

Figure 3. Reaction time as a function of the number of alternatives in a trial block. Either the first stroke or the complete pattern was written. The patterns, i.e. the graphemes or letters, that were written are shown.

explanation in terms of perceptual processes rather unlikely.

The significant interaction between the number of alternatives and the type of drawing pattern (grapheme or letter) defies a simple explanation. The finding that this interaction also occurred in the conditions in which only a single stroke had to be written, suggests that perceptual processes may be involved. But an alternative explanation is equally plausible. Therefore it must be assumed that in the letter-conditions the subject searches through a pattern memory or through a motor memory, which will take more time if the search involves more alternatives. In the grapheme conditions the subject will probably follow another strategy, i.e. to copy the stimulus pattern or its first stroke not from memory but from the screen. Such a difference in strategy explains the interaction. In addition, the latter explanation is in line with the supposition that the subject, when he or she has to write only the first stroke of a letter, retrieves the program for the entire letter from memory and programs an extra stop after the first stroke, resulting in an even longer reaction time for a more simple movement sequence.

The most important finding of this study is that it confirmed the large effect of practice that was found already in the second experiment of Study 2. The study had a disadvantage, however, since movement complexity was not varied over systematically increasing values, but only between its two extremes, i.e. as one stroke or as the complete pattern. Single strokes may be programmed in a completely different way from patterns. Therefore, in the next experiment symbols were employed that varied over a wider range in their number of strokes.

Study 4

In the former experiments practice was varied on two levels. Overlearned movement patterns like letters are perceptually very familiar as well as motorically well trained. In the next experiment an attempt was made to separate both effects. Perceptually familiar symbols were chosen that varied in their number of strokes. These symbols were contrasted with letters or letter combinations which were roughly equivalent in movement complexity, and with novel patterns that were constructed by transforming the symbols. As a result there was a condition in which the movement patterns were perceptually as well as motorically very familiar (letters), a condition in which the movement sequence was never trained (symbols) and a condition with patterns that were unfamiliar at both levels (graphemes).

Method

The 6 student subjects participated in all three conditions. In each condition ten different stimuli were presented. These stimuli are displayed in Figure 4. In order to allow the effect of pre-experimental practice to be as large as possible and not to be confounded with experience during the experiment, the stimuli were presented only three times and were shown only once during the instruction. Within a condition, the ten stimuli were randomly presented in three blocks of ten trials. The points in Figure 4 are averaged over 18 values only, i.e. 3 repetitions and 6 subjects. The conditions were presented in balanced order.

The subjects were instructed to "write" the patterns as fast and accurately as possible. They were told to make the movements without pauses and without looking up from the writing paper back to the stimulus on the screen. However, particularly halfway through the more complex patterns, some subjects could not complete the pattern without reinspecting the stimulus.

Further procedural details, as well as equipment and data analysis, were simiiar to Study 3.

Results and Discussion

Figure 4 presents the letters, symbols and novel graphemes that were used in this experiment, as well as the average reaction times in starting to write or draw these patterns. Probably due to the small number of trials and subjects that were used and possibly as a result of unexpected peculiarities of some of the symbols and graphemes, the points in Figure 4 show considerable variation. Despite these limitations these data reveal an interesting picture that nicely fits with the earlier results. The reaction time for symbols was considerably larger than for letters and the time to initiate unfamiliar graphemes was slightly longer than for symbols. But that is not very surprising; the more interesting finding was that the reaction time tended to increase with the number of elements much more strongly in the symbol and grapheme conditions, while the best fitting straight line through the letter data is nearly horizontal.

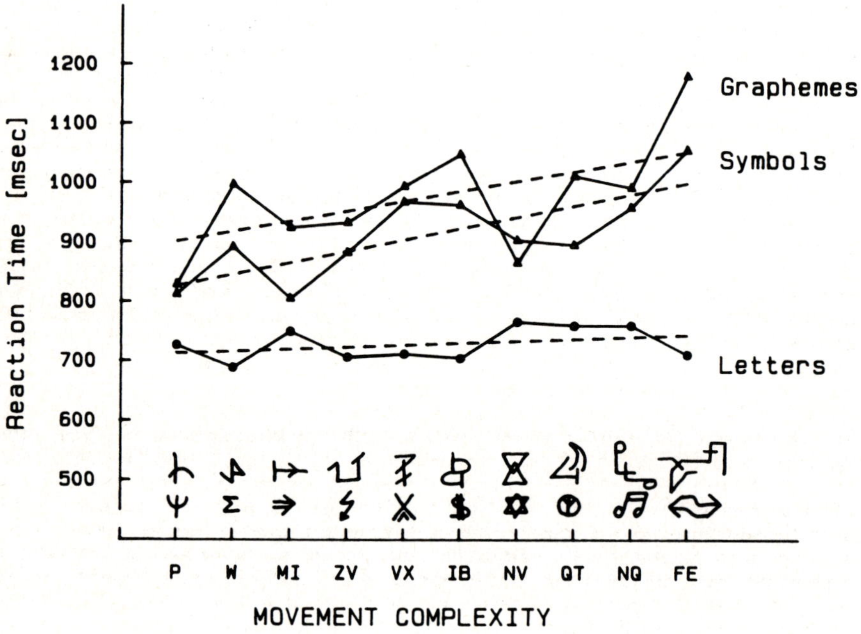

Figure 4. Reaction time as a function of movement complexity for letters, symbols and new patterns (graphemes).

It has been stated before that this was only a pilot experiment. However, the data of a large scale replication experiment, that was completed very recently, significantly confirmed the picture presented in Figure 4. But although this picture has been replicated, and although it fits well with the results of earlier studies, it does not give a definite answer to the question of how far the phenomena that were observed are due to differences in motor programming only. Letters differ from well-known symbols not only in the amount of motor training but also in the frequency with which they are encountered. As a result, even in a perceptual experiment, letters will be recognized after a shorter reaction time, and the increase in reaction time with complexity will be smaller. One solution to this experimental problem was tried in the next and final study.

Study 5

In this final study, practice was again manipulated. This time it was not done by comparing groups of patterns, like the letters and symbols of the previous experiment, but by manipulating the way in which the same patterns had to be written. In a way, this final study may be viewed as a modification and extension of the digits experiment that was reported as Experiment 2 in Study 2. One modification was that the digits were changed for capital letters. The reason for this change was to avoid curved line segments, since curved strokes can be considered as either one or two programming units. The second and more important modification was that in the unfamiliar condition the order of the strokes was not changed, as was done previously, but that the letters had to be written in a "spaced" way. This meant that the individual straight strokes had not to be connected but had to be drawn apart with a clear space in between. It was hoped that in this condition the normal way of writing would be broken up into separable elements. This manipulation can be considered equivalent to the unfamiliar condition in the digits experiment, but the advantage of the spaced condition was that the first stroke was the same in the spaced and in the normal condition. Previous experiments proved that the direction of the first stroke was an important determinant of the length of the reaction time. The extension to the digits experiment was that both types of reaction time task were used.

In the light of our earlier results the predictions were that the number of strokes is not an important variable if the capitals had to be written normally. A letter is retrieved as a unit, irrespective of its number of strokes. In the spaced condition, however, one might assume that the motor program can not simply be retrieved from a long term store, but should be assembled each trial, just like the programs for symbols or novel graphemes. This would mean that, in the spaced condition the number of strokes would influence reaction time. It should, however, only influence reaction time in a choice reaction task, since the unfamiliar movement pattern can probably be prepared in advance in a simple reaction paradigm, as was found in the digits experiment.

Method

The experiment consisted of four conditions, which were presented to all eight student subjects in a counterbalanced order. The conditions were formed by combining one of two ways of performing the writing task – normal or spaced, with one of two paradigms – simple or choice.

A trial in the simple reaction task started with a warning signal – a 500 ms, 500 Hz tone – followed by a "preview" period of 600 ms. During this period the letter that had to be written was presented on a video monitor. After a foreperiod that varied with steps of 500 ms between 500 and 2500 ms, the letter was again presented on the monitor for 4000 ms. The subject had to write the letter as fast as possible after this second presentation. No visual feedback was allowed, the subject had to keep watching the screen. In the spaced condition the various strokes of a letter could not be connected but had to be made apart with a space of at least half the size of a normal stroke. A trial in the choice reaction task differed from a simple task trial only by virtue of the fact that the 600 ms preview period was left out.

The four conditions were presented in four blocks of 72 trials: 12 repetitions of 6 different letters. Each experimental block was preceded by 18 practice trials in the same condition. The 6 letters were of two types: continuous letters – "V", "Z" and "W" – normally made without lifting the pen, and discontinuous letters – "T", "H" and "E" – in which the pen is normally lifted between strokes. In both groups of three letters the number of strokes varied from two to four.

Stimulus presentation and pen movement recording were controlled by an Apple IIe microcomputer. Subjects wrote on normal paper that was lying on an Apple X-Y tablet, with a specially-made pen that was very much like an ordinary ballpoint pen. The X- and Y-coordinates, as well as the pen pressure, were digitized and sampled at 100 Hz, the error being approximately 0.2 mm, and later analyzed on a VAX computer, as described earlier.

Results and Discussion

The mean reaction times in the four conditions are displayed in Figure 5, as a function of movement complexity. In this figure the continuous and discontinuous letters are combined, since both types of letters produced similar results. In an analysis of variance on the reaction times, the difference between both types was far from significant. Of the other three factors in this analysis only two were significant and none of the interactions was significant. Inspecting Figure 5 reveals that choice reactions were larger than simple reactions ($\underline{F}(1,7) = 152.89$, $\underline{p} < .001$). More interestingly, the effect of spacing, i.e. of an unfamiliar way of writing, was considerable ($\underline{F}(1,7) = 6.70$, $\underline{p} < .05$): about 50 ms in the choice task and about 20 ms in the simple task. These latter data suggest that the interaction between the type of task and the way of writing should be significant. This was not the case, however ($\underline{F}(1,7) = 2.02$, $\underline{p} < .20$). A larger reaction time in the simple reaction task due to spacing was not expected. It may have something to do with the extra programming required to make an unusual stop at the end of the first stroke. The effect is of the same size as the unexpectedly longer simple RT's for single strokes and letters that were found earlier.

The main hypothesis in this experiment focussed on the effect of movement complexity. In the analysis of variance, movement complexity, measured in number of strokes, was not significant. As is clear in Figure 5, the reaction times did not increase with the number of strokes, which was contrary to expectations. It seems that in the writing of letters an increase in the number of strokes does not produce any effect upon reaction time, even if an unfamiliar strategy of writing is used. Possibly, spacing did not have the effect of isolating each separate stroke. The spaced movement pattern was probably not as unfamiliar as originally was assumed. The spaced capital may have been programmed like the normal capital, but with only one extra feature: spacing. This extra feature required some extra time, but this time was constant irrespective of the letter length.

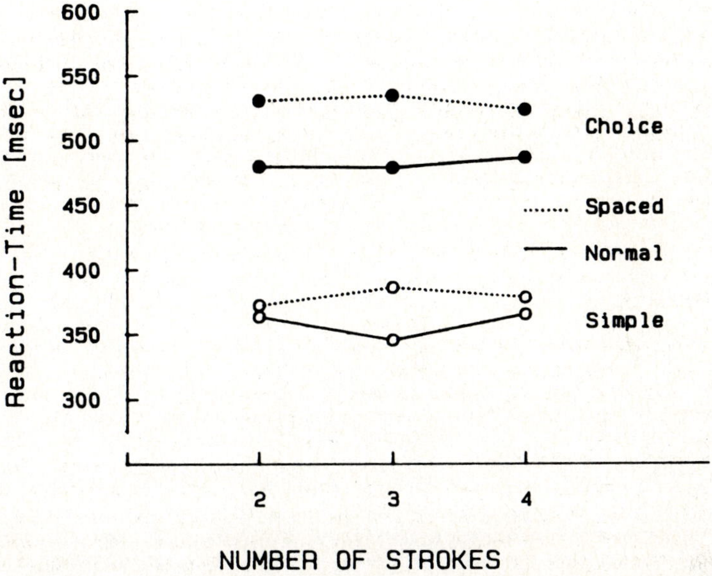

Figure 5. Reaction time in the simple and choice reaction task, given separately for normal and unpracticed, spaced, writing. Reaction times are averaged over continuous and discontinuous letters, and are presented as a function of the number of strokes.

General Discussion

The series of studies presented here was originally set up to find the basic unit of motor programming in handwriting. Study 1 varied the number of strokes of the movement sequence. Study 2 varied the number of letters. In both studies the reaction time increased with sequence length. However, this increase was very small: 5 ms per stroke in Study 1 and from 12 ms to 1.5 ms per letter in Study 2. Moreover, this increase in reaction time occurred only after an initial decrease for very short sequences. Although a reasonable explanation was put forward for this initial decrease, the data from these first two studies do not provide definitive evidence for either the stroke, or the letter, as the programming unit.

Much more striking than the effects of sequence length were the effects of practice. One type of practice effect was demonstrated in Study 2, in which practice within and across experiments resulted in a decreasing reaction time slope. The other type of practice effect resulted from learning that took place outside the laboratory. Its first manifestation occurred in Experiment 2 of Study 2, where the introduction of an unusual way of writing digits had a large effect on the duration of the time interval between writing these digits. This effect was replicated in the choice reaction experiment of Study 3, in which novel graphemes were initiated much later than equally complex letter pairs. In Study 4 similar results were found in that novel graphemes, as well as symbols, if compared with letters, were not only initiated after a longer reaction time but also showed a greater rise in reaction time if the number of their strokes increased. Finally in Study 5, in which no perceptually or motorically unfamiliar graphemes were used, but in which overlearned capitals had to be written in an unusual, spaced, way, this relatively unpracticed way of writing resulted in a considerable increase in reaction time. All these practice effects were much larger (110 ms in Study 2, 87 ms in Study 3, about 110 or 140 ms in Study 4, and 50 or 20 ms in Study 5) than the very small effects of sequence length in Study 1 and 2 (5 ms and 12 to 1.5 ms respectively).

These results, taken together, suggest that the unit of programming is not a fixed motorically-defined entity, but that it is chosen flexibly depending on the nature of the task and the amount of practice the subjects have with the movements. In the sawtooth movement of Study 1, the subjects may have chosen the stroke as the element, although other strategies may have been used also; for example, to code the two-stroke and four-stroke patterns as the letters "V" or "U" and "W". In Study 2 the optimal strategy was to code the movement sequences as letter strings. Unfamiliar patterns, like the ones used in Studies 3 and 4, were probably programmed as sequences of straight and curved line segments. Writing digits in an unusual way probably caused the movements to be programmed as a sequence of individual strokes. Finally, the "spaced" writing of capital letters was probably programmed with the letter as the unit to which one extra feature, i.e. spacing, was added.

The foregoing view implies that the programming of motor commands proceeds at least on two levels. The higher level is the one on which the subject chooses the units. It is a cognitive level where "controlled programming", analogous to "controlled processing" as defined by Shiffrin and Schneider (1977), takes place. The lower level is the domain of automatic processes in which the movement plan, that was set up at the higher level, is translated into muscle commands. This conception of motor programming as a hierarchical and flexible process is not new (see Keele, 1981; van Galen & Wing, 1984). In a recent study on the concurrency of motoric preparation and retrieval processes, van Galen, Smyth and Meulenbroek (1987) proposed a psychomotor model of handwriting in which linguistic, semantic, allographic and motor programming is done by parallel processors. Although parallel, these processors work in a hierarchy in that the lower level processors have to wait for input from higher processors. At the lower levels the elements of programming are smaller and less abstract. Learning, or the effect of extended practice, is conceived in this view as the formation of more efficient codes in motor memory. As a result of the formation of these codes the element of programming will change between conditions in which letters or novel graphemes are written, and between tasks in which practiced or unpracticed movement trajectories have to be followed. According to this view, the search for the basic unit, or the fundamental inflexible element, of programming is bound to fail, since the nature of the task, the training of the subject, the strategy that the subject has chosen and the level at which the unit is searched, all influence the outcome.

These speculations do not derive directly from the data that were presented. However, one safe conclusion that can be drawn is that the amount of practice had a large effect on reaction time. This conclusion reaches far beyond the skill of writing. Most reaction time experiments on motor programming have used non-automatized, unfamiliar, tasks like finger-tapping (Semjen & Garcia-Colera, 1986), finger pressing at different forces (Ivry, 1986), key-press responses (Zelaznik & Hahn, 1985), pushing bars, buttons and plates (Harrington & Haaland, 1987) or pointing to targets laid out in an accidental way (Fischman, 1984). So it might well be that most of the effects that were found had not so much to do with the programming at a motor level, but more with the planning of the recently learned, not yet automatized, sequence at a higher, cognitive level. This reasoning leads to the conjecture that Klapp's (1977) well-known dit-dah results will not be replicated if experienced morse key operators are used as subjects and if these operators are required not to press "dah" or "dit" but to press the corresponding letters "T" or "E", or the words "The" "End".

References

Fischman, M.G. (1984). Programming time as a function of number of movement parts and changes in movement direction. Journal of Motor Behavior, 16, 405-423.

Harrington, D.L. & Haaland, K.Y. (1987). Programming sequences hand postures. Journal of Motor Behavior, 19, 77-95.

Henry, F.M. & Rogers, D.E. (1960). Increased response latency for complicated movements and a "memory drum" theory of neuromotor reaction. Research Quarterly, 31, 448-458.

Hullstijn, W. (1987). Programming of speech and nonspeech motor activity. In H.F.M. Peters & W. Hulstijn (Eds.), Speech Motor Dynamics in Stuttering (pp.41-55). New York: Springer-Verlag.

Hulstijn, W. & van Galen, G.P. (1983). Programming in handwriting: Reaction time and movement time as a function of sequence length. Acta Psychologica, 54, 23-49.

Ivry, R.B. (1986). Force and timing components of the motor program. Journal of Motor Behavior, 18, 449-474.

Kao, H.S.R., van Galen, G.P., & Hoosain, R. (Eds.) (1986). Graphonomics: Contemporary research in handwriting. Amsterdam: North-Holland.

Keele, S.W. (1968). Movement control in skilled motor performance. Psychological Bulletin, 70, 387-403.

Keele, S.W. (1981). Behavioral analysis of movement. In V.B. Brooks (Ed.), Handbook of physiology: Sec.1. The nervous system: Vol.2. Motor control (pp.1391-1414). Bethesda, MD: American Physiological Society.

Keele, S.W. (1982). Learning and control of coordinated motor patterns: The programming perspective. In J.A.S. Kelso (Ed.), Human motor behavior: An introduction (pp.161-186). Hillsdale, NJ: Lawrence Erlbaum Associates.

Klapp, S.T. (1977). Reaction time analysis of programmed control. Exercise and Sports Sciences Reviews, 5, 231-253.

Plamondon, R., Suen, C.Y., Deschenes, J., & Poulin, G. (Eds.), (1987). Proceedings of the Third International Symposium on Handwriting and Computer Applications. Montreal: Editions de l'Ecole Polytechnique de Montreal.

Rosenbaum, D.A., Inhoff, A.W., & Gordon, A.M. (1984). Choosing between movement sequences: A hierarchical editor model. Journal of Experimental Psychology: General, 113, 372-393.

Schmidt, R.A. (1982a). More on motor programs. In J.A.S. Kelso Human motor behavior: An introduction (pp.189-217). Hillsdale, NJ: Lawrence Erlbaum Associates.

Schmidt, R.A. (1982b). Motor control and learning: A behavioural emphasis. Champaign, IL: Human Kinetics.

Semjen, A., & Garcia-Colera, A. (1986). Planning and timing of finger-tapping sequences with a stressed element. Journal of Motor Behavior, 18, 287-322.

Shiffrin, R.M. & Schneider, W. (1977). Controlled and automatic human information processing: II. Perceptual learning, automatic attending and a general theory. Psychological Review, 84, 127-190.

Stelmach, G.E., Mullins, P.A., & Teulings, H.L. (1984). Response programming, temporal patterns and response characteristics. Annals of New York Academy of Science, 423, 144-157.

Sternberg, S., Monsell, S., Knoll, R.L., & Wright, C.E. (1978). The latency and duration of rapid movement sequences: Comparisons of speech and typewriting. In G. Stelmach (Ed.), Information processing in motor control and learning. New York: Academic Press.

Teulings, H.L., Mullins, P.A., & Stelmach, G.E. (1986). The elementary units of programming in handwriting. In H.S.R. Kao, G.P. van Galen, & R. Hoosain (Eds.), Graphonomics: Contemporary research in handwriting (pp.21-32). Amsterdam: North-Holland.

Thomassen, A.J.W.M., Keuss, P.J.G., & van Galen, G. (Eds.) (1984). Motor aspects of handwriting. Amsterdam: North-Holland.

van Galen, G.P. (1980). Handwriting and drawing: A two stage model of complex motor behavior. In G.E. Stelmach & J. Requin (Eds.), Tutorials in motor behavior. Amsterdam: North-Holland.

van Galen, G.P., Smyth, M.M., & Meulenbroek, R.G.J. (1987). The monitoring of repetitive stroking patterns under visual and non visual guidance of handwriting. In R. Plamondon, C.Y. Suen, J. Deschenes, & G. Poulin (Eds.), Proceedings of the third international symposium on handwriting and computer applications (pp.30-32). Montreal: Editions de l'Ecole Polytechnique de Montreal.

van Galen, G.P. & Teulings, H.L. (1983). The independent monitoring of form and scale factors in handwriting of sequence length. Acta Psychologica, 54, 9-22.

van Galen, G.P. & Wing, A.M. (1984). The sequencing of movements.

In M.M. Smyth & A.M. Wing (Eds.), The psychology of human movement (pp.153-181). London: Academic Press.

Zelaznik, H.N. & Hahn, R. (1985). Reaction time methods in the study of motor programming: The precuing of hand, digit, and duration. Journal of Motor Behavior, 17, 190-218.

Cognition and Action in Skilled Behaviour
A.M. Colley and J.R. Beech (Editors)

A MOVEMENT CONSTRAINT INTERPRETATION OF THE RESPONSE COMPLEXITY EFFECT ON PROGRAMMING TIME

Ben Sidaway, Robert W. Christina
and John B. Shea
The Pennsylvania State University

This paper reinterprets data from five recently published experiments on response complexity and programming time in which number of movement parts of rapidly executed limb responses was advanced as the principal element influencing length of response programming time. Alternatively it is argued here that programming time, in these experiments, was predominantly a function of the constraints placed upon the output of the motor system by the demand for movement accuracy. The quantification of this accuracy demand is achieved by using the metric of Index of Difficulty (Fitts, 1954). In discrete and straight-line tapping responses to circular targets, response complexity may be conceptualized in terms of the angular constraint imposed on movement initiation at the start key. When responses require changes of direction between movement parts it is proposed that programming time may be a function of the cumulative movement constraints imposed by the task. The discussion focuses on the process by which an increased accuracy demand requires a more constrained motor system output which is brought about by a larger and/or more precise muscle synergy recruitment pattern, resulting in an increase in programming time.

According to Henry and Rogers' (1960) original theory of neuromotor reaction, well learned rapid movements were thought to be executed under the control of previously stored neuromotor programs. They proposed that when a program is needed, it is selected and read out to the appropriate neuromotor coordination centers where it is translated into efferent commands to the muscles to initiate the desired movement. This translation was believed to take place mainly during the simple reaction time (RT) interval and was termed programming. According to this interpretation a more complex movement requires greater involvement of neuromotor coordination centers, and greater use of previously stored neuromotor information, which results in a longer duration for the complex distribution of neural impulses through the coordination centers. A consequent prediction of the Henry and Rogers' theory was that the time to prepare a movement, as measured by simple RT, becomes longer as the movement becomes more complex because the programming process is also more complex (Henry, 1980). The original theory has not gone unchallenged these past 28 years and some parts of it may have to be modified in the light of what is known today. However, the central idea of the theory and its consequent prediction are still being used as the basis for many current investigations. More recent elaborations of this theory and discussions of the methods used for testing it can be found in numerous publications (e.g. Hayes & Marteniuk, 1976; Henry, 1980, 1981; Kerr, 1978; Klapp, 1978, 1980, 1981; Marteniuk & MacKenzie, 1981; Sternberg, Monsell, Knoll, & Wright, 1978).

Since the Henry and Rogers' (1960) paper, many studies (e.g. Anson, 1982; Glencross, 1972, 1973, 1976; Klapp, 1976; Klapp & Erwin, 1976; Lagasse & Hayes, 1973; Norrie, 1967, 1974) have been conducted in which response demands were varied in order to observe the effects of movement complexity on programming time. The main purposes of these studies were to identify the crucial elements of the complexity effect and to determine how much of a modification in complexity was required to generate a noticeable change in programming time. Some of the response elements examined have included movement duration; movement velocity; number of connected movement parts; movement distance; movement accuracy; changes in movement direction, and force. Recently, Christina and his colleagues (Christina, Fischman, Lambert, & Moore, 1985; Christina, Fischman, Vercruyssen, & Anson, 1982; Christina & Rose, 1985; Fischman, 1984) identified the number of movement parts in a response as the principal element influencing programming time. Essentially, they concluded that programming time increased as the number of movement parts increased, although Christina et al. (1985) did acknowledge that a very small portion of the RT increase could be attributed to an increase in the demand for movement accuracy. Furthermore, Christina and Rose (1985) concluded that the combined influence of number of movement parts and accuracy demand increased programming time more than either of these elements did separately. Nonetheless, Christina and his colleagues maintained that programming time was more a function of number of movement parts than accuracy demand. However, when the evidence produced by Christina and his associates is re-examined and interpreted in terms of movement constraints as quantified by Fitts' (1954) Index of Difficulty (ID), a much stronger case can be made for movement accuracy as a crucial element of the complexity effect.

The purpose of this paper is to present an alternative explanation for the effects of movement complexity on programming time that were found by Christina and his colleagues. This explanation holds that the underlying cause of the lengthened programming time in their experiments was the increased constraint placed upon the motor system that resulted when the number of movement parts and movement accuracy were manipulated. The motor system in the present case is defined as the distributed network of neurological processing and control systems responsible for governing muscle action and hence movement (Pew, 1984). This paper begins with an explanation of how ID may reflect the complexity of the response programming process. A mathematical expression of Fitts' (1954) ID as a function of one variable, namely the angle subtended at the start position by a circular target, is derived to explain how the output of the motor system and hence programming time may vary with the ID of a response. Next, the evidence produced by Christina and his colleagues is re-examined in terms of ID to demonstrate that the accuracy content in rapidly executed target striking responses correlates highly with programming time as measured by RT[1]. The paper concludes with a theoretical explanation of how the programming time may be a function of the increased demand for movement accuracy. It is proposed that a greater demand for accuracy reduces the degrees of freedom of movement and hence a successful response will only be achieved by the motor system reducing the degrees of freedom of its output. This is achieved through the inhibition of unwanted muscle synergies and motor units and a more precise temporal and spatial recruitment pattern of the necessary synergies.

ID, Movement Constraints and Programming Time

Fitts (1954) formulated an index that specified the minimum information required, on average, for controlling a series of movements of given amplitude (A) to targets of a certain width (W). Fitts defined his index of movement difficulty as ID = Log2 (2A/W) and found that average movement time (MT) was linearly related to ID as given by the following equation: MT = a+b (ID), where the values a and b are empirical constants. Essentially then average MT increases as ID increases, and, within certain limits, remains constant for different values of amplitude and width as long as ID is held constant. Crossman (1957) and Welford (1968) have suggested a slight modification of Fitts' ID. They proposed that instead of actual target width a corrected estimate of W, adjusted for errors, should be used in computing ID values. This has been referred to as the effective target width and has been shown to provide a slightly greater correlation between ID and MT. Fitts proposed that the major factor limiting MT or the rate of motor performance was the degree of control over the organization of a response. His information theory interpretation has been criticized by several authors who have proposed alternative explanations to explain the ID-MT correlation (e.g. Crossman & Goodeve, 1963; Keele, 1968, 1981; Howarth, Beggs, & Bowden, 1971; Schmidt, Zelaznik, Hawkins, Frank, & Quinn, 1979; Wright & Meyer, 1983). The correlation of MT and ID, however, is still considered to be one of the most reliable relationships in perceptual-motor control. It is proposed in this paper that under certain conditions programming time, as measured by simple RT, also may be a function of ID since it, too, is a function of response organization.

Since Fitts' ID is a ratio of the amplitude of a target to its width, ID for an aiming response may be mathematically expressed as a function of the angle subtended, at the start key, by a given circular target[2]. This geometric relationship is shown diagrammatically in Figure 1. Fitts' ID may be thought of as a function of the angle (θ) subtended at the start key by the diameter of the target which is given by the following equation: Log2 (2A/W), dividing both sides of the term in brackets by 2 gives: Log2 (A/R) = ID, where R is the radius of the target. Using trigonometry one can substitute cotangent (cot) $\theta/2$ for A/R which results in the

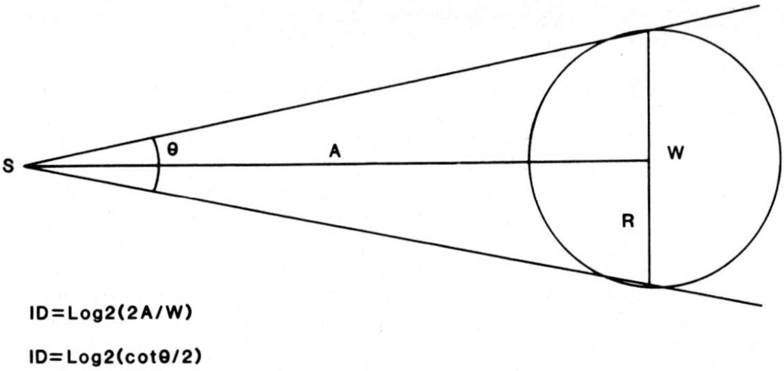

Figure 1. The relationship between ID and subtended angle where: S = the start position; θ = the subtended angle; A = amplitude; W = width (diameter) of the target; and R = radius of the target.

following equation: Log2 (cot θ/2) = ID, where θ represents the subtended angle. Thus ID for a rapid aiming response to contact a circular target can be expressed as a function of just one variable, the subtended angle. The relationship between ID and subtended angle is shown graphically in Figure 2. It is clear that ID increases as the subtended angle decreases and that any two circles whose diameters subtend the same angle at the start key will have the same ID.

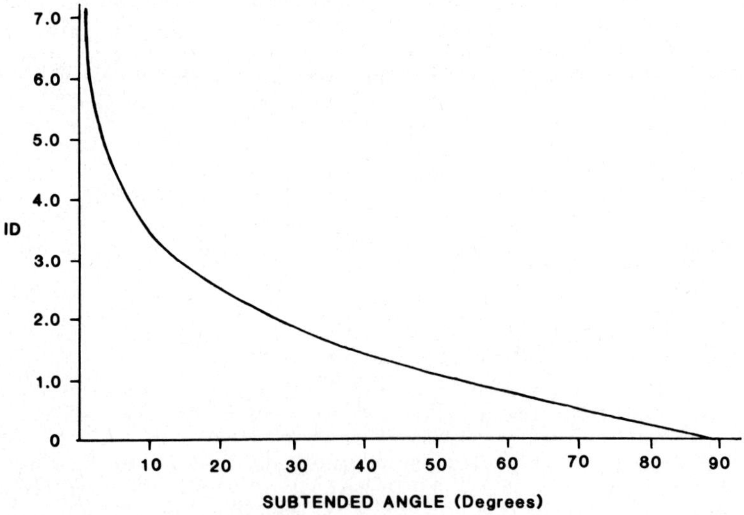

Figure 2. The function relating ID and subtended angle.

Unidirectional Movement Constraints

The circular target tapping task shown in Figure 3 illustrates the constraints placed upon the output of the motor system by the demand for movement accuracy. The two lines arising from the starting position, point 2, can be thought of as the planar directional limits that a movement must be kept within, in order to successfully hit target A. The smaller the angle subtended at the start key, the greater the restriction of the degrees of freedom of that movement, whereas the larger the subtended angle the less the restriction of the degrees of freedom of that movement. In other words, the greater the degrees of freedom, the more variable the movement may be and yet still successfully hit the target. In a discrete tapping response one may equate the angular restriction in the subtended angle with the restriction in the degrees of freedom of that movement. Just as one can think of a movement demanding a certain restriction in the degrees of freedom available, one can conceptualize the motor system that produces the movement as also having a number of degrees of freedom with which to work. The motor system is capable of producing an almost infinite number of responses, but the experimental instructions requiring the subject to hit the target as rapidly and as accurately as possible necessitate that the various distributed neural control centers in the motor system constrain their enormous capability for variable output. In such a way, the final output of the system allows only a narrow band-width of responses, all of which are capable of successfully accomplishing the experimental task. This band-width increases in tolerance as the ID of the target decreases or the experimental instructions become more lenient. If programming time, as measured by simple RT, is a function of response organization which in turn is a function of the degrees of freedom of that response, then RT will be proportional to the Log2 $(\cot\theta/2)$ function of the subtended angle of a circular target. Another prediction is that since the circular Targets A, B and C in Figure 3 share a common subtended angle, the RTs of discrete responses to hit any of these targets will be essentially the same.

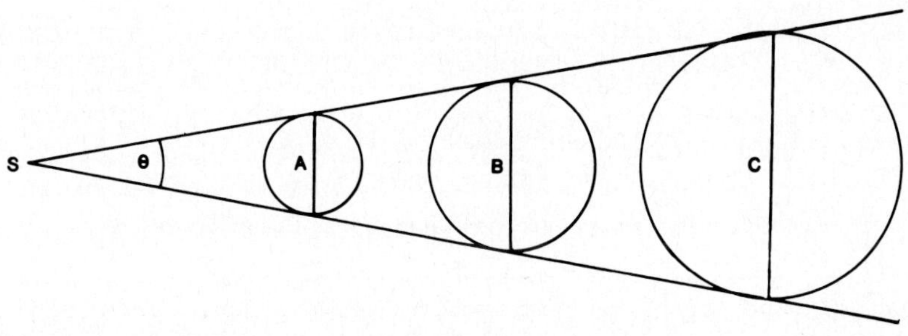

Figure 3. A series of targets subtending a common angle where S = the start position; θ = the subtended angle; and A, B, C = circular targets.

Turning to responses with more than one target, it is hypothesized that, given a task with successive targets all constrained by the same two lines arising from the start position, that is subtending a common angle as shown in Figure 3, the RTs to strike two or more of these targets in sequence should be very similar. This is due to the fact that when targets are positioned in a straight line all the directional constraints on the movement can occur at only one point, namely the start position. The movement can be thought of as being constrained along the same path throughout the series of taps. Consequently it is hypothesized that programming time in this serial task is a function of the target that imposes the greatest constraint upon the movement path. That target will be the target within the series of targets with the highest ID as measured from the start position. Just as in the case of discrete responses the demand for accuracy in a movement, imposed by the task and experimental instructions, forces the motor system to produce a more constrained or precise output. A more precisely controlled movement requires a more complex program and hence results in a lengthened programming time.

Cumulative Movement Constraints

If the targets are in a straight line, the ID of one target may be responsible for most of the constraints placed on the movement for the whole sequence of taps. However, this may not be the case for responses in which direction changes are required. If subjects are required to make changes in direction of their movement path in order to accurately complete a response, the ID of a single target in that sequence will not be representative of the total difficulty of that response. In these responses the constraints on the trajectory of the movement must change as a function of the ID of that movement component and thus the constraints on the motor system differ from component to component. It is possible that, in this situation, programming time is a function of the cumulative series of movement constraints. In order to arrive at some measure of the accuracy demand in these situations, ID from the start key to the first target may be added to the ID from the first to second target, and so on. This additive ID calculation will become less valid as more movement parts are added to the response, thus increasing the duration of the response. As the duration of the response increases, the assumption that the whole response is programmed during the RT interval becomes less likely. The control of the later components of the response, particularly if they are of a long duration, may be influenced by feedback, particularly that from the visual system.

Evidence for Programming Time as a Function of ID

Fitts and Peterson (1964) were the first to report a relationship between ID and RT. In their simple RT condition, which had 50% catch trials, they found a correlation of .79. However, the slope of the linear function relating the two variables was only 5.4 msec per 1-bit change in ID. This fact, together with the clearer effect of ID on MT, has resulted in little research being published on the effect of ID on RT, and even less using ID as a measure of response complexity in response programming.

Recent studies by Christina and colleagues have examined rapidly executed limb responses, with and without changes in movement direction, that required subjects to hit a series of various sized targets. The authors proposed in all the papers that the most important element contributing to increased RT was the number of movement parts of the response. However, they did not measure the ID of the different elements contained within the responses they used. As a result, they did not consider interpreting their results with reference to ID and the concept of movement constraint, as has been done for this paper and which is presented next.

Fischman (1984) conducted an experiment to examine the effect of number of movement parts and changes in movement direction on programming time. Two groups of subjects had to tap a series of targets, ranging in number from one to five, positioned in a straight line or in a zig-zag movement pattern. Since there was no significant difference between RTs for the changes in direction and the straight line movement patterns, Fischman combined the two sets of data and reported that the increases in RT were significantly linear across the range of movement parts. However, the greatest effect was found as the number of movements within the response increased from one to two taps. Following the single tap response, the number of connected taps had to increase by at least two before a significant increase in RT occurred. Fischman also fractionated RT in order to examine premotor time (PMT) which Lagasse and Hayes (1973) argued is a more valid indicator of programming time than RT. However, the findings for PMT essentially paralleled those of RT.

Fischman's data on the number of taps is confounded by the concomitant increase in the distance the hand had to travel from the start position. Fischman assumed that it was the number of intermediate taps between the start position and the final target that caused the increase in RT. The geometric relationship proposed earlier in this paper predicts that, when a series of targets in a straight line are to be contacted, it is the target that imposes the greatest constraint on the movement path that dictates programming time. Since in Fischman's task all the targets were the same size, the last target always had the highest ID as measured from the start key and hence imposed the greatest constraint on the movement path.

To examine the validity of this prediction, ID was calculated in Fischman's straight line pattern for the last target in all the tapping sequences. The calculated ID value is plotted against RT in Figure 4. A correlation between ID and RT resulted in a coefficient of $\underline{r}=.994$. This lends support to the hypothesis that programming time is a function of the movement constraints imposed by the most difficult target. This hypothesis is further strengthened by some recently collected data by the first author (Sidaway, 1986), using the Fischman apparatus. Three subjects performed 40 trials in each of three conditions, the last 10 trials being statistically analyzed. Using a simple RT paradigm, subjects had to either hit the first, third or fifth target on the Fischman apparatus. The intermediate targets were removed and so no taps were required before the final target. Thus, the number of movement parts was held constant at one and only the amplitude of the movement varied. Reaction time means for each of the three responses are presented as a function of ID in Figure 4. The data from these subjects is

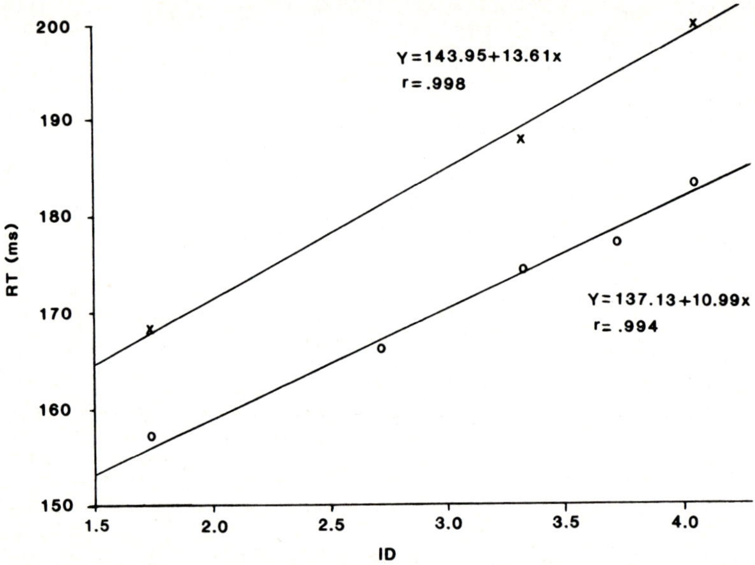

Figure 4. Mean reaction time as a function of the ID of one target. The circles plot mean reaction time against the ID of the last target in Fischman's (1984) straight-line tapping condition. The crosses plot mean reaction time against the ID of a single target in a discrete one tap response (Sidaway, 1986).

similar and closely parallels the data from Fischman's study. These data support the contention that in Fischman's task the most important variable in determining RT was the ID of the last target and not the number of taps.

Christina et al. (1982) investigated responses that were very similar to those originally used by Henry and Rogers (1960). They examined four responses. One response consisted of a tennis ball grasp, while the three other responses consisted of striking one, two or three targets in different planes of motion. Since in its present form ID is insensitive to the information required for specifying additional manipulatory acts, such as finger movements required to grasp objects, the tennis ball grasp was not included in this analysis. Using the target sizes and positions reported by Christina et al. (1982), additive ID was calculated. Reaction time from Experiment 3 was plotted as a function of ID for the three target striking responses and is shown in Figure 5a. The regression equation calculated for these data reveals that, as more targets are required to be hit, and as additive ID increases, RT also increases.

In Christina et al. (1982) it is difficult to separate the effect of ID

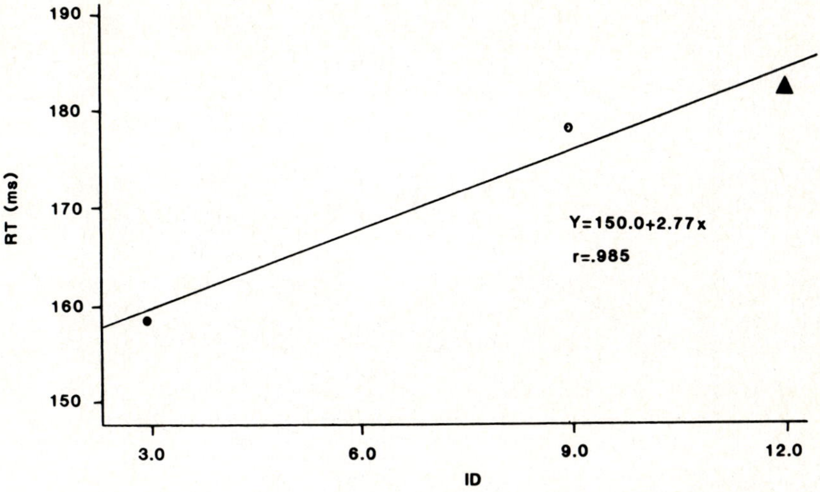

Figure 5a

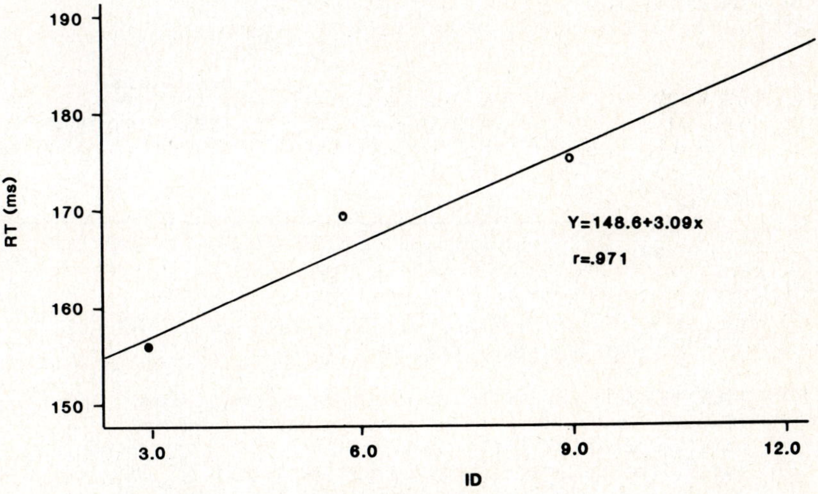

Figure 5b

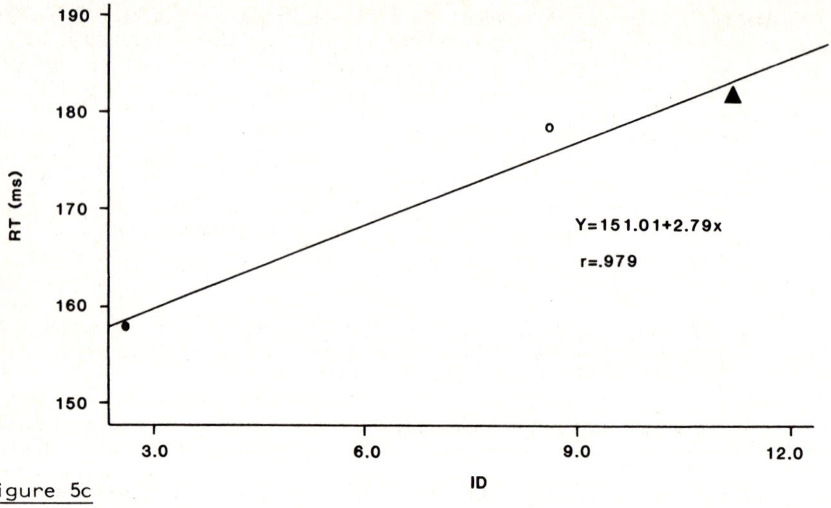

Figure 5c

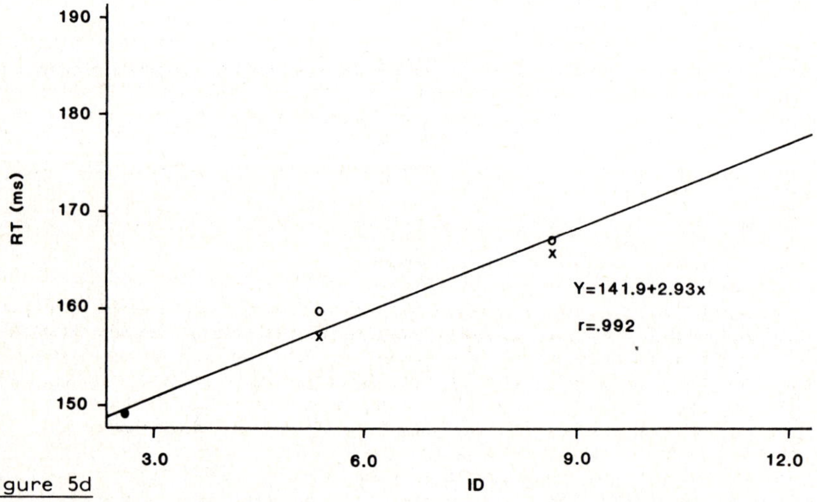

Figure 5d

Figure 5. Mean reaction time as a function of additive ID. Christina et al., 1982 (Exp.3) is in 5a; Christina et al., 1985 (Exp.2) is in 5b; Christina and Rose, 1985 (Exp.1) is in 5c; and Christina and Rose, 1985 (Exp.2) is in 5d. The filled circles represent one-part responses. The crosses represent two-part responses in which there was a downward but no forward change in direction between the two parts of the response. The open circles represent two-part responses in which there was a forward and downward change in direction between the two parts of the response. The filled triangles represent responses in which there were three movement parts.

from that of number of movement parts, but in Christina et al. (1985), Experiment 2, a one-element response and two different two-element responses were examined. In the two-part responses, the first target size was kept constant but the final target size was either 0.79 cm or 8.5 cm in diameter. Therefore, additive ID is different between these two two-part responses. Reaction time for the one-part and two-part responses is plotted in Figure 5b as a function of additive ID. Although the number of movement parts remains at two, as shown in Figure 5b, there is a difference in ID between the two-part response culminating in an 8.5 cm target and the two-part response with a final target size of 0.79 cm. This extra difficulty is reflected in RT.

Christina and Rose (1985), Experiment 1, replicated the work of Christina et al. (1982) with one-, two-, and three-part movements. Reaction time for these responses is plotted as a function of additive ID and the calculated regression equation is shown in Figure 5c. Their second experiment was very similar to that of Christina et al. (1985) in that the final target size of the two-movement part responses was changed. Christina and Rose also altered the type of change in direction required between the two elements of these responses. There was very little effect of type of change in direction on RT, but, as Christina et al. (1985) found, there was a significant increase in RT when the target size in the second element was reduced from 8.5 cm to 0.79 cm. Reaction time for the five responses examined is plotted against additive ID and shown in Figure 5d, along with the calculated regression equation and correlation coefficient for the line of best fit. The increase in additive ID when the 8.5 cm second target is replaced with a 0.79 cm target results in a consistent increase in RT.

Discussion

Re-examination of the evidence produced by Christina and his colleagues, and interpretation of it with reference to ID, revealed that a stronger case could be made for the accuracy content of a response being a crucial element of the complexity effect on programming time than was previously thought by these investigators. A target to be hit, either by itself or within a series of targets, has a certain accuracy demand which can be measured by ID. The higher the accuracy demand, the greater the demand for constraint that is placed upon the motor system. In responses where only one target is to be hit, or a series of targets arranged in a straight line are to be struck, programming time as measured by RT will be a function of the restrictions placed upon the angle of take-off at the start position. The wider that angle, the less is the accuracy content of that response and hence fewer constraints are placed upon the degrees of freedom of the motor system. When ID is higher, the subject must leave the start position with a less tolerant trajectory than when ID is smaller. This narrow angle of take-off, resulting in a reduction in the degrees of freedom in the motor system output, may be effected by a more complex and precise pattern of muscle synergy and motor unit activation. When large-scale direction changes are required within a response, the necessity for pathway constraint of the moving limb also occurs after the initiation of movement. Each target to be hit imposes a degree of constraint proportional to its ID as calculated from the previous target. With an increasing demand for response organization and motor system constraint, the number and/or precision of muscle synergies required for effecting the response will change, as will their temporal and spatial recruitment pattern. As the ID of a response increases, the bandwidth of possible successful responses becomes smaller, necessitating a more constrained motor system output. While the motor system must recruit a temporally and spatially precise pattern of muscle synergies and motor units, it must also increasingly inhibit unwanted motor activity as response accuracy content increases. The motor system is inherently noisy: this neural noise results in unwanted movement variability and contributes to inaccuracy. Increasing the accuracy requirement of a response and hence movement constraint forces the motor system to increase the signal to noise ratio of its output. Unwanted neural activity is the noise in the system whereas required neural-motor activity can be thought of as the signal. Responses to low ID targets can tolerate a higher degree of noise in the output of the motor system, a lower signal to noise ratio, and still be successful since the movement can be more variable and yet still hit the target. Successful responses to targets with a high ID cannot tolerate a noisy output because error would occur. The requirement, in high accuracy content responses, for inhibition of unwanted neural noise, along with necessity for temporal and spatial precision in the neural activity that is allowed, results in a greater complexity and hence increased duration of motor programming. The stage at which this increased program complexity affects RT is probably at the translation of the stored motor program into efferent commands to the muscles through the distributed and partially parallel motor system. It is the degree of organization or complexity of motor system output that is the major factor limiting the speed of the translation process and consequently the length of RT.

There are at least two alternative hypotheses that may be proposed to explain the high relationship between RT and ID (accuracy content). The first would simply hold that as response accuracy content increases the velocity at which the subject leaves the RT key decreases. In other words, a greater demand for accuracy slows down the response. Falkenberg and Newell (1980), and Newell, Hoshizaki, Carlton, and Halbert (1979) have reported that RT tends to vary as an inverse function of average movement velocity. However this explanation is not supported by the data on PMT that was obtained in two of the studies examined in this paper. Christina and Rose (1985), and Fischman (1984) found that nearly all the increases in RT, as responses increased in complexity, were due to increases in PMT with very little effect on motor time. If the increases in RT were due to a slower velocity off the key, one would expect to find increases in the motor time component of RT with decreasing velocity. Also contradicting the velocity hypothesis is the finding in many of the studies examined, that RT increased as the demand for accuracy within the responses increased, but the movement times of the initial segment of the responses were essentially the same. This suggests that, although RT changed significantly, the velocity of the initial movement off the key remained the same.

This paper hypothesizes that programming time lengthens because of the increase in the number and/or precision of muscle synergies and motor units recruited along with the increased inhibition of unwanted motor activity as the accuracy content within a response increases. A somewhat different interpretation may be offered by those who hypothesize that movement duration is the key parameter affecting programming time (Klapp & Erwin, 1976; Quinn, Schmidt, Zelaznik, Hawkins, & McFaquhar, 1980). As response accuracy content increases so does the time taken to complete the response. It is possible that it is the increase in movement time that is responsible for the lengthened programming time. Keele (1981) suggested that longer duration movements require smaller stopping and starting forces which results in an increase in the interval between accelerative and decelerative forces. Keele proposed that it is this increase in demand for timing that increases programming time. Essentially this explanation holds that when a response has to be executed as rapidly and as accurately as possible, programming time for that response is a function of the variation in the forthcoming MT and not a function of the underlying cause of the increase in MT (i.e. the increase in the accuracy content of the response). However, as Christina et al. (1985) have argued, this explanation is weakened by evidence showing that certain response elements can increase MT without affecting RT, such as movement distance (Brown & Slater-Hammel, 1949; Lagasse & Hayes, 1973) or changes in movement direction (Fischman, 1984; Glencross, 1973). It appears that the most likely cause of the increased RT, in the studies examined, was a lengthened programming time which resulted from a greater demand for output precision placed upon the motor system by increases in the accuracy content of the response.

Footnotes

[1]Throughout this paper, the abbreviation RT refers to the mean simple reaction time. Although premotor time (PMT) is a more exact estimate of programming time than RT (Lagasse & Hayes, 1973), PMT was not analyzed in this chapter because most of the studies examined did not fractionate RT and the few that did found an almost identical pattern of results for both measures.

[2]This relationship does not hold for noncircular targets since movement constraints are not directionally constant.

Acknowledgements

The authors wish to thank Greg Anson, Mark Fischman, and Merrill Noble for their comments on an earlier version of this paper.

References

Anson, J.G. (1982). Memory drum theory. Alternative tests and explanations for the complexity effects on simple reaction time. Journal of Motor Behavior, 14, 228-246.

Brown, J.S., & Slater-Hammel, A.T. (1949). Discrete movements in the horizontal plane as a function of their length and direction. Journal of Experimental Psychology, 34, 86-95.

Christina, R.W., Fischman, M.G., Lambert, A.L., & Moore, J.F. (1985). Simple reaction time as a function of response complexity: Christina et al., (1982) revisited. Research Quarterly for Exercise and Sport, 56, 316-322.

Christina, R.W., Fischman, M.G., Vercruyssen, M.J.P., & Anson, J.G. (1982). Simple reaction time as a function of response complexity: Memory drum theory revisited. Journal of Motor Behavior, 14, 301-321.

Christina, R.W., & Rose, D.J. (1985). Premotor and motor reaction time as function of response complexity. Research Quarterly for Exercise and Sport, 56, 306-315.

Crossman, E.R.F.W. (1957). The speed and accuracy of simple hand movements. In E.R.F.W. Crossman, & W.D. Seymour (Eds.), The nature and acquisition of industrial skills. Report to M.R.C. and D.S.I.R. Joint Committee on Individual Efficiency in Industry.

Crossman, E.R.F.W., & Goodeve, P.J. (1963). Feedback control of hand-movement and Fitt's Law. Paper presented at the meeting of the Experimental Psychology Society, Oxford, 1963. Quarterly Journal of Experimental Psychology, 1983, 35A, 251-278.

Falkenberg, L.E., & Newell, K.M. (1980). Relative contribution of movement time, amplitude and velocity to response initiation. Journal of Experimental Psychology: Human Perception and Performance, 6, 760-768.

Fischman, M.G. (1984). Programming time as a function of number of movement parts and changes in movement direction. Journal of Motor Behavior, 16, 405-423.

Fitts, P.M. (1954). The information capacity of the human motor system in controlling the amplitude of movement. Journal of Experimental Psychology, 47, 381-391.

Fitts, P.M., & Peterson, J.R. (1964). Information capacity of discrete motor responses. Journal of Experimental Psychology, 67, 103-112.

Glencross, D.J. (1972). Latency and response complexity. Journal of Motor Behavior, 4, 241-256.

Glencross, D.J. (1973). Response complexity and latency of different movement patterns. Journal of Motor Behavior, 5, 95-104.

Glencross, D.J. (1976). The latency of aiming movements. Journal of Motor Behavior, 8, 27-34.

Hayes, K.C., & Marteniuk, R.G. (1976). Dimensions of motor task complexity. In G.E. Stelmach (Ed.), Motor control: Issues and trends. New York: Academic Press.

Henry, F.M. (1980). Use of simple reaction time in motor programming studies: A reply to Klapp, Wyatt, and Lingo. Journal of Motor Behavior, 12, 163-168.

Henry, F.M. (1981). The evolution of the memory drum theory of neuromotor reaction. In George A. Brooks (Ed.), Perspectives on the academic discipline of Physical Education. Champaign,

IL.: Human Kinetics Publishers.
Henry, F.M., & Rogers, D.E. (1960). Increased response latency for complicated movements and a "memory drum" theory of neuromotor reaction. Research Quarterly, 31, 448-458.
Howarth, C.I., Beggs, W.D.A., & Bowden, J. (1971). The relationship between speed and accuracy of movement aimed at a target. Acta Psychologica, 35, 207-218.
Keele, S.W. (1968). Movement control in skilled motor performance. Psychological Bulletin, 70, 387-403.
Keele, S.W. (1981). Behavioral analysis of movement. In V. Brooks (Ed.), Handbook of physiology: Motor control. Washington, D.C.: American Physiological Society.
Kerr, B. (1978). Task factors that influence selection and preparation for voluntary movements. In G.E. Stelmach (Ed.), Information processing in motor control and learning. New York: Academic Press.
Klapp, S.T. (1976). Short-term memory as a response preparation state. Memory and Cognition, 4, 721-724.
Klapp, S.T. (1978). Reaction time analysis of programmed control. In R.S. Hutton (Ed.), Exercise and sport science reviews. Santa Barbara, C.A.: Journal Publishing Affiliates.
Klapp, S.T. (1980). The memory drum theory after twenty years: Comments on Henry's note. Journal of Motor Behavior, 12, 169-171.
Klapp, S.T. (1981). Motor programming is not the only process which can influence RT: Some thoughts on the Marteniuk and MacKenzie Analysis. Journal of Motor Behavior, 13, 320-328.
Klapp, S.T., & Erwin, I. (1976). Relation between programming time and the duration of the response being programmed. Journal of Experimental Psychology, 100, 368-374.
Lagasse, P.P., & Hayes, K.C. (1973). Premotor and motor reaction time as a function of movement extent. Journal of Motor Behavior, 5, 25-32.
Marteniuk, R.G., & MacKenzie, C.L. (1981). Methods in the study of motor programming: Is it just a matter of simple vs. choice reaction time? A comment on Klapp et al. (1979). Journal of Motor Behavior, 13, 313-319.
Newell, K.M., Hoshizaki, L.E.F., Carlton, M.J., & Halbert, J.A. (1979). Movement time and velocity as determiners of movement timing accuracy. Journal of Motor Behavior, 11, 49-58.
Norrie, M.L. (1967). Practice effects on reaction latency for simple and complex movements. Research Quarterly, 38, 79-85.
Norrie, M.L. (1974). Effects of movement complexity on choice reaction and movement times. Research Quarterly, 65, 154-161.
Pew, R.W. (1984). A distributed processing view of human control. In W. Prinz & A.F. Sanders (Eds.), Cognition and motor processes. Berlin: Springer.
Quinn, J.T., Schmidt, R.A., Zelaznik, H.W., Hawkins, R., & McFarquhar, R. (1980). Target-size influences on reaction time with movement time controlled. Journal of Motor Behavior, 12, 239-261.
Schmidt, R.A., Zelaznik, H., Hawkins, B., Frank, J.S., & Quinn, J.T. (1979). Motor output variability: A theory for the accuracy of rapid motor acts. Psychological Review, 86, 415-451.
Sidaway, B. (1986). Reaction time of discrete tapping responses. Unpublished raw data.
Sternberg, S., Monsell, S., Knoll, R.L., & Wright, C.E. (1978). The

latency and duration of rapid movement sequences. Comparisons of speech and typewriting. In G.E. Stelmach (Ed.), Information processing in motor control and learning. New York: Academic Press.

Welford, A.T. (1968). Fundamentals of skill. London: Methuen.

Wright, C.E., & Meyer, D.E. (1983). Conditions for a linear speed-accuracy trade-off in aimed movements. Quarterly Journal of Experimental Psychology, 35A, 279-296.

Cognition and Action in Skilled Behaviour
A.M. Colley and J.R. Beech (Editors)

THE ACQUISITION OF BIMANUAL COORDINATION IN AN INTERACTIVE GRAPHICS TASK

David M. Frohlich
University of Surrey

The problems of multi-limb coordination and environmental control are identified as important to any theory of skilled action. It is argued that these problems are well recognised yet unrelated in the research literature and would benefit from integration. Data are presented on the acquisition of bimanual coordination showing how both problems are solved together in a manipulative task. Subjects were required to steer a screen-displayed cursor along a variety of tilted tracks using two control knobs. Analysis of the knob and cursor movements used by subjects on the task shows that with practice, movement tends to become faster, more coordinated, continuous, accurate and economical; although the exact combination of these improvements depends upon individual differences in movement strategy. The implications of these findings for theories of coordination and control are discussed.

Purpose of the paper

Coordination and control are central concepts for any theory of skilled movement organisation to explain. In fact skill can be defined in terms of these concepts; as the optimal control of coordinations to achieve some goal (Kelso, 1982, pp.28-29).

In this paper I present data relevant to the acquisition of coordination and control in human action. The data come from a study of bimanual coordination in an interactive graphics task in which subjects learned to control the movement of a screen-displayed cursor using two control knobs. I argue that the data have a bearing on two problems which appear unrelated in current theory and research; the problem of multi-limb coordination and what might be called the problem of environmental control. The purpose of the paper in presenting these data is to juxtapose both problems by showing how they are solved together in a single task. Towards the end of the paper I present a preliminary account of the findings in terms of the learning and application of effector function knowledge (Frohlich, 1985; Frohlich & Elliott, 1984), and suggest that accounts of this kind will become increasingly necessary to explain the development of multi-limb coordination in manipulative tasks.

The paper begins by defining the problems of multi-limb coordination and environmental control, and outlining some theoretical ideas advanced to explain how each problem might be solved in the organisation of purposeful movements.

The problem of multi-limb coordination

It was the Soviet physiologist Bernstein (1967) who first drew attention to the fact that the possibilities for movement are very much greater than the actual movements arising in human skilled performance, especially in gross motor skills involving many parts of the body. This appears to present a "degrees of freedom" problem to the human motor system to the effect that with so many possibilities for movement available, how do movements ever become coordinated to achieve the goals of particular tasks? The sheer scale of the problem is challenging for those theories of skill are based on the central control of movements. Literally hundreds of separate instructions to individual muscles would be required, simultaneously and continuously, to produce the kind of coordination observed in even the simplest of gross motor acts.

Bernstein's answer to this problem was to turn the prevailing "executive control" approach on its head and suggest that coordination is the result of constraints on possible movements. In this view, coordinated movement could be seen as the result of controlling what movements were "left over" after most possibilities had been ruled out. Coordination was thereby conceived as an exercise in reducing the number of degrees of freedom for movement to within manageable proportions, and the notion of the coordinative structure was advanced to refer to such manageable collections of muscles as are constrained to act together in a single unit.

Subsequent research has been conducted which supports this view. For example, Easton (1972) has reviewed evidence for a hierarchy of reflexes which can be seen as "basic coordinative structures" underlying normal voluntary movement in man. Furthermore, a mechanism for controlling the operation and combination of reflexes has been found in the pre-tuning of segmental interneurons in the spinal cord (e.g. Gurfinkel, Kots, Krinskiy, Pal'tsev, Feldman, Tsetlin, & Shik, 1971; see Turvey 1977 for a review). Various self-correcting and oscillatory properties of human limb movements have been proposed as examples of coordinative structures in operation (e.g. Kelso, 1977; Kelso, Holt, Kugler, & Turvey, 1980; Kelso, Southard, & Goodman, 1979), and a growing body of theory is now concerned to explain how coordination can result from the modulation and control of constraints on action (e.g. Greene, 1972, 1982; Turvey, 1977; Kugler, Kelso, & Turvey, 1980, 1982; Turvey, Shaw, & Mace, 1978).

A key consideration for this theory is to account for the development of task-dependent coordinations. Evidence of natural task-dependent constraints on interlimb coordination is not enough, in itself, to promote the concept of the coordinative structure as central to an explanation of human skilled action. For the concept to have this kind of generality it must be shown that new and appropriate kinds of coordinative structures can arise in the context of performing particular tasks under particular environmental conditions.

This fact has been clearly appreciated for some time now. Fowler and Turvey, writing in 1978, spoke of the actor "making of himself a 'special-purpose device' designed optimally for the task at hand" (p.23), while Kelso, Southard and Goodman in 1979 state that coordinative structures are "not necessarily prefabricated, as Easton (1972) has argued in the case of reflexes. Rather, they are functional and can be marshalled temporarily and expressly for the purpose of accomplishing a particular behavioural goal" (p.236). Research into this issue has focussed primarily on the role of visual perception in the organisation of action, following Turvey's (1977) thesis that vision serves to tune coordinative structures to environmental demands. This, in turn, has led to a renewed interest in the work of Gibson, Lee and others on ecological optics (e.g. Gibson, 1958, 1966, 1979; Lee, 1977, 1980a, 1980b; Lee, Lishman, & Thomson, 1982; Lee & Reddish, 1981), and to the development of an ecological approach to skilled action (see Turvey, this volume).

Although this work is important in showing how organisms might use various invariant properties of the optic array to control their behaviour, it gives few clues as to the way in which behaviour, particularly human behaviour, is structured initially and becomes re-structured over time. The focus on the tuning of pre-existing or pre-selected coordinative structures begs the question of how people learn to assemble or recall appropriate coordinations with practice. In fact the whole business of learning is somewhat neglected within the ecological framework (see Martenuik, this volume). This is unfortunate since data on the learning of multi-limb coordination might provide important insights into the way in which different kinds of coordinations arise in different performance contexts, where each is adapted to the skilful attainment of task goals.

The problem of environmental control

About the same time as the publication of Bernstein's work on "The Coordination and Regulation of Movements" another book was being prepared on the topic of "Manual and Automatic Control" (Kelley, 1968). Kelley's book had to do with how it is possible for people to regulate changes in the state of environmental control systems with which they interact. Although Kelley's primary concern was to determine better ways of designing control systems, the problem he discusses is an important one for understanding human skilled performance; how do people organise manipulative movements to effect changes in the state of the environment? I have chosen to call this the problem of environmental control since it can be contrasted with problems of motor control directed towards effecting changes in the state of the performer's own limb system.

Kelley suggests that two things are required to organise manipulative movements. The first is a knowledge by the performer of the correspondence between movement and its effect on the world. The second is an ability to use this knowledge predictively so as to generate only those movements which will have the desired effect. This observation has been illustrated beautifully by Pew (1974) in relation to a problem faced by engineers early in the NASA space program.

They had to generate a very loud tone in order to measure the effect of high intensity noise on rocket booster materials. The problem was not easy as Pew recalls:

> Everyone knew that if they started with a sine wave signal, any sound transmission or loudspeaker system would severely distort it, and the actual sound produced would hardly be a high-fidelity pure tone. The solution was obtained by working backwards. The engineers asked, in effect, what kind of wave shape must we put in such that the distortions introduced by the system will leave us with a pure sine wave at the output?

Pew argued that the human motor system makes a similar calculation when manipulating objects, because the "transmission" properties of the objects themselves will affect the outcome of any body movements applied to them. A performer may ask, in effect, what kind of movements must I execute such that when they are applied to the object they leave the object in the desired state? In order to answer this question the performer needs to know about the interaction between limb movement and the movement of objects in the world; information which effectively describes the control dynamics of environmental objects or systems.

Empirical support for the operation of a mechanism of this kind is provided somewhat indirectly by certain tests of Schmidt's (1975) motor schema theory. The theory itself can be interpreted as an account of the learning and application of knowledge about control system dynamics, since it proposes that performers learn a variety of response-outcome relationships during the execution of patterned movements (Frohlich & Elliott, 1984). However, the evidence is equivocal because some tests of the theory are invalid and the theory proposes only a limited kind of response-outcome learning related to the parameterisation of generalised motor programs (see Chapter 2 in Frohlich, 1985, for a detailed discussion). More direct evidence for the learning of control system dynamics comes from two tests of a revision of Schmidt's theory (Frohlich & Elliott, 1984). We suggested that the kind of response-outcome learning referred to in motor schema theory might be specific to the system being controlled rather than to some generalised pattern of movement applied to it. In an initial experiment we were able to show that such learning occurred under conditions of movement pattern variability and could itself account for the organisation of patterned movements on the experimental equipment. A subsequent experiment showed this skill to be specific to the dynamics of this equipment, since practiced subjects were not able to perform the same task any better than naive subjects when the control dynamics were changed. These findings imply that people can indeed learn something about the dynamics of environmental control systems with which they interact, and use this knowledge to organise skilful manipulations of those systems. We coined the term effector function to refer to the performer's acquired representation of a system's control dynamics. Similar concepts have been advanced in the areas of process control (e.g. Bainbridge, 1981; Jagacinski & Miller, 1978; Veldhuyzen & Stassen, 1976), human-computer interaction (e.g. Owen, 1986; Young, 1981), cognitive psychology (e.g. Gentner & Stevens, 1983; Johnson-Laird, 1983) and artificial intelligence (e.g. Hayes, 1978, 1985).

Despite this demonstration of effector function learning and some convergence of opinion on its general importance in environmental interactions, relatively little is known about how exactly it works in practice. Such ignorance applies particularly to the nature of the dynamic information represented in the effector function for any system, and to the way in which this information is abstracted through practice and applied in performance. These issues cannot be addressed without collecting further data on the development of environmental control over specific objects or systems. Experiments on the transfer of learning across tasks and control systems are needed to investigate the content of effector function representations, while studies of the re-organisation of manipulative movements over time are required to illuminate effector function learning and application.

The acquisition of multi-limb coordination in manipulative tasks

To summarise, I have described two problems for any theory of skill which are well recognised yet unrelated in the research literature. Some promising ideas have been proposed to explain how each problem might be solved in organising movements, although, to date, the ideas relating to multi-limb coordination make no reference to those relating to environmental control and vice versa.

This state of affairs is clearly unsatisfactory since both problems are solved together in the majority of human performance skills. Environmental control is required in any action whose goal involves changing the state of the environment in some way. Such actions include displacing objects relative to each other as in throwing, or to oneself, as in feeding; altering the structure of objects as in constructive and destructive acts of all kinds; and using objects as tools in any of the above activities and others besides. Multi-limb coordination is required wherever more than one body part is used in the performance of these actions. Thus theories of multi-limb coordination and environmental control must eventually address a common concern: the acquisition of multi-limb coordination in manipulative tasks.

This concern is investigated in the present study by examining the organisation of bimanual manipulative movements in an interactive graphics task. The task and control system is the same as that used by Frohlich and Elliott (1984) to demonstrate effector function learning. The study aims to discover what movement strategies are used by subjects under these conditions and how these strategies change with learning. The data are relevant to an understanding of the learning and application of effector function knowledge, to the origin of task-dependent coordinations, and to the relationship between the two.

Methods

Apparatus and control system

The equipment comprised a Data General Nova 840 mini-computer, a Hewlett Packard 1310A CRT and a Megatek BP271 refreshed graphics interface. These were used to administer an interactive graphics task in which subjects were required to steer a cursor around the CRT using two control knobs. Details of the task conditions are given below. The cursor moved in direct proportion to the position of each control knob as shown in Figure 1. Rotation of the right-hand knob away from its midposition moved the cursor up to the right or down to the left on a 45° axis drawn through the centre of the screen. Conversely, rotation of the left-hand knob moved the cursor up to the left or down to the right, i.e. orthogonally. Any combination of knob turns moved the cursor directly to the sum of the two vectors given by each knob.

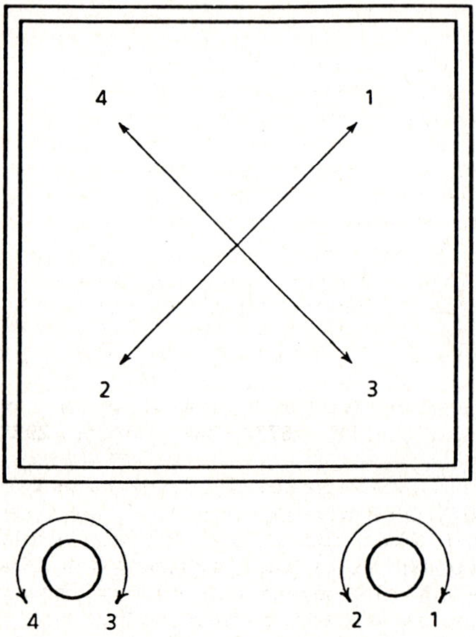

Figure 1. The effect of each control knob on the cursor (centre) in the experimental control system.

The task

The system described above is useful for investigating the acquisition of multi-limb coordination because subjects must usually combine the rotation of both the left and right control knobs to steer the cursor in any desired direction. Subjects cannot do this very skilfully at first because the control dynamics governing the relationship between knob and cursor movement are arbitrary and unknown to them. The task given to subjects was to steer the cursor along several 15mm wide tracks displayed within a circle 230mm in diameter. The cursor was made to slide alongside of each track if its next position was calculated to lie outside it. Tracks were tilted at 22°, 67°, 112° and 157° from vertical. These angles were chosen to encourage a range of asymmetric coordinations involving all possible combinations of left and right, clockwise and anti-clockwise knob rotations.

Subjects and measures of performance

Four naive subjects and the author performed the task. Their initials, sex and age were as follows: NA, female, 24 years; PA, male, 26 years; GR, female, 23 years; KQ, male, 22 years; DF, male, 24 years.

Task performance was recorded by storing the position of each control knob and the x,y coordinates of the virtual cursor position every 20 milliseconds throughout each trial.

Procedure

All subjects were informed that the study was an investigation of movement coordination in which they would be required to steer a small dot along a tilted track with two control knobs, as quickly and accurately as possible. The equal importance of minimising both time and error on the task was indicated by telling subjects that both would be measured. Subjects were warned that the computer itself might interrupt a trial if it calculated that the subject had had enough practice on the current direction and track. Otherwise they were to continue steering the cursor until it left the far end of the current track.

Within each session, tracks tilted at 22°, 67°, 112° and 157° were displayed to all subjects in that order. Each subject was required to perform on each track in a left-to-right and right-to-left direction before proceeding to the next track. This meant that each subject was required to approximate the following vectors of cursor displacement respectively: 22°, 202°, 67°, 247°, 112°, 292°, 157° and 337°.

During each trial subjects attempted to steer the cursor from one end of the track to the other without allowing it to touch the track sides. A trial ended either when the cursor left the track at its target end or when the calculated on-track distance travelled by the cursor equalled or exceeded 1300 pixels (about $1\frac{1}{2}$ times its length). In either case the display would be reset to the next direction or track in the presentation sequence. Each subject performed about 16 trials in all (exactly 10400 pixels of forwards on-track cursor movement).

Results

Data analysis

The knob and cursor position data was used to produce a graphical trace of knob and cursor movement for each subject over the duration of each trial. Limb movement organisation on the task was illustrated by a graph of left and right control knob position over time, while its outcome on the system was illustrated by a graph of cursor position per se.

The results now to be described are based on an analysis of six different movement parameters calculated for each subject's first and last (complete) trial. Examination of the change in parameters across these trials, both within and between subjects, gives some indication of the trends in movement reorganisation exhibited by subjects, and

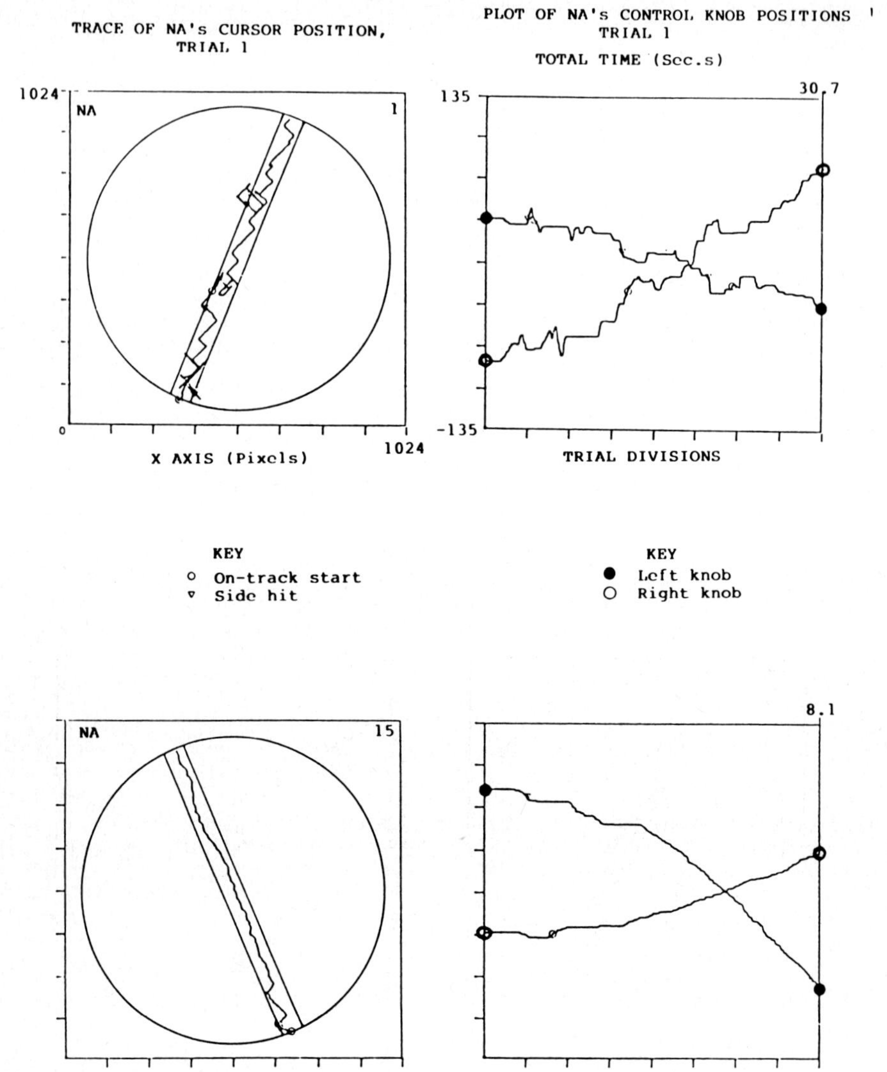

Figure 2. Knob and cursor movement profiles for subject NA on her first and last (complete) trial.

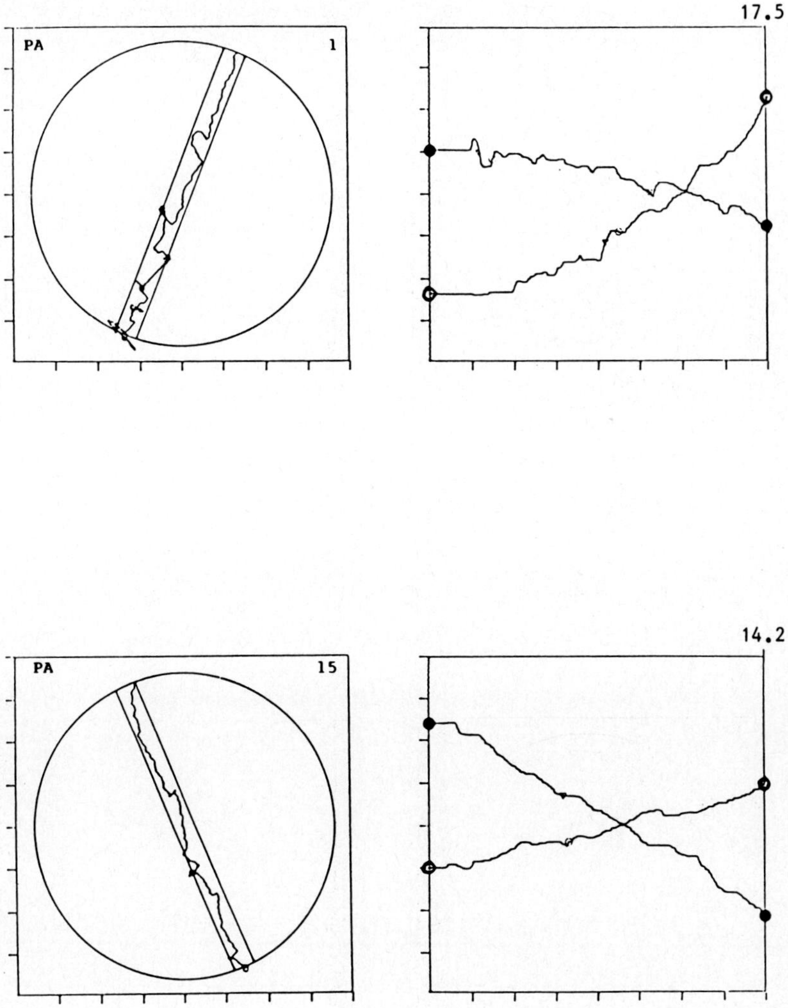

<u>Figure 3.</u> Knob and cursor movement profiles for subject PA on his first and last (complete) trial.

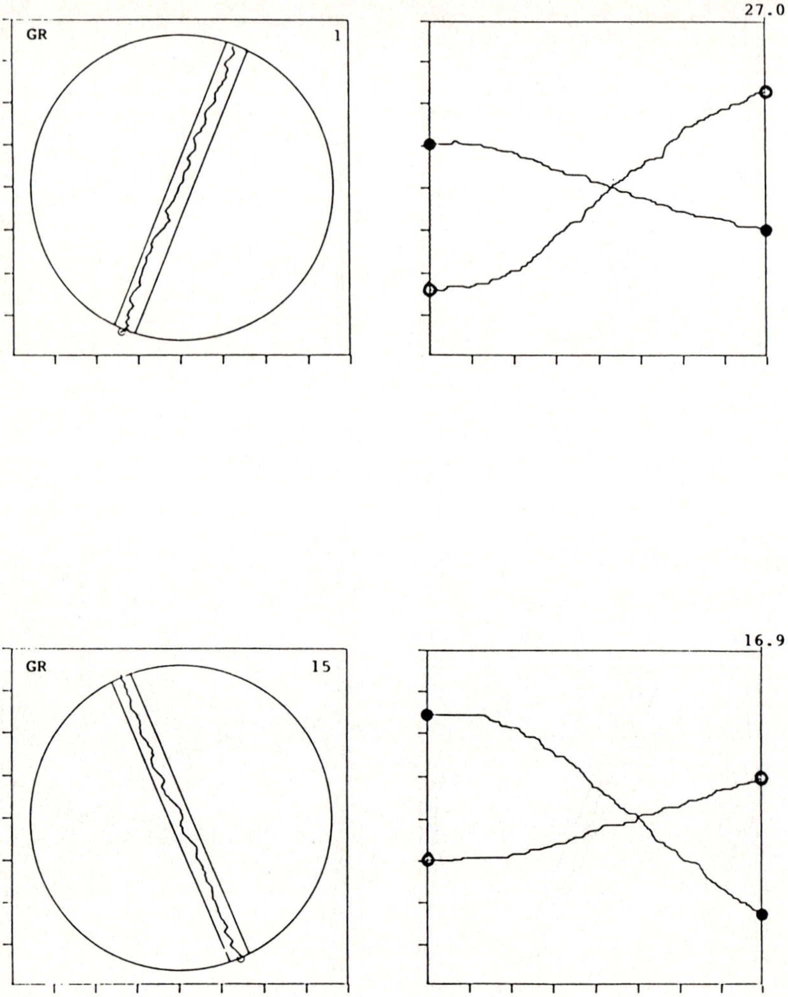

Figure 4. Knob and cursor movement profiles for subject GR on her first and last (complete) trial.

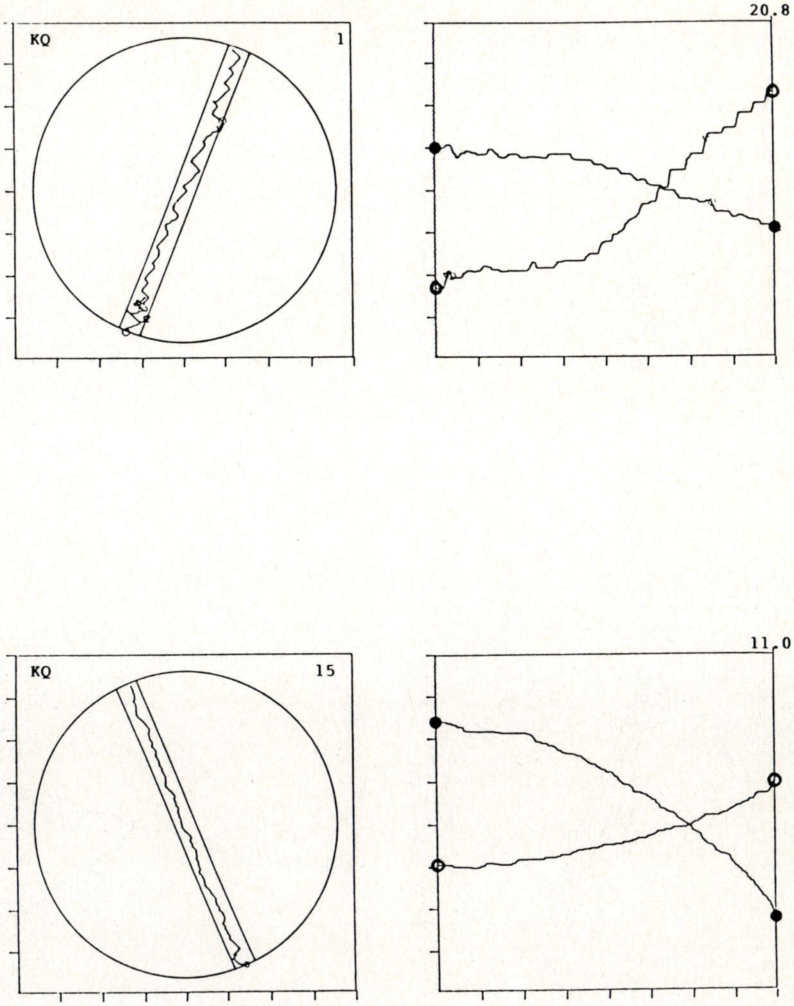

Figure 5. Knob and cursor movement profiles for subject KQ on his first and last (complete) trial.

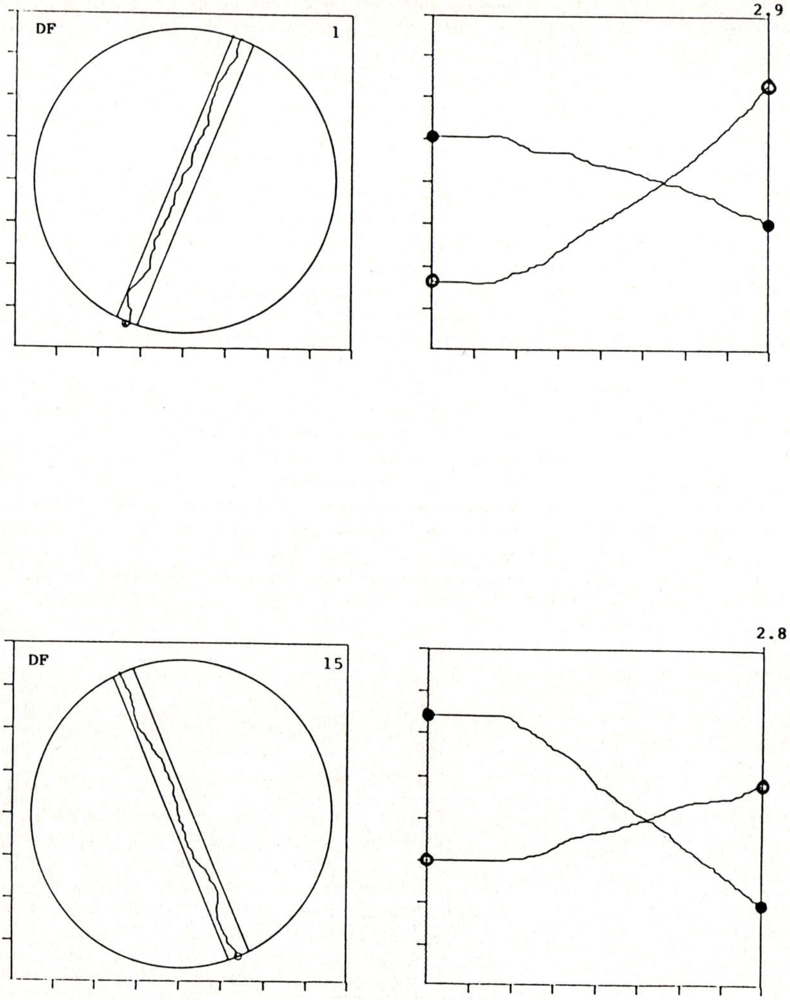

Figure 6. Knob and cursor movement profiles for subject DF on his first and last (complete) trial.

of the differences in individual movement strategies employed. The interpretation of this quantitative analysis is informed by an unreported qualitative analysis of about 160 graphs.

Movement reorganisation with learning

Changes in movement organisation with learning are apparent across the performance of all trials by naive subjects. These changes are illustrated most dramatically in Figures 2, 3, 4 and 5 which contrast these subjects' first and last (complete) trial performance. Furthermore, the performance of all trials by subject DF represents a highly advanced form of movement organisation based on extensive task practice. The relative stability of DF's performance can be seen from Figure 6 which also contrasts his first and last (complete) trial performance. The nature of the changes in movement organisation with learning can be simply determined by quantifying a number of salient movement parameters for the trials shown in Figures 2 to 6. The results and implications of these various calculations are now described.

Bimanual coordination

Although the nature of the task was such as to encourage the bimanual coordination of control knobs, the graphs of subjects NA and KQ at least, suggest that this was something which developed over time. Sequential alternation of left and right control knobs can be seen most clearly in the first trial graphs of these subjects, but is also evident in most other graphs to a lesser extent.

Table 1 shows the exact proportions of bimanual movement produced by each subject on trials 1 and 15. This was calculated by measuring the amount of time spent moving both knobs simultaneously during a trial, and expressing the result as a percentage of the total time (excluding initial reaction time). A pause in the movement of either knob greater than 250 milliseconds was taken to indicate non-simultaneous movement.

Table 1

Percentage time spent in bimanual movement excluding reaction time, for each subject on trials 1 and 15.

SUBJECT	TRIAL 1	TRIAL 15
NA	10	61
PA	44	48
GR	40	41
KQ	8	57
DF	76	100

The greatest improvement in control knob coordination was exhibited by subjects NA and KQ, whose first trial performances were based almost exclusively on alternating unimanual movements. Subjects PA and GR began performing by rotating both control knobs together for just less than half the time, but improved very little over 15 trials. The extremely high degree of bimanual coordination in the performance of subject DF suggests that this aspect of movement organisation tends to become literally perfected with extensive practice.

Movement continuity

In addition to improvement in the overlapping of right and left control knob rotation in time, rotation of each knob itself appears to become smoother or more continuous with learning. This is indicated in Table 2 by a decline in the number of pauses greater than about 250 milliseconds, in each subject's left and right control knob rotation on trials 1 and 15.

Table 2

Number of pauses greater than 250 msec in individual knob rotation, for each subject on trials 1 and 15.

SUBJECT	TRIAL 1		TRIAL 15	
	Left	Right	Left	Right
NA	23	19	3	4
PA	12	16	8	15
GR	20	19	9	14
KQ	25	23	6	12
DF	1	0	0	0

The improvements in movement continuity across subjects were broadly similar to those in bimanual coordination shown in Table 1. Thus subjects NA and KQ improved most while subject DF exhibited almost completely continuous movement throughout. However the movements of subject GR also became substantially smoother with practice, despite a negligible improvement in bimanual coordination. This suggests that the organisation of individual limb movements can change in ways which do not necessarily affect their integration over time.

Finally, it appears that irrespective of the trend towards less pauses with practice, subjects usually paused most when rotating the left knob in trial 1, whereas they paused least when rotating this knob on trial 15. This may be related to the absolute distance moved by the left and right hands on these trials. To move the cursor along the 22° track on trial 1, required subjects to rotate the right knob further than the left. To move the cursor along the 157° track on trial 15, required subjects to rotate the left knob further than the right. The fact that most subjects exhibit smoother movement of the knob rotated furthest on the trial, suggests a distinct performance strategy. Subjects use the "lagging" hand on each trial to apply discrete corrections to continuous movement of the "leading" hand. This strategy appears to be more typical of trial 15 performance by subjects GR and KQ.

Errors in cursor movement

A simple count of the number of times the cursor hit the track sides is shown in Table 3, for each subject on trials 1 and 15. This indicates that the gross accuracy of performance improves with practice wherever possible.

Table 3

Number of track side hits by each subject on trials 1 and 15

SUBJECT	TRIAL 1	TRIAL 15
NA	3	1
PA	3	1
GR	0	0
KQ	2	0
DF	0	0

What is not clear from this table is how easily errors are corrected once they occur. Although the graphs in Figures 2, 3 and 5 suggest that the errors shown are quickly and easily corrected, this may be because these errors are of shallow penetration. That is, the virtual position of the cursor in these instances is only a short perpendicular distance from the track side. Where penetration is deeper, subjects have much more trouble retrieving the cursor from the track side. Such errors result in more serious degradation of visual feedback of cursor position, and are particularly disturbing to subjects early in practice. This may be because the organisation of initial task performance is more reliant on the correction of visible error in cursor position.

Reversals of direction in knob rotation

Further insight into the improvement of performance accuracy with practice, is revealed by examining the frequency with which the direction of knob rotation is reversed. The frequency of right and left knob reversal for each subject on trials 1 and 15 is shown in Table 4.

Table 4

Number of reversals in the direction of knob rotation by each subject on trials 1 and 15.

SUBJECT	TRIAL 1		TRIAL 15	
	Left	Right	Left	Right
NA	10	6	0	1
PA	9	7	0	5
GR	1	0	0	0
KQ	6	4	0	3
DF	0	0	0	0

Subjects NA, PA and KQ exhibit a relatively large number of reversals on trial 1 which are considerably reduced by trial 15. It is interesting to note that the remaining reversals occurring on trial 15 apply to right knob rotation. This is in keeping with the error correction strategy suggested above, confirming that movement is less continuous in the lagging hand.

Examination of the distribution of knob reversals within trials reveals that they are most likely to occur either at the beginning of a trial or at a collision of the cursor with the track sides. Their function appears to be to introduce a change in knob manipulation when its current effect is unsatisfactory. Occasionally knob reversals occur for no apparent reason when the cursor is well clear of the track sides, but more often they produce a "knotted" cursor trace close to the track side itself.

Movement redundancy

Inspection of cursor movement across trials shows that the line taken by the cursor towards the target track end becomes less tortuous with practice. This trend can be quantified by measuring the actual distance travelled by the cursor and expressing it as a proportion of the track length. This measure was calculated as shown in Table 5 for each subject on trials 1 and 15. These figures represent movement redundancy in performance.

Table 5

Proportion of actual to ideal cursor movement (%) for each subject on trials 1 and 15.

SUBJECT	TRIAL 1	TRIAL 15
NA	231	110
PA	214	121
GR	121	106
KQ	168	110
DF	108	105

The tsable shows how movement redundancy decreases for all subjects by trial 15. In general, movement organisation becomes more economical with practice. However, there are large individual differences in the amount of movement redundancy exhibited by subjects on their first trial. These may reflect differences in the relative importance subjects attach to speed and accuracy in performance. By trial 15, the variation in redundancy scores is substantially reduced as an optimum score of about 105% is approached. This suggests that all subjects have compensated for their initial inaccuracy over this number of trials.

Total time taken

The overall speed of performance is indicated by the total time taken by each subject to complete an uninterrupted trial. The changes in the total time taken by each subject to perform trials 1 and 15 can be seen in Table 6.

As with movement redundancy, there are large individual differences in the total time taken by naive subjects to complete trial 1 which have largely disappeared by trial 15. Thus all subjects increased their speed of performance with practice, but with widely different savings in movement time. The relative size of these and other improvements in performance made by individual subjects will now be considered.

Table 6

Total time (secs) taken by each subject to perform trials 1 and 15.

SUBJECT	TRIAL 1	TRIAL 15
NA	30.7	8.1
PA	17.5	14.2
GR	27.0	16.9
KQ	20.8	11.0
DF	2.9	2.8

Individual differences in movement strategy

A number of individual differences in the organisation of movements over time have already been mentioned. Such observations are drawn together in this section, for each subject respectively. The observations are made from the combination of each subject's movement parameter scores recorded across Tables 1 to 6.

Subject NA
Of all subjects, NA exhibited the greatest improvement in performance. Her initial strategy was to steer the cursor along the 22° track in diagonal steps resulting from the alternation of left and right control knob rotation. This approach was relatively effective in allowing her to move the cursor towards the appropriate track end, while keeping it off the track sides. For example, early error correction by NA consisted in simply reversing the direction of the knob currently being rotated, before moving the other knob. However, its disadvantage was that it limited the speed with which a trial could be correctly completed.

Although evidence of bimanual coordination was apparent in trial 7, it was not until trial 10 that NA abandoned control knob alternation as her major strategy. Only then was it possible for her to attain fast performance times on trials free of error.

Subject PA
The approach of subject PA to the task was quite different. From the outset, he exhibited considerable bimanual coordination and a respectable performance time. This was at the expense of movement accuracy and economy. The rest of his performance appeared to involve an effort to improve these latter movement parameters.

PA's cursor traces were typified by short bursts of well-coordinated and economical movement separated by "knots" localized on or near a track side. These knots appear to represent choice points in how to rectify unacceptable cursor drift. Each involved at least one knob reversal as can be seen in Figure 3. Improvement in PA's performance simply resulted from an increase in the length of uninterrupted periods of cursor manipulation on any given track.

Subject GR
The organisation of movements by subject GR was remarkably consistent throughout practice. Only movement time and movement continuity

improved considerably over time. It seems that subject GR initially achieved the high degree of movement accuracy shown, by slowly edging round one control knob at a time in a direction found to be appropriate to the current track. In this connection, it is notable that the only knob reversal on GR's first trial occurred at its very beginning. This was a small clockwise rotation of the left knob, which appeared to establish that its anti-clockwise rotation was required for the rest of the trial. Thereafter, both control knobs were rotated in the appropriate direction, either bimanually at about the same rates or unimanually to correct cursor drift. This caused the cursor to move in roughly vertical and diagonal steps towards the target track end on the trials shown in Figure 4. Thus GR employed a strategy of unimanual correction of equivalent bimanual coordination. This appeared, from careful inspection of all her performance graphs, to persist throughout practice. Its speed of execution simply increased over trials.

Subject KQ

This subject exhibited similar performance to that of subject NA; achieving large improvements in most of the movement parameters shown in Tables 1 to 6. Like subject NA, KQ began with a strategy of control knob alternation which eventually gave way to more continuous bimanual coordination. Only the scale of the strategy was different; with KQ employing smaller alternate movements, and therefore pausing more often. These were replaced rather suddenly on trial 5 by simultaneous movements which became progressively faster with practice.

Subject DF

The performance of subject DF is likely to represent an optimum strategy of movement organisation on the task. This is because it is based upon about two years' practice of cursor manipulation on the system, experienced at frequent intervals within that period. A striking feature of DF's cursor traces is their oscillation about the axis of the track. This indicates that both control knobs are not rotated at a constant ratio. Inspection of the graphs of knob movement shows that only one knob is rotated at a relatively constant speed, while the other applies a continuous but oscillating influence to the cursor. The control knob rotated at a constant speed is always the leading knob for the current track. This is effectively a continuous version of the strategy first observed in the section on movement continuity, in which discrete error corrections are applied by one hand to continuous movement of the other. In DF's case, cursor drift is corrected not by discrete movements of the lagging hand, but by increasing or decreasing the speed of its continuous rotation. This strategy appears to be a particularly elegant way of accommodating variability in the accuracy of cursor manipulation, resulting from the continuous rotation of control knobs at high speed.

Discussion

It was argued in the introduction that the above data are relevant to an understanding of both multi-limb coordination and environmental control. In this section, I explore the implications of the findings for each issue in turn. To begin, let us consider what the findings tell us about the origin of bimanual coordination on the task and how this fits with current ideas about coordinative structures.

Coordination of hand movements was encouraged by the demands of the experimental task. To get the cursor to travel quickly and efficiently along any of the displayed tracks, subjects really had to rotate the control knobs together in the right directions and at different speeds. Although this kind of coordination could be seen in the performance of subject DF, it was absent from the initial performance of each naive subject. Early task performance by these subjects was typified by alternating movements of the left and right control knobs, or by periods of intermittent bimanual and unimanual knob rotation. Movement became coordinated gradually, as subjects increased the proportion of bimanual to unimanual movements and began to control the relative rates of left and right knob rotations. The continuity or smoothness of these movements improved in a similar way; with subjects initially performing faltering and discrete rotations of each knob, before stringing together longer sequences of rotations in shorter amounts of time. In short, smooth coordinated movement arose out of a period of practice in which movements became progressively smoother and more coordinated. What is interesting about this is that it happened in different ways for different subjects, depending on their choice of initial movement strategy and their modification of this strategy over time.

Two aspects of these findings can be related rather well to the learning of a coordinative structure. In the first place, the early performance strategies exhibited by subjects can be seen as ways of constraining the number of degrees of freedom for movement on the task (Turvey, Fitch, & Tuller, 1982). For example, by rotating the left and right knobs alternatively, subjects need only decide at any moment on the direction of rotation for a single control knob; by rotating both knobs at about the same rate, subjects manage to avoid decisions about the relative speed of rotation of each knob; and by correcting continuous rotations of the leading knob with movements of the lagging hand, subjects have only to decide on the direction and speed of leading hand movement, once, at the beginning of each trial. In the second place, transitions to more sophisticated strategies can be seen as the result of increasing sensitivity or "attunement" to higher order variables of stimulation (Fitch, Tuller, & Turvey, 1982). Subjects seem to begin the task by attempting to control the cursor's position on the track by altering individual control knob positions. Over time, as cursor position changes, subjects may execute control knob rotations to control cursor movement. With further learning, combinations of rotations may be used to control the direction of cursor movement, and various ratios of control knob rotations may be introduced to control cursor drift (or change in the direction of cursor movement).

In other respects, the findings are difficult to explain in these terms. Individual differences in performance strategy are impossible to explain normatively, with recourse to the perception of some "organisational invariance" specific to the task at hand. Strategies themselves are difficult to equate with the traditional concept of a coordinative structure. Although they constrain the movement of a collection of muscles to act in a particular way, the style of performance arising from such constraints is only loosely related to success on the task. What is crucial for skilful performance here is the ability to make correct decisions about control movement activity, direction and speed, whatever strategy is employed. Coordinative strategies may simply be the result of an inability to make reliable decisions about such parameters. Coordinative structures are not usually considered in this way.

Strategic performance is best understood in terms of the learning of effector function knowledge. If people do indeed learn about the dynamic properties of objects by manipulating them, we might expect any collection of subjects faced with the experimental task to attribute varying kinds and amounts of such knowledge to the experimental equipment. This could account for initial differences in performance strategy. Given such differences, we might further expect subjects to learn different things about the cursor control system since their practice experience is in fact unique in each case. This could account for the perseverance of individual differences in control movement organisation despite general improvements in skill.

The fact that subjects might learn different things about the same control system is an interesting implication of the findings for understanding effector function learning. It suggests that performers may acquire quite different representations of control system properties, depending on the transfer of existing knowledge and its continuous effect on the quality of practice experience. Such differences may be akin to differences in the perception of the same visual scene by two observers. Although the objects in the scene are the same for both observers, their appearance differs according to the perspective of each observer to the scene. Additional differences in perception are introduced by what the observers make of what they see, i.e. by what interpretation they give to it. In short, the current findings can be taken to imply that in the action domain also, differences in perspective and interpretation operate to affect the representation and manipulation of control systems.

At a rather abstract level then, it is possible to explain strategic differences in performance in terms of the learning of individual views of the same cursor control system. Whether or not this explanation can be extended to account for the particular strategies observed in subject performance remains an open question. The beginnings of an answer to this question can be seen in the operation of a computer simulation of task performance called CONTROLLER which Paul Luff and I have constructed recently[1]. The simulation is based on the learning and application of production rules relating control knob rotation to cursor displacement and can account for a good deal of subject performance. It is worth mentioning briefly here because it shows how knowledge of control system dynamics can be acquired and used to organise increasingly effective coordinations of the two hands.

CONTROLLER works in cycles by firing condition-action rules. The conditions of each rule specify a range of possible cursor movements and are represented by angular sectors. For example, one rule has a condition for cursor movements "to the right", characterised by a sector ranging from 0° to 180°. The actions of each rule are discrete control knob rotations, represented by labelled knob displacements of variable direction and extent. The rule mentioned above has an action for "clockwise rotation of the right knob by 10 units", given by the expression: left (0), right (+10). Since each rule describes a mapping between cursor displacement and knob rotation, it can be seen as a piece of knowledge about control system dynamics. In the example given, the rule effectively says "to move the cursor to the right, move the right knob clockwise". The total set of rules available to CONTROLLER corresponds to its effector function for the experimental equipment.

The firing of rules depends upon the current position of the cursor in relation to the target track end. This is given by a "cursor-goal sector" usually drawn between the cursor and each target end of the displayed track. By matching the current cursor-goal sector with the cursor movement conditions of each available rule CONTROLLER determines which rules are relevant to the current situation. If more than one rule is satisfied, CONTROLLER fires the rule which comes first in a specified order, and the resulting action changes the cursor-goal sector for the next cycle. In this way, control knob movements are generated directly from the cursor-knob movement mappings represented in the available rules.

Finally, by storing a trace of fired rules and inspecting the trace for repeated patterns of movements, it is possible for CONTROLLER to learn new rules and add them to the available rules. This causes CONTROLLER to modify its performance on the basis of changes to the set of available rules; through a kind of effector function learning.

So far it has been possible to simulate most of the observed performance strategies using very few rules. Thus we have found CONTROLLER successfully negotiating a variety of displayed tracks by executing alternate unimanual knob rotations, by correcting equal bimanual rotations with unimanual ones and by producing unequal bimanual rotations without error. In all these cases, strategic performance emerged incidentally, as a result of the application of particular combinations of rules arranged in a particular order in the rule set. Improvements in performance occurred as CONTROLLER added new rules to those already available, changing both the combination and the order of rules in the set. The fact that new rules are always generated from local track experience, means that learning is highly dependent on task practice. However, the rules themselves are not task specific since they always relate to the dynamics of the controlled system. This arrangement is consistent with the findings of Frohlich and Elliott (1984), and shows how the variability of practice might affect the quality of an effector function rule set representing control system dynamics.

Conclusion

In conclusion, the observed acquisition of bimanual coordination is difficult to explain in terms of the development of coordinative structures for left and right knob rotation. A clear understanding of subject performance is only attained by considering the manipulative as well as the coordinative nature of the task. Improvements in manipulating the experimental equipment can be explained in terms of the learning of effector function information about its control dynamics.

What is challenging about this explanation for theories of multi-limb coordination is that coordination can itself be modelled by the application of effector function knowledge. It will be interesting to see how this challenge is taken up by those committed to an ecological approach to skill who have so far reserved comment on the role of cognition in action. I suggest that if they continue to do so in this case, they may find themselves forced to exclude from study, many self-paced manipulative skills at which humans seem particularly adept.

Notes

[1]Frohlich and Luff (1987). "The acquisition of bimanual coordination in an interactive graphics task: A computer simulation. Paper presented to the conference from which these proceedings are taken.

Acknowledgements

The data were collected during a doctoral programme of research sponsored by the British Science and Engineering Research Council and conducted at the Department of Psychology, University of Sheffield. Thanks are due to John Elliott for his support throughout this period; to Kevin Connolly and David Lee for their encouragement to publish these findings; and to the Department of Sociology, University of Surrey, for the opportunity to complete the work.

References

Bainbridge, L. (1981). Mathematical equations or processing routines? In J. Rasmussen & W.B. Rouse (Eds.), Human detection and diagnosis of system failure. New York: Plenum Press.

Bernstein, N. (1967). The coordination and regulation of movements. London: Pergamon Press.

Easton, T.A. (1972). On the normal use of reflexes. American Scientist, 60, 591-599.

Fitch, H.L., Tuller, B., & Turvey, M.T. (1982). The Bernstein perspective III. Tuning of coordinative structures with special reference to perception. In J.A.S. Kelso (Ed.), Human motor behavior: An introduction. Hillsdale, New Jersey: Erlbaum.

Fowler, C.A. & Turvey, M.T. (1978). Skill acquisition: An event approach with special reference to searching for the optimum of a function of several variables. In G. Stelmach (Ed.), Information processing in motor control and learning. New York: Academic Press.

Frohlich, D.M. (1985). The acquisition of environmental control in skilled movement organisation. Unpublished Ph.D. thesis, University of Sheffield.

Frohlich, D.M. & Elliott, J.M. (1984). The schematic representation of effector function underlying perceptual-motor skill. Journal of Motor Behavior, 16, 40-60.

Gentner, D. & Stevens, A.L. (Eds.), (1983). Mental models. Hillsdale, New Jersey: Erlbaum.

Gibson, J.J. (1958). Visually controlled locomotion and orientation in animals. British Journal of Psychology, 49, 182-194.

Gibson, J.J. (1966). The senses considered as perceptual systems. Boston: Houghton-Mifflin.

Gibson, J.J. (1979). The ecological approach to visual perception. Boston: Houghton-Mifflin.

Greene, P.H. (1972). Problems of organisation in motor systems. In R. Rosen & F.M. Snell (Eds.), Progress in theoretical biology. New York: Academic Press.

Greene, P.H. (1982). Why is it easy to control your arms? Journal of Motor Behavior, 14, 260-286.

Gurfinkel, V.S., Kots, Ya M., Krinskiy, V.I., Pal'tsev, Ye. I., Fel'dman, A.G., Tsetlin, M.L., & Shik, M.L. (1971). Concerning tuning before movement. In I.M. Gelfand, V.S. Gurfinkel, S.V. Fomin, & M.L. Tsetlin (Eds.), Models of the structural-functional organisation of certain biological systems. Cambridge, Massachusetts: MIT Press.

Hayes, P.J. (1978). The naive physics manifesto. In D. Michie (Ed.), Expert systems in the microelectronic age. Edinburgh: Edinburgh University Press.

Hayes, P.J. (1985). The second naive physics manifesto. In J.R. Hobbs & R.C. Moore (Eds.), Formal theories of the common sense world. New York: Ablex.

Jagacinski, R.J. & Miller, R.A. (1978). Describing the human operator's internal model of a dynamic system. Human Factors, 20, 425-433.

Johnson-Laird, P.N. (1983). Mental models. Cambridge University Press.

Kelley, C.R. (1968). Manual and automatic control. New York: Wiley.

Kelso, J.A.S. (1977). Coding processes and motor control: an integrated approach. In D.M. Landers & R.W. Christina (Eds.), Psychology of motor behavior and sport. Volume 1. Illinois: Human Kinetics.

Kelso, J.A.S. (1982). Concepts and issues in human motor behavior: coming to grips with the jargon. In J.A.S. Kelso (Ed.), Human motor behavior: An introduction. Hillsdale, New Jersey: Erlbaum.

Kelso, J.A.S., Holt, K.G., Kugler, P.N., & Turvey, M.T. (1980). Empirical lines of convergence. In G.E. Stelmach & J. Requin (Eds.), Tutorials in motor behaviour. Amsterdam: North Holland.

Kelso, J.A.S., Southard, D.L., & Goodman, D. (1979). On the coordination of two-handed movements. Journal of Experimental Psychology: Human perception and performance, 5, 229-238.

Kugler, P.N., Kelso, J.A.S., & Turvey, M.T. (1980). On the concept of coordinative structures as dissipative structures: I Theoretical lines of convergence. In G.E. Stelmach & J. Requin (Eds.), Tutorials in motor behaviour. Amsterdam: North Holland.

Kugler, P.N., Kelso, J.A.S., & Turvey, M.T. (1982). On the control and coordination of naturally developing systems. In J.A.S. Kelso & J.E. Clarke (Eds.), The development of movement control and coordination. New York: Wiley.

Lee, D.N. (1977). The functions of vision. In H. Pick & E.L. Saltzman (Eds.), Modes of perceiving and processing information. Hillsdale, New Jersey: Erlbaum.

Lee, D.N. (1980a). The optic flow field: The foundation of Vision. Philosophical Transactions of the Royal Society of London, Series B, 290, 169-179.

Lee, D.N. (1980b). Visuo-motor coordination in space-time. In G. E. Stelmach & J. Requin (Eds.), Tutorials in motor behaviour. Amsterdam: North Holland.

Lee, D.N., Lishman, J.R., & Thomson, J.A. (1982). Regulation of gait in long jumping. Journal of Experimental Psychology: Human perception and performance, 8, 448-459.

Lee, D.N. & Reddish, P. (1982). Plummeting gannets: A paradigm of ecological optics. Nature, 293, 293-294.

Owen, D. (1986). Naive theories of computation. In D.A. Norman & S. Draper (Eds.), User centered system design: New perspectives on human-computer interaction. Hillsdale, New Jersey: Erlbaum.

Pew, R.W. (1974). Human perceptual-motor performance. In B.H. Kantowitz (Ed.), Human information processing: Tutorials in performance and cognition. New York: Halstead Press.

Schmidt, R.A. (1975). A schema theory of discrete motor skill learning. Psychological Review, 82, 225-260.

Turvey, M.T. (1977). Preliminaries to a theory of action with reference to vision. In R.E. Shaw & J. Bransford (Ed.), Perceiving, acting and knowing: Toward an ecological psychology. Hillsdale, New Jersey: Erlbaum.

Turvey, M.T., Fitch, H.L., & Tuller, B. (1982). The Bernstein perspective 1. The problems of degrees of freedom and context-conditioned variability. In J.A.S. Kelso (Ed.), Human motor behavior: An introduction. Hillsdale, New jersey: Erlbaum.

Turvey, M.T., Shaw, R.E., & Mace, W. (1978). Issues in the theory of action: degrees of freedom, coordinative structures and coalitions. In J. Requin (Ed.), Attention and performance VII. Hillsdale, New Jersey: Erlbaum.

Veldhuyzen, W. & Stassen, H.G. (1976). The internal model. What does it mean in human control? In T.B. Sheridan & G. Johanssen (Eds.), Monitoring behavior and supervisory control. New York: Plenum Press.

Young, R.M. (1981). The machine inside the machine: User's models of pocket calculators. International Journal of Man-Machine Studies, 15, 87-134.

Cognition and Action in Skilled Behaviour
A.M. Colley and J.R. Beech (Editors)

CONSTRAINTS IN COORDINATING LIMB MOVEMENTS

S.P. Swinnen and C.B. Walter
Catholic University of Leuven, and
University of Illinois at Chicago.

When coordinating movements of the limbs or fingers, constraints emerge that impose limits on our ability to perform different actions concurrently. For example, it is a common observation that one action pattern tries to impose its spatiotemporal characteristics on the other, or that both actions mutually affect each other. This has been denoted as structural or specific interference within information processing accounts. It has been argued to result from a fundamental limitation in the division of attention. Rather than a limitation, action theoretical accounts regard this phenomenon, called entrainment, as evidence for an economical control model in which an optimal solution to the degrees of freedom problem is explored. Entrainment is considered an important feature of coordinative structures. In acquiring new skills, humans often attempt to overcome the constraints imposed by entrainment. We discuss experimental evidence showing that practice enables subjects to inhibit or repress the resulting superfluous muscle activity. Moreover, in coordinating differing movements, the human control system manages to delay the initiation of one activity with reference to the other (possibly through inhibitory processes), thereby preventing the occurrence of interference. This delay mechanism allows functionally-related effector systems to perform concurrent actions largely independently. The generality of this mechanism needs to be further explored.

Information processing accounts of bimanual coordination

For a number of years, scientists have addressed the limitations in performing tasks concurrently and the possible role of the nature of the tasks therein. In a number of these studies, use has been made of motor tasks. On the one hand, the simultaneous performance of cognitive-motor activities has received substantial attention. For example, evidence has been advanced that speaking interferes more with motor activities (e.g. tapping) performed in the right than in the left hand in right-handed persons, congruent with the left-hemisphere's presumed lateralization for language (Clark, Guitar, & Hoffman, 1985; Hicks, 1975; Hicks, Bradshaw, Kinsbourne, & Feigin,

1978; Hicks, Provenzano, & Rybstein, 1975; Hiscock, 1982; Keefe, 1985; Kinsbourne & Cook, 1971; Kinsbourne & Hiscock, 1983; Lomas & Kimura, 1976; McFarland & Ashton, 1978; but see Chang & Hammond, 1987, and Kelso, Tuller, & Harris, 1983 for a critique). The findings of this work are also consistent with the predictions of the model of functional cerebral distance or space which was proposed by Kinsbourne and Hicks (1978). According to this model, it is difficult to control activity simultaneously to brain centers that are functionally close. The distance between centers is mainly determined by their degree of interconnectedness. More is said about this model later in this chapter.

On the other hand, some studies have attempted to determine the limitations in the simultaneous performance of repetitive or nonrepetitive hand or finger movements (Cohen, 1970; Duncan, 1979; Klapp, 1979; Peters, 1977, 1985a, 1985b). The general finding that has emerged from this work is that motor activities can be performed concurrently as long as they are temporally compatible. For example, Deutsch (1983) studied the accuracy in producing simple rhythms (in which the intervals associated with one sequence are equal to or an integer multiple of the interval associated with the other, e.g. a 1-to-1 or 2-to-1 tap = temporally compatible) in comparison to polyrhythms (when there is no such relationship, e.g. 3-against-2, 5-against-3 tap = temporally incompatible). Subjects were found to be less accurate in producing polyrhythms compared to the simple rhythms. In other words, interference emerged when incompatible rhythms had to be produced. Under these circumstances, interference is often a result of one rhythm trying to impose its tempo on another or both rhythms mutually affecting each other, leading to errors in timing and consistency. The explanation advanced here by many is that when tasks are very similar, both compete for the same structures or mechanisms of perception or response and this has come to be known as "structural interference" (Kahneman, 1973). Structural interference is distinguished from capacity interference that is a result of a competition for a general limited capacity (Kahneman, 1973; Kerr, 1973; Wickens, 1980). The observed interference is said to be specific in the former case while it is rather nonspecific in the latter. Both models of interference have sometimes been integrated into a common conceptual framework (e.g. Kahneman, 1973; Navon & Gopher, 1979).

Where motor activities have to be performed concurrently, the emergence of specific or structural interference is most likely to be predominant. Recently, Allport (1980) has even proposed the working hypothesis that all interference is specific. Kinsbourne and Hicks (1978) also reserve an important role for specific interference in their model of functional cerebral space. They argue that interference is a result of the spread of whatever is the dominant activity within a highly linked cerebral space. This spread of activity makes it difficult for another activity to be performed at the same time. When tasks are more similar, i.e. their loci of control are functionally close, more interference has to be overcome. Because the degree of similarity between tasks is a major concern here, the major source of interference is structural (Kinsbourne, 1981; Kinsbourne & Hiscock, 1983). All together, there appears to be a limitation in dividing attention to similar (but not the same) tasks, while tasks involving differing modalities of perception or response can be performed concurrently more easily, sometimes without impairment of either task (Allport, Antonis, & Reynolds, 1972). When interference emerges, the type of errors that occur in one task reflect the nature of the concurrent task, also referred to as neural cross-talk (Allport, 1987; Kinsbourne, 1981; MacKenzie & Marteniuk, 1985; Neumann, 1987).

Some researchers have tried to ascertain the locus of interference more specifically. In bimanual finger tapping, Klapp (1979) ascribed the observed interference to a limitation in response generation or the stage in which response commands are programmed or organized. Conversely, Cohen (1970) suggested that right-left interference in the upper limbs is a result of excessive attentional demands for the processing of response-produced feedback coming from both limbs. Following this reasoning, the subject would attempt to reduce the amount of information to be processed by reducing the generation of motor commands or by synchronizing the movements. Cohen's explanation was mainly inspired by the finding that passive movements in one limb were not found to induce interference in the other limb's activity. However, it should be noted that passive movements also differ from active movements in that they do not have to be programmed and generated.

In sum, the information processing accounts of bimanual coordination seem to be based upon the premise that "attention is limited". Nevertheless, they contain several conceptually different explanations for the limitations ranging from limited general capacity to limitations due to competition for specific structures or a combination thereof (the hybrid concepts, see Wickens, 1980). When motor tasks have to be performed simultaneously, the concept of structural interference prevails. Unless disparate activities can be integrated into a higher order action plan, their concurrent performance often fails as reflected through interference. Nested within these information-processing accounts of dual-task performance is the question of where along the sequence of processing stages the limitations occur. In this respect, response programming or organization may be a valid candidate.

Action theoretical accounts of bimanual coordination

The concurrent performance of motor tasks has also been addressed from an action theoretical perspective (Kelso, Southard, & Goodman, 1979a, 1979b; Kelso, Putnam, & Goodman, 1983). For example, Kelso et al. (1979a, 1979b) asked subjects to move one index finger over a long distance to a small target (difficult movement) and another one over a short distance to a large target (easy movement). They wondered what would happen if subjects were to perform these movements concurrently. Findings indicated that, although subjects were not instructed to do so, they performed these movements together, i.e. the movements were initiated and terminated virtually simultaneously although they had a markedly different duration when performed in isolation. Simultaneity of action was achieved through a rescaling of both movement times towards a common or unitary timing basis. This was discussed in support of an economical control model that tries to handle the multiple degrees of freedom problem by controlling functional groupings of muscles, also called synergies or "coordinative structures". Synergies are "those classes of movements which have similar kinematic characteristics, coinciding active muscle groups and conducting types of afferentation" (Gelfand, Gurfinkel, Tsetlin, & Shik, 1971). Easton (1972, 1978) and Turvey (1977) prefer the term coordinative structures which they consider to be mainly reflex based. Kelso and Tuller (1982) do not necessarily see coordinative structures as reflex based. They think of coordinative structures as the significant units of action "not by virtue of their shared degrees of freedom, but by their capability of achieving a common goal" (p.326). In any case, the coordinative structure concept serves to preserve economy in the control system by use of a common underlying activity pattern for the different limbs involved in the movement. This process of rescaling towards a common timing basis has been denoted by action theorists as mutual entrainment [1], a feature that also characterizes coupled non-linear oscillators (Kelso, 1981; Kelso, Holt, Rubin, & Kugler, 1981; Kelso et al., 1983; Kugler, Kelso, & Turvey, 1980). Entrainment is seen as an emergent property of a system of non-linear oscillators and it is held responsible for self-organization within that system. The observed functional coupling of the limbs is noteworthy especially when it is compared with the functional independence among segments in intramanual coordination despite the strong mechanical coupling in the latter case (Morasso, 1983). Although functional coupling has been predominantly documented in the upper limbs, it has also been demonstrated for voluntary movements of the ipsilateral limbs (Baldissera, Cavallari, & Civaschi, 1983).

While action theorists have not greatly elaborated on the underlying neurological substrate for these coordinative structures, concepts in neurophysiology have emerged that appear to fit in with these ideas, e.g. coupled neural oscillators (Yamanishi, Kawato, & Suzuki, 1979, 1980), central pattern generators (CPG), etc. (Grillner, 1975, 1985). These concepts refer to autonomous neural circuits that are responsible for coordinating the activity patterns of different muscles to produce rhythmical behaviour. According to Grillner (1985), these neural networks can not only be made responsible for complex coordinations but also for the production of more specific movements. In order for locomotion to occur, the entire CPG ensemble network, responsible for foot, ankle, knee and hip movement, needs to be activated. But, only parts of the total unit can be activated for the volitional control of more specific ankle, knee, or foot movements. Within this viewpoint, production of new movements may require "learning to combine and sequence specific fractions of the neuronal apparatus used to control the innate movement patterns in a novel way" (Grillner, 1985, p.148).

Mutual interference or mutual entrainment?

The principle of (mutual) entrainment or the tendency of one rhythm to impose its tempo on another is considered an important feature of coordinative structures. This principle may underlie our tendency to move both hands together, to tap compatible rhythms with the fingers, to move our hands when we talk (Kimura, 1973), to synchronize vocal activities and finger movements, etc.. Action theorists have determined the behavioural and kinematic concomitants of this organizational principle. These appear to be very similar to the consequences of what advocates of the information-processing approach have called structural interference. Structural or specific interference has a rather negative connotation because it is seen as a consequence of fundamental limitations in the division of attention. Action theorists consider mutual entrainment as an important organizational principle in the human control system that enables coordinated movement without the need for excessive computation. It provides a solution to the degrees of freedom problem (Bernstein, 1967). Von Holst (1939, 1973) discovered a similar phenomenon some fifty years ago in the coordination of fin movements among a variety of fish species. He used the term "magnet effect" to denote the (mutual) phasic attraction of fin movements.

Thus, we find two differing approaches to a related phenomenon. One approach considers entrainment as evidence for a limitation in attention. The other one sees it as a principled solution to the degrees of freedom problem. The question is not whether one of these approaches should receive priority. Both stress different aspects of the same phenomenon. Under certain conditions, movements of the limbs do need to have a common underlying pattern of innervation. But, when the movements to be performed concurrently in functionally related effector systems differ in spatiotemporal features, entrainment needs to be overcome because now it is a source of interference. Information-processing scientists have elaborated on this latter aspect.

Mutual interference, entrainment and skill acquisition

In this section, the question arises of whether human subjects can learn to overcome mutual interference, or to prevent the intrusions of one motor program into the execution of the other; can we divide attention among similar tasks or tasks requiring functionally related effector systems? From the stance of action theory, the question can be put differently: Is it possible to get released from the constraints imposed by coordinative structures? A well-trained pianist can apparently time the finger movements of both hands independently (Shaffer, 1982). However, the question can be raised whether there is real independence between the pianist's finger movements or whether both action patterns are integrated into a less obvious action plan of higher order.

The idea that functional groupings of muscles may be the building blocks of volitional acts is appealing. Nevertheless, in performing everyday activities and highly specialized sports skills, these synergies or coordinative structures are often undesirable. A major goal of learning then becomes the dissociation of coordinative structures. What is the evidence in favour of such a viewpoint?

Follow-up studies to the Kelso et al. (1979a, 1979b) work have indicated that the strong interlimb coupling may be somewhat distorted when the spatiotemporal and force specification characteristics of the movements to be coordinated diverge. For example, in one of their later experiments, Kelso et al. (1983) put an obstacle in the path of one limb and found that some subjects displayed preservance of synchrony between both limb movements while other subjects displayed some disruption of the synchrony. Furthermore, Marteniuk, MacKenzie, and Baba (1984) had subjects move different distances with styli of different weights in both hands (thereby making the tasks more disparate than in the Kelso et al. study). They observed differences in movement time for the right and left limb when the differences in task requirements became larger. Corcos (1984) also noted movement time differences for two-handed stylus aiming when the ratio of the distance travelled by both limbs was four to one. In sum, these studies suggest that some subjects start to uncouple the limbs (as reflected by differing movement times) when the task requirements of the activities to be coordinated become more dissimilar. The question as to what extent learning can affect the degree of interlimb coupling has remained unanswered so far.

Swinnen, Walter and Shapiro (in press) investigated the acquisition of two movements in the upper limbs that were considerably different in spatiotemporal features. Subjects put their forearms on a double horizontal lever system and moved the levers together towards the body midline. There were two performance sessions, consisting of 75 trials each. In the first session, subjects performed unidirectional movements towards the body midline in both limbs concurrently. The target movement time was 500 ms and subjects moved to a specified endpoint (72 deg.). In the second session, subjects were to perform the same unidirectional movement in the left limb while making a new "double reversal" movement in the right limb (see Figure 1). Time and target-position were kept the same for both limb movements (500 ms, 72 deg.). Subjects were informed about their movement time after each trial. The major goal was to determine the degree of interlimb coupling between these differing movements across practice. More specifically, the possible changes in the left limb movement as a result of performing a different movement in the right limb (in session 2) were studied. A kinematic and electromyographic analysis of the data was considered appropriate for this purpose.

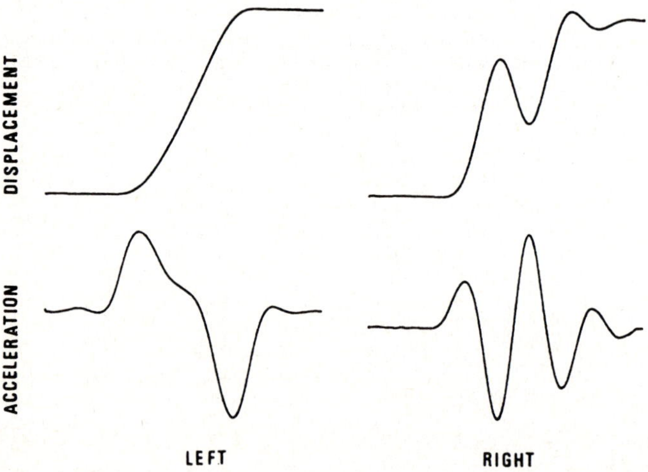

Figure 1. The required displacement and acceleration traces in the right and left limb during session 2.

2a. **Displacement Subject 4 - Session 2**

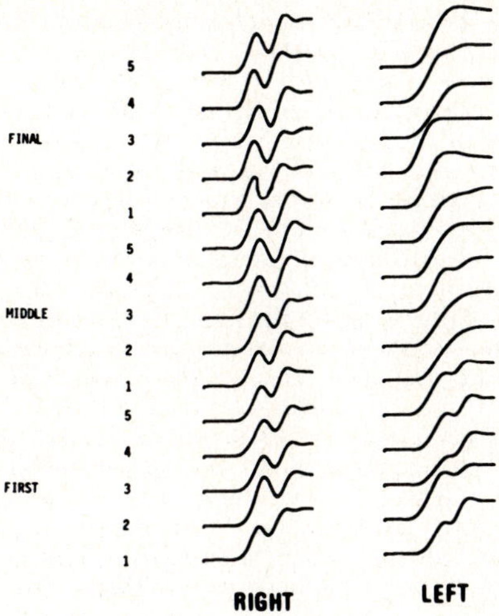

2b. **Displacement Subject 5 - Session 2**

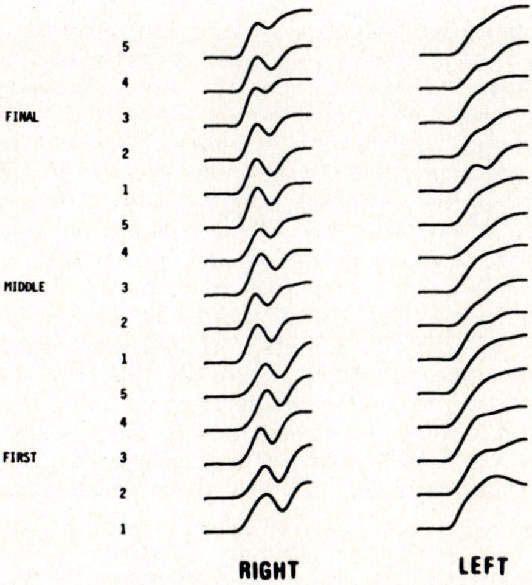

Figure 2. Some examples of displacement patterns produced by the subjects in session 2.

In order to reflect the changes in interlimb relationships across practice, the first, middle, and final five trials of session 2 are presented.

Some examples of displacement patterns that were actually produced by two subjects are presented in Figure 2. These need to be compared to the displacement patterns of right and left limb movements performed in isolation (Figure 1). As can be seen from these patterns, subjects did not always perform the required movement patterns in the left limb. Interference in the left limb movement was mainly evident at the beginning of practice. It appeared as if there was a strong tendency for one action pattern (for the right limb) to impose its spatiotemporal characteristics on the other (the left limb). Some subjects actually made reversal movements in the left limb. Others lined up the left displacement pattern with the first or final portion of the right displacement pattern. Nevertheless, at the end of the second session, subjects (except for one) were successful in performing both limb movements, i.e. a reversal movement was made in the right limb and not in the left. That most of the subjects managed to reduce superfluous muscle activity through practice also became evident from the analysis of EMG activity in the left biceps and triceps. A significant reduction in left biceps and triceps activity took place across practice in session 2. This is consistent with the viewpoint that skill acquisition involves the selective inhibition of unnecessary muscular activity rather than simply the activation of additional motor units (Basmajian, 1977; Kinsbourne, 1981, 1982). Coordination emerges here through progressive inhibition of the superfluous and even disturbing surplus of muscular activity. It is this irradiation or spread of activity that often leads to observable patterns of specific interference. However, there is more to the problem of reducing interference or crosstalk as will become evident later in this section.

To further determine interlimb relationships, the acceleration patterns of both movements were compared[2]. Cross correlations were computed between the right and left limb acceleration patterns. Higher positive cross correlations were considered to reflect a higher degree of coupling[3] between limbs. Findings revealed large inter-individual differences. Some subjects were able to make the right and left limb movement independently or to uncouple both movements almost completely by the end of session 2. This was inferred from the low correlations between left and right acceleration traces. Others still displayed high relationships at the end of practice. Some examples are demonstrated in Figure 3. The top left pattern looks like a "figure eight" form. This configuration is to be expected in the case of independent performance of the right and left limb movement (=reference pattern). The correlation between both patterns is low. The other patterns show some examples of plots of right-left accelerations of movements that were actually performed together by the subjects at the end of session 2. These need to be compared to the upper-left pattern.

In sum, these findings suggest that some subjects learned to uncouple the limb movements or to break down the coordinative structure when the spatiotemporal demands of the movements (to be coordinated) were considerably different. There were high intra- and inter-individual differences through practice. Some subjects appeared highly coupled at the beginning of the second session and succeeded in uncoupling the limb movements through practice (see Figure 2). Others became more coupled towards the end.

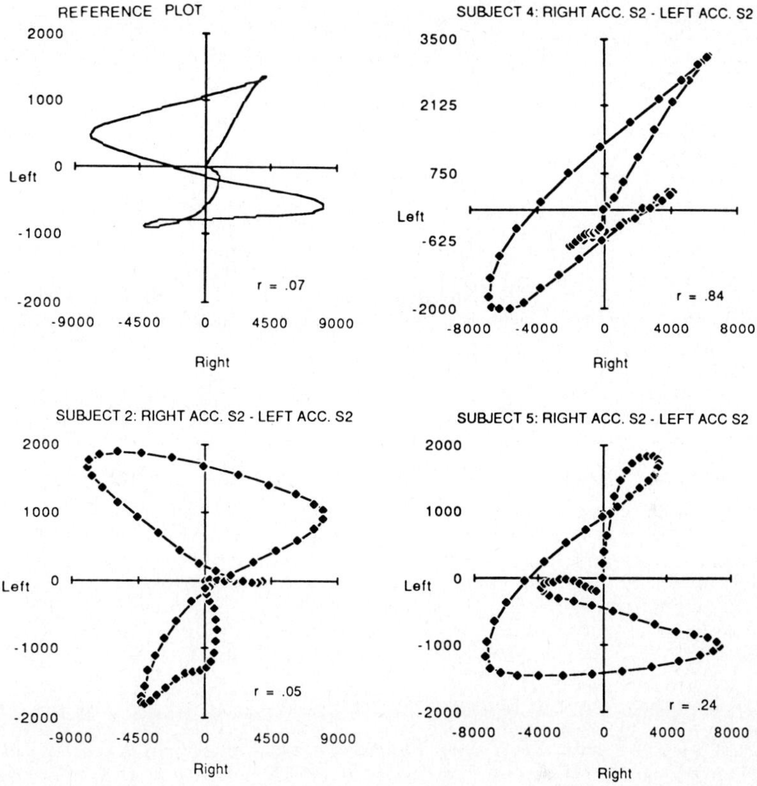

Figure 3. The acceleration patterns of the left limb plotted against the acceleration pattern of the right limb (from Swinnen et al., in press).

The right acceleration values are presented in the abscissa, the left acceleration values in the ordinate. The reference plot (upper-left) is the configuration to be expected when the right and left limb movements are performed in isolation. The correlation is low. Subject A demonstrates a high linear relationship between right and left acceleration patterns. Subjects B and C display a low relationship. The lower the correlation between right and left acceleration patterns, the higher the independence or uncoupling achieved. The upper-right pattern demonstrates two important effects that were identified by Von Holst as the "magnet" and the "super position" effect. One movement (the right) attracts the other (the left). The former imposes its temporal structure on the latter and also has an additive effect on the other.

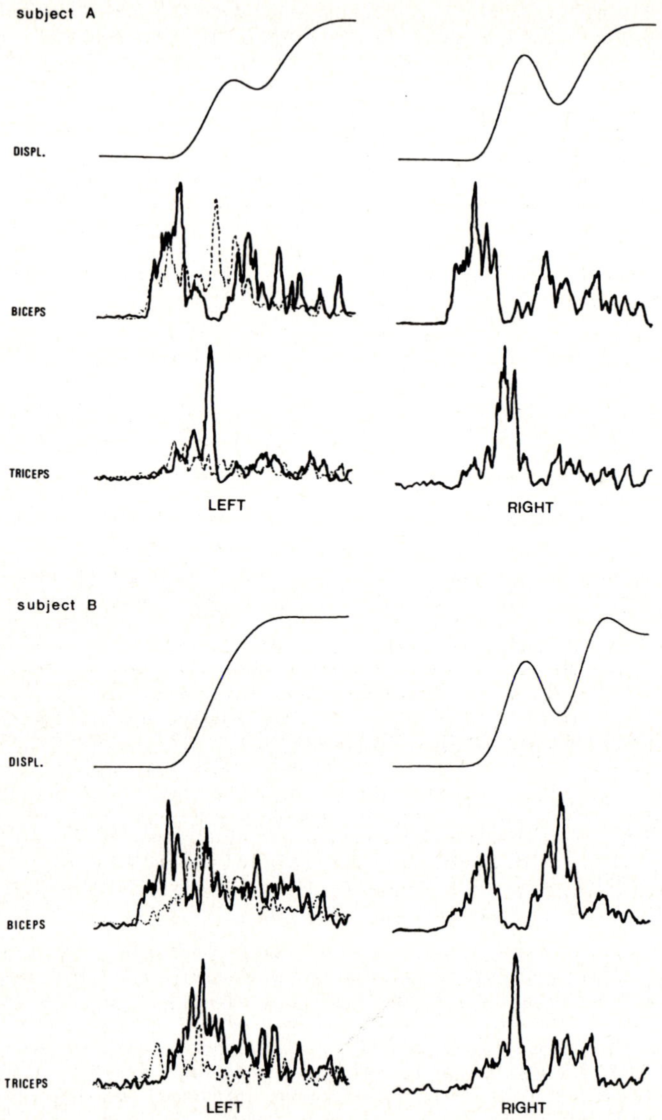

Figure 4. Electromyographic activity in the left and right biceps at the end of session 2 for a successful and less successful subject.

Average electrical activity for the unidirectional movement in the left limb at the end of session 1. Session 1 and session 2 data of the left limb are matched at the onset of overt movement. Subject A is not able to produce the correct unidirectional displacement pattern in the left limb but instead makes a small reversal. The patterns of electrical activity in the left biceps and triceps line up in time with the activity patterns of the corresponding muscles in the contralateral limb. Both movement patterns are initiated simultaneously. Subject B succeeds in performing the correct unidirectional movement in the left limb independent of the right reversal movement. Here the movements are not initiated simultaneously. It is also evident that, compared to the electrical activity for biceps and triceps at the end of session 1 (dashed lines), electrical activity in both muscles is increased.

Observe in both examples the decreased EMG activity in the left biceps (for the movement of session 2 in reference to session 1) at the time a major burst of activity occurs in the left triceps. This is probably a result of "reciprocal antagonistic inhibition". It is more prevalent in Session 2 because muscle activity in both the agonist and antagonist is generally higher.

The observed variability could partly be explained by the following observation: the more subjects delayed the initiation of one movement with reference to the other, the more the limb movements appeared to be uncoupled. In the previous section, we proposed cross correlations between right and left acceleration patterns as a means to determine the degree of coupling between limbs. When these values were correlated with the absolute time difference between initiation of the right and left limb movement, moderate to high negative correlations emerged ($r = -.75, -.42, -.23, -.57, -.84$ for subjects1 to 5). In other words, the greater the difference between interlimb initiation times, the lower the magnitude of dynamical coupling between the limbs (see Walter & Swinnen, 1987, for a replication of this finding). Initiation delays ranged from about 28 to 70 ms on average. This method may be one way to relate the degree of coupling between limbs with events that occur before overt movement takes place.

The EMG activity in biceps and triceps of a successful and less successful trial is displayed in Figure 4. Subject A initiated the right and left limb movement simultaneously and a high degree of interference is evident. Subject B produced the required displacement pattern in the left limb more successfully. While subjects who made use of a delay mechanism initiated the right limb movement usually before the left, Subject B initiated the left limb movement first. It is also evident from the latter example that biceps as well as triceps activity for producing the left displacement pattern was still elevated in comparison to the corresponding activity at the end of session 1. Thus, although limb uncoupling was successful, muscle activity was still increased. It remains to be seen if more extensive practice could lead to lower levels of activity or if some concurrence cost would be inevitable.

One is prompted to ask what the initiation delay means and how it affects interlimb coupling. Some hypothetical explanations will now be explored and these pertain to the psychological, as well as the neurobiological level of explanation. From an information-processing perspective, one might propose that successive movement initiation enables the subjects to divide attention between both tasks. It can possibly be viewed as an effort to safeguard against interference. Subjects appear to invoke this delay mechanism at variable times during practice and this appears to account for the observed inter- as well as intra-individual differences in degree of interlimb dependence. Kinsbourne (1981) refers to this phenomenon as staggered processing. In a more general way, it may be an important function of attention to prevent interference by selecting one action out of a number of possible actions. Allport (1987) refers to this as selection for-action. Because effector systems are typically limited to carrying out just one action of a given kind at a time, he considers selection-for-action as a biological necessity of theoretical importance. For example, in order to maximize prey capture, a predator needs to focus on only one prey out of the group. Certain neurological mechanisms may subserve the assignment of relative priority among actions. In this respect, Allport (1987) suggests that this can be achieved by either selective enhancement (i.e. the cueing or prioritization of favoured information) or by selective inhibition or attenuation (i.e. the suppression or exclusion of information). However, he goes on to favour selection by selective enhancement because of a lack of evidence for inhibitory mechanisms. Nevertheless, inhibitory mechanisms may intervene here as well. Inhibitory processes of several kinds are an essential part of functional considerations of the human nervous system. An obvious example is "reciprocal antagonistic inhibition" in which the activity of the antagonist is depressed when the agonist is active through connections with inhibitory interneurons. More generally, the brain can be understood as a highly linked neural network consisting of countless connections. The simultaneous performance of differentiated action patterns is possible through inhibitory synapses that serve to limit the spread of whatever is the dominant activity at a particular time.

Evidence for delay mechanisms in movement organization has been provided by Cordo and Nashner (1982; Nashner & Cordo, 1981). They proposed a model for action prioritization in which inhibitory mechanisms figure predominantly. They studied the interactions between rapid arm actions (pushing or pulling a handle) and postural adjustments needed to maintain equilibrium. Under most circumstances, they found the arm movements to be preceded by postural reactions and they hypothesized the operation of some kind of delay mechanism affecting the arm action. Following a tone stimulus, the average of subjects' reaction times (measured as the earliest detectable increase in biceps brachii EMG) was 155 ms +/-37 while the gastrocnemius muscle was already active after 111ms +/-27; i.e. 44 ms earlier. Furthermore, increased postural requirements were accompanied by a greater delay of activation of the arm musculature. Similar findings were generated earlier by Belen'kii, Gurfinkel', and Pal'tsev (1967) and by Pal'tsev and El'ner (1967). They investigated the interactions between arm lifting and lowering, and postural activity. The deltoid muscle (responsible for the arm action) showed an increase in activity 130 to 140 ms after the sound signal. Again, the postural muscles were activated sooner: the biceps femoris on the ipsilateral side was activated 40 to 50 ms before detection of deltoid activity while the biceps femoris on the contralateral side displayed increased electrical activity up to 30-40 ms before its contralateral counterpart. Hubbard and Seng (1954) investigated the relationship between the stepping and swing action in baseball batters and found that 40 ms after planting the forward foot, the batswing was initiated. The precedence of associated postural actions has a functional significance in that it prevents loss of balance due to focal arm activity. But, it may also serve to prevent interference between focal and postural activity in much the same way as interference between the right and left limb movement was relieved through movement initiation delays in the Swinnen et al. (in press) study.

Cordo and Nashner (1982) presented a model to account for their findings in which inhibitory mechanisms play a dominant role. They hypothesized that temporal sequencing of the postural movements in advance of the arm movement would occur via two parametric signals, one which would inhibit the focal arm activity, and another which would release it after initiation of the postural adjustment. This would enable changes in body orientation without having the requirements of postural stability to interfere with the accurate completion of the focal movement. The hypothesis that temporal sequencing of actions takes place through inhibitory mechanisms gains strength in view of the following observation: in certain exceptions, Cordo and Nashner found biceps activity to be initiated before the postural muscles were activated. However, biceps activity remained at a low level prior to gastrochemius activity while vigorous biceps activity occurred only following gastrocnemius activity. Although the physiological basis of inhibitory processes is not well understood, several authors have hinted to its role in the organization of action (Arbib, 1981; Kinsbourne, 1981; Neumann, 1987; Shallice, 1978).

To summarize, when certain actions have to be performed simultaneously, temporal sequencing of the actions may take place through an inhibition mechanism which allows the initiation of one activity and results in the delay of the other activity. Its major goal is apparently to prevent interference between concurrent actions. although the actions to be combined appear to be initiated consecutively, the remaining portions of these actions run off concurrently and independent of each other. As a consequence, functionally related effector systems can indeed perform simultaneous actions largely independently. Action uncoupling requires practice. A provocative hypothesis in this respect is that learning implies a release from entrainment through the recruitment of inhibitory networks.

Footnotes

[1]Kelso et al. (1981) makes a distinction between entrainment and synchronization, although they note that these terms are often used interchangeably in the literature. They refer to synchronization as "that state which occurs when both interval and phase of coupled oscillators are matched exactly; entrainment refers to the matching of intervals, but one oscillator may lead or lag the other" (p.234).

There are two types of entrainment. When coupled oscillators of slightly different frequencies will tend to accomplish a common frequency (rescaling), the term mutual entrainment is used. If the frequency of one of two coupled oscillators is an integer multiple of the other one, it is denoted as subharmonic entrainment or frequency demultiplication.

[2]Acceleration was chosen as the primary kinematic variable for analysis because it provides a much more sensitive measure than displacement. The determination of cross correlations between right and left acceleration patterns may be a valuable way to quantify topological interactions.

[3]Higher coupling implies here that the left limb undergoes interference from the right limb movement; in other words, the left limb displays the features of the right limb movement.

Acknowledgements

The authors are indebted to two anonymous referees for their helpful suggestions.

References

Allport, D.A. (1980). Attention and performance. In G. Claxton (Ed.), Cognitive Psychology. New directions. London: Routledge and Kegan Paul.

Allport, A. (1987). Selection for action: some behavioral and neurophysiological considerations of attention and action. In H. Heuer & A.F. Sanders (Eds.), Perspectives on perception and action. Hillsdale, N.J.: Erlbaum.

Allport, D.A., Antonis, B., & Reynolds, P. (1972). On the division of attention: a disproof of the single channel hypothesis. Quarterly Journal of Experimental Psychology, 24, 225-235.

Arbib, M.A. (1981). Perceptual structures and distributed motor control. In V.B. Brooks (Ed.), Handbook of Physiology: the nervous system (section 1), Vol.2: Motor control. Bethesda, Maryland: American Physiological Society.

Baldissera, F., Cavallari, P., & Civaschi, P. (1983). Preferential coupling between voluntary movements of ipsilateral limbs. Neuroscience Letters, 34, 95-100.

Basmajian, J.V. (1977). Motor learning and control: a working hypothesis. Archives of Physical Medicine and Rehabilitation, 58, 38-41.

Belenkii, V.Y., Gurfinkel, V.S., & Paltsev, Y.I. (1967). Elements of control of voluntary movements. Biofizika, 12, 135-141.

Bernstein, N. (1967). The co-ordination and regulation of movements.

Oxford: Pergamon Press.

Chang, P., & Hammond, G.R. (1987). Mutual interactions between speech and finger movements. Journal of Motor Behavior, 19, 265-274.

Clark, D.G., Guitar, B., & Hoffman, P.R. (1985). Reliability of verbal-manual interference. Brain and Cognition, 4, 486-491.

Cohen, L. (1970). Interaction between limbs during bimanual voluntary activity. Brain, 93, 259-272.

Corcos, D.M. (1984). Two-handed movement control. Research Quarterly for Exercise and Sport, 55, 117-122.

Cordo, P.J., & Nashner, L.M. (1982). Properties of postural adjustments associated with rapid arm movements. Journal of Neurophysiology, 45, 287-302.

Deutsch, D. (1983). The generation of two isochronous sequences in parallel. Perception and Psychophysics, 34, 331-337.

Duncan, J. (1979). Divided attention: the whole is more than the sum of its parts. Journal of Experimental Psychology: Human Perception and Performance, 5, 216-228.

Easton, T.A. (1972). On the normal use of reflexes. American Scientist, 60, 591-599.

Easton, T.A. (1978). Coordinative structures - the basis for a motor program. In D. Landers & R.W. Christina (Eds.), Psychology of motor behavior and sport. Champaign, IL.: Human Kinetics Publishers.

Gelfand, I.M., Gurfinkel, V.S., Tsetlin, M.L., & Shik, M.L. (1971). Some problems in the analysis of movements. In I.M. Gelfand, V.S. Gurfinkel, S.V. Fomin, & M.L. Tsetlin (Eds.), Models of the structural-functional organization of certain biological systems. Cambridge: MIT.

Grillner, S. (1975). Locomotion in vertebrates: central mechanisms and reflex interaction. Physiological Reviews, 55, 247-306.

Grillner, S. (1985). Neurobiological bases of rhythmic motor acts in vertebrates. Science, 228, 143-149.

Hicks, R.E. (1975). Intrahemispheric response competition between vocal and unimanual performance in normal adult human males. Journal of Comparative and Physiological Psychology, 89, 50-60.

Hicks, R.E., Bradshaw, G.J., Kinsbourne, M., & Feigin, D.S. (1978). Vocal-manual trade-offs in hemispheric sharing of human performance control. Journal of Motor Behavior, 10, 1-6.

Hicks, R.E., Provenzano, F.J., & Rybstein, E.D. (1975). Generalized and laterilized effects of concurrent verbal rehearsal upon performance of sequential movements of the fingers by the left and right hands. Acta Psychologica, 39, 119-130.

Hiscock, M. (1982). Verbal-manual time sharing in children as a function of task priority. Brain and Cognition, 1, 119-131.

Holst, E. von (1939). Die relative Koordination als Phanomen und als Methode zentralnervoser Funktionsanalyse. Ergebnisse der Physiologie, 42, 228-306.

Holst, E. von (1973). The behavioral physiology of animals and man: The collected papers of Erich von Holst (Vol.1). (R. Martin, Trans.). London: Methuen. (Original work published 1937.)

Hubbard, A.W., & Seng, C.N. (1954). Visual movements of batters. Research Quarterly, 25, 42-57.

Kahneman, D. (1973). Attention and effort. Englewood Cliffs, N.J.: Prentice-Hall.

Keefe, K. (1985). Motor and cognitive interference effects on

unimanual tapping rates. Brain and Cognition, 4, 165-170.
Kelso, J.A.S. (1981). Contrasting perspectives on order and regulation in movement. In J. Long & A. Baddeley (Eds.), Attention and performance IX. Hillsdale, N.J.: Erlbaum.
Kelso, J.A.S., Holt, K.G., Rubin, P., & Kugler, P.N. (1981). Patterns of human interlimb coordination emerge from the properties of non-linear, limit cycle oscillatory processes: theory and data. Journal of Motor Behavior, 13, 226-261.
Kelso, J.A.S., Putnam, C.A., & Goodman, D. (1983). On the space-time structure of human interlimb coordination. Quarterly Journal of Experimental Psychology, 35A, 347-375.
Kelso, J.A.S., Southard, D.L., & Goodman, D. (1979a). On the coordination of two-handed movements. Journal of Experimental Psychology: Human Perception and Performance, 2, 229-238.
Kelso, J.A.S., Southard, D.L., & Goodman, D. (1979b). On the nature of human interlimb coordination. Science, 203, 1029-1031.
Kelso, J.A.S., & Tuller, B. (1982). A dynamical basis for action systems. In M.S. Gazzaniga (Ed.), Handbook of Cognitive Neuroscience. New York: Plenum Press.
Kelso, J.A.S., Tuller, B., & Harris, K.S. (1983). A "dynamic pattern" perspective on the control and coordination of movement. In P.F. MacNeilage (Ed.), The production of speech. New York: Springer-Verlag.
Kerr, B. (1973). Processing demands during mental operations. Memory and Cognition, 1, 401-412.
Kimura, D. (1973). Manual activity during speaking— 1. Right-handers. Neuropsychologia, 11, 45-50.
Kinsbourne, M. (1981). Single-channel theory. In D. Holding (Ed.), Human Skills. Chichester: Wiley.
Kinsbourne, M. (1982). Hemispheric specialization and the growth of human understanding. American Psychologist, 37, 411-420.
Kinsbourne, M. & Cook, J. (1971). Generalized and lateralized effects of concurrent verbalization on a unimanual skill. Quarterly Journal of Experimental Psychology, 23, 341-345.
Kinsbourne, M. & Hicks, R.E. (1978). Functional cerebral space: a model for overflow, transfer and interference effects in human performance: a tutorial review. In J. Requin (Ed.), Attention and performance VII. Hillsdale: Erlbaum.
Kinsbourne, M. & Hiscock, M. (1983). Asymmetries of dual-task performance. In J.B. Hellige (Ed.), Cerebral hemisphere asymmetry. Method, theory, and application. New York: Praeger.
Klapp, S.T. (1979). Doing two things at once: the role of temporal compatibility. Memory and Cognition, 7, 375-381.
Kugler, P.N., Kelso, J.A.S., & Turvey, M.T. (1980). On the concept of coordinative structures as dissipative structures: 1 Theoretical lines of convergence. In G.E. Stelmach & J. Requin (Eds.), Tutorials in motor behavior. Amsterdam: North Holland.
Lomas, J. & Kimura, D. (1976). Intrahemispheric interaction between speaking and sequential manual activity. Neuropsychologia, 14, 23-33.
MacKenzie, C.L. & Marteniuk, R.G. (1985). Motor skill: feedback, knowledge, and structural issues. Canadian Journal of Psychology, 39, 313-337.
Marteniuk, R.G., MacKenzie, C.L., & Baba, D.M. (1984). Bimanual movement control: information processing and interaction

effects. Quarterly Journal of Experimental Psychology, 36A, 335-365.

McFarland, K., & Ashton, R. (1978). The lateralized effects of concurrent cognitive and motor performance. Perception & Psychophysics, 23, 344-349.

Morasso, P. (1983). Coordination aspects of arm trajectory formation. Human Movement Science, 2, 197-210.

Navon, D. & Gopher, D. (1979). On the economy of the human-processing system. Psychological Review, 86, 214-255.

Nashner, L.M. & Cordo, P.J. (1981). Relation of automatic postural responses and reaction-time voluntary movements of human leg muscles. Experimental Brain Research, 43, 395-405.

Neumann, O. (1987). Beyond capacity: a functional view of attention. In H. Heuer & A.F. Sanders (Eds.), Perspectives on perception and action. Hillsdale, N.J.: Erlbaum.

Paltsev, Y.I. & Elner, A.M. (1967). Preparatory and compensatory period during voluntary movement in patients with involvement of the brain of different localization. Biofizika, 12, 142-147.

Peters, M. (1977). Simultaneous performance of two motor activities: the factor of timing. Neuropsychologia, 15, 461-465.

Peters, M. (1985a). Constraints in the performance of bimanual tasks and their expression in unskilled and skilled subjects. Quarterly Journal of Experimental Psychology, 37A, 171-196.

Peters, M. (1985b). Performance of a Rubato-like task: when two things cannot be done at the same time. Music Perception, 2, 471-482.

Shaffer, L.H. (1982). Rhythm and timing in skill. Psychological Review, 89, 109-122.

Shallice, T. (1978). The dominant action system: an information-processing approach to consciousness. In K.S. Pope & J.L. Singer (Eds.), The stream of consciousness. New York: Plenum Press.

Swinnen, S.P., Walter, C.B., & Shapiro, D.C. (in press). The coordination of limb movements with different kinematic patterns. Brain and Cognition.

Turvey, M.T. (1977). Preliminaries to a theory of action with reference to vision. In R. Shaw & J. Bransford (Eds.), Perceiving, acting, and knowing. Toward an ecological psychology. Hillsdale, N.J.: Erlbaum.

Walter, C.B. & Swinnen, S.P. (1987). The nature of coupling during bimanual actions. Paper presented at the Fourth Mid-Central Ergonomics/Human Factors Conference, Champaign, Illinois; July.

Wickens, C.D. (1980). The structure of attentional resources. In R.S. Nickerson (Ed.), Attention and performance VIII. Hillsdale, N.J.: Erlbaum.

Yamanishi, J., Kawato, M., & Suzuki, R. (1979). Studies on human finger tapping neural networks by phase transition curves. Biological Cybernetics, 33, 199-208.

Yamanishi, J., Kawato, M., & Suzuki, R. (1980). Two coupled oscillators as a model for the coordinated finger tapping by both hands. Biological Cybernetics, 37, 219-225.

Cognition and Action in Skilled Behaviour
A.M. Colley and J.R. Beech (Editors)

DISCUSSION : PROGRAMMING AND COORDINATION

John Annett
University of Warwick

It is nearly ninety years since Woodworth in his classic monograph (Woodworth, 1899) deplored the fact that there was then "no psychophysics of voluntary movement". Although, in the manner of the times, he talked of the "conscious content of movement" as being the proper subject matter of this psychophysical study his experimental programme was in fact almost entirely devoted to investigations of "the relative accuracy of movement under the control of different senses".

The seven papers in this symposium represent a sample of current work in the field established by Woodworth, and, in particular, some recurrent issues foreshadowed in Woodworth's monograph and still awaiting resolution. The computer has displaced the stopwatch but the methods remain much the same, with the emphasis on the analysis of fast visually aimed movements, and fine manual control tasks, including handwriting.

As in Woodworth's day the nature of mechanisms underlying the relationship between speed and accuracy is a central theme. So too is the question of internal and sensory control, that is the extent to which an action is generated from a memory store or motor program and how much it depends on processing sensory information. This was the problem which Woodworth explored by comparing movements made under visual control, or blindfold, or when the subject's attention was directed to something else. Woodworth was also aware of the effects of practice on the ability to make fast and accurate movements and this topic also features in our symposium. I propose, therefore, to direct my comments on the present papers primarily to these issues.

A series of experiments by Fitts (Fitts, 1954) was a landmark in the study of voluntary movement. Between Woodworth and Fitts a great deal of normative data on the speed of movements of different amplitudes, directions and loads had been collected, primarily for the purpose of work study engineering, but the impact of Fitts' work lay in his demonstration of a logarithmic relationship between movement time and the ratio of movement amplitude to terminal accuracy. It was "information load" rather than physical load which determined movement time. This in itself justified the interest of psychologists who might otherwise have abandoned the study of movement to the engineers and physiologists. The idea that motor skill is a function of perceptual limitations was not new. Woodworth had tried, and failed, to fit his data to Weber's Law but Fitts' new law, based on an analogy with the Shannon-Weaver theory of information, provided a much closer fit not only to the data but to the new conceptual underpinnings of what was to become cognitive psychology.

Fitts' results showed that the perceptual-motor system can best be understood as an information-processing device, and the debate since 1954 has been about what kind of information-processing device is needed to generate the movements of which humans are capable. Fitts himself was cautious about the detailed interpretation of his law and did not go beyond the suggestion that perceptual information was needed to overcome the inherent "noise" in the "channel", in other words he saw the speed/accuracy trade-off as essentially a transmission problem. An alternative interpretation proposed by Crossman (Crossman & Goodeve, 1963) was based on Craik's intermittent servo model of the human operator. This assumes an initial (pre-programmed) output followed by a number of discrete corrections with a minimum interval (or refractory period) between corrections of something less than half a second. Howarth and Beggs have refined the model in a series of papers of which we have the latest here (4). Its principal rival is the impulse-variability model by Schmidt et al. (1979). This goes further than Fitts in ascribing the principal source of "noise", or variability, to the force required to initiate the movement and proposing that variability is proportioned to the magnitude of the initial force, but it generates a linear rather than a logarithmic relation between speed and accuracy for movements of short duration.

Standing back a little from these alternative models and the data collected in support of each, there seem to be two related problems. First, curve fitting is one of the psychologically most appealing but least powerful means of testing theories. Typical research reports in this field offer sets of data which are claimed to fit a specific model better than their competitors. Second, apparently minor differences in experimental technique generate data which fit different mathematical functions (Wright & Meyer, 1983). Although it was one of the strengths of Fitts' 1954 paper that he used a range of different tasks all of which produced data to fit the law, it has since become clear (as Beggs has pointed out) that variations in the equipment used, and in the requirements for spatial or temporal accuracy, and hence in the demand characteristics of the task, can generate different subject strategies. It is inappropriate to test for "best fit" under conditions where the mathematical model is at variance with the underlying physical model, that is the mechanism or strategy for producing the movement. Wherever possible we need supplementary evidence from a detailed examination of individual subjects' performance in order to understand which strategy is being used.

Annett, Golby and Kay (1958) used film analysis to show that in the Fitts peg-moving task almost all of the variance in movement time attributable to Index of Difficulty was to be found in the last half inch of an eight inch movement. Subjects were making the gross movement at much the same speed but were slowing down to make the final corrections just before hitting the target. This confirmed Woodworth's account of the biphasic nature of these rapid aiming movements. What happens towards the end of the movement may, however, vary with the task. Beggs and Howarth, for example, have typically required their subjects to hit a target perpendicular to the direction of movement in the saggital plane, a dart-throwing action, as compared with inserting a peg in a hole on the horizontal plane used by Fitts, or unconstrained knob or lever movement transmitted to a cursor on a screen as used by Crossman and Goodeve (1963), and Wright and Meyer (1983).

A discrete correction model fits the qualitative features of the 1958 film analysis quite well. However, a more detailed analysis can reveal the different strategies used by subjects. Annett, Annett, Hudson and Turner (1979) looking at differences between preferred and non-preferred hands found that by far the biggest percentage difference between left and right was in the final corrective movement, that is in just the place where movement time is most sensitive to Index of Difficulty. However it was not a simple matter of the non-preferred hand slowing down more in its final phase in order to make a single correction. Rather, the non-preferred hand missed the target more often and had to make a second or even a third movement before getting the peg safely into the hole. Moreover each of these corrective movements was of about the same duration (approximately 120 ms for either hand) thus the relative slowness of the non-preferred hand is related to the probability of hitting the target in one shot rather than to having a longer minimum correction time. Of course in the Beggs and Howarth task the physical constraints are different and hence the appropriate strategy is different. Each trial ends with the first contact on the target board so subjects necessarily have to make any corrections whilst still "in flight", and no doubt have to make some trade-off between the rate of approach and the likelihood of hitting the required target first time. If this is the case then the Crossman model matches the process quite well, but for the peg-board task the strategy of allowing oneself a number of discrete corrections (with a good chance of a "hole in one") matches the impulse variability model rather better. There are other data which are relevant to the choice of explanatory model such as actual variability in velocity and angular error (in two dimensions) at various stages of the movement which require rather more sophisticated recording equipment than is used by many experimenters. The sheer technical economy of Woodworth's original experiments can lead us astray. It should not be necessary to make deductions about the fine structure of motor performance on the basis of aggregated movement times when kinematic methods are readily available.

Fitts' Law is primarily to do with the accurate termination of a movement. Research on motor programs, by contrast, is about the initiation of movements. The motor program is a theoretical construct of somewhat variable meaning. Some authors use the term to refer to the process of preparation which goes on before there is any detectable muscular activity whilst others use it to refer to a stored set of instructions, a memory trace or engram. Of course both versions imply an entity or process which is, by definition, independent of feedback and so the classical method of investigating motor programs is to deprive the subject of some or all feedback. Woodworth did this by comparing the accuracy of movement with and without vision, and more subtly by directing the subject's attention elsewhere. Deafferentiation due to disease or injury (Lashley,

1917), or by surgical intervention (Taub & Berman, 1968) or ischemia (Laszlo, 1966) has been used to distinguish sensory (closed-loop) control from central (open-loop) or programmed control. The interpretation of results using these feedback deprivation techniques is far from straightforward and they shed little light on the nature of the motor programs or the programming process in normal conditions.

If motor programming is presumed to be a process, such as specifying the parameters of a movement, and this process is expected to occupy a finite amount of time, then reaction time seems to provide the appropriate methodology. If motor programs are conceived as sets of instructions resident in motor memory (as in the "memory drum" theory, Henry & Rogers, 1960) to be retrieved on appropriate occasions, for example in writing a familiar letter or words, reaction time methods are appropriate only if one is prepared to make additional assumptions about retrieval, for instance that it takes longer to retrieve a more complex program. The use of reaction time depends on the use of the subtraction method with its implication of serial processing, an assumption which it is increasingly difficult to make without the support of independent evidence (see Annett, 1969; Rabbitt, 1981).

The memory drum concept of a motor program would lead one to look for signs of automatisation such as uniformity over a number of repetitions, indifference to potentially interfering stimuli and dissociation from new environmental information, so patterns of the early part of the response should provide important cues. Bairstow's (3) results suggest that a close examination of the acceleration patterns of the first 50 ms or so of a rapid interception movement shows that it is scaled to certain characteristics of the target motion, evidence of a programming process taking 270 ms at most. It would appear that the direction of the initial part of the movement is not related to any target parameters and is presumably not specified in the initial programming process. There are several points which should be made about this. At first sight it seems odd that instructions for speed and direction should be separated. If this were generally the case it would certainly make nonsense of Sidaway, Christina and Shea's (6) contention that programming time is partly determined by the angle subtended by the target at the point of origin of the movement. However, Bairstow's targets are moving and may be intercepted at any point before they disappear from the screen whilst Sidaway's targets are at fixed locations, known in advance. Bairstow's subjects usually approach the target through a curvilinear path, apparently adopting the strategy of first getting started and then making directional corrections en route, a strategy quite appropriate to the task demands. The speed of a movement is strongly affected by the force of agonist contraction whilst movement direction depends on agonist-antagonist balance which can be adapted en route. This provides reason enough for a strategy in which they are separated. Target interception can probably be regarded as a well-practised skill yet it would be useful to know more about practice effects with this particular task. For example, if target presentation is blocked such that the speed and direction become highly predictable, is the initial movement scaled for direction as well as speed, does spatio-temporal patterning become more uniform and is the reaction time affected?

Bairstow does not find significant variation in reaction time with features of the target, such as distance from the subject's start point, so are the doubts about the value of reaction time studies mentioned above justified by these results? Sidaway, Christina and Shea (6) fail to confirm Sternberg's finding (Sternberg, Monsell, Knoll, & Wright, 1978) that reaction time is related to the number of discrete elements in a response pattern, but we have to bear in mind possible differences between the emission of linguistic strings and a string of arbitrary hand movements. What they do find is an effect due to more than one response component which adds up to 20 ms to RT and a smaller effect of target size, about 10 ms for the smaller of two targets. Fitts and Peterson (1964), incidentally, found an addition of about 5 ms per Index of Difficulty "bit". Taken overall this is not particularly strong evidence for a "response constraints" (or Fitts' Law) interpretation of movement initiation time.

Hulstijn and van Galen (5) also employ reaction time methodology in their studies of the effects of familiarity and practice, by having subjects write either nonsense graphemes, familiar but not frequently produced symbols and normal letters. Both familiarity and practice are presumed to be operating on the programming process but their relationship with response initiation time is found to be far from straightforward. Again Sternberg's finding on the relationship between number of elements and reaction time is only weakly confirmed in the case of unfamiliar graphemes. Truncated versions of familiar letter patterns yield longer reaction times although comprising fewer elements, and only unfamiliar graphemes show a positive relation between reaction time and number of elements. Whilst plausible reasons for these discrepancies can be offered it seems that reaction time methodology is not being very successful in elucidating the response programming process without the introduction of ad hoc assumptions.

Three of the papers address issues in motor learning. Harvey (2) asks how regularities in task-related information are learned, Swinnen and Walter (8) ask how practice affects the ability to perform two tasks at once, and Frohlich (7) provides a detailed examination of the development of two-hand coordination. Probably the bulk of the literature on motor learning has been concerned with the manipulation of independent variables such as practice schedules (massed vs. spaced, part vs. whole), and instructional techniques such as providing guidance and knowledge of results. The simplest possible dependent variables, response probability, accuracy or latency, are used in a classical psychophysical paradigm. The papers in this symposium, however, reflect an old but less commonly used tradition of keeping the independent variable simple, e.g. amount of practice, but providing a detailed analysis of a number of dependent variables. This hypothesis-forming rather than hypothesis-testing research mode is a particularly fruitful way of freshening up stale theories because it offers an opportunity to reconsider just what are the phenomena to be explained.

The questions addressed by Harvey (2) concern the nature of the presumed internal model of external world regularities and his intriguing result is that the learner appears to have more than one model, or at least use different aspects of whatever record of past experience is stored, in order to be able to carry out two distinctly different "memory" tasks. The first of these, associated with every learning trial, is the motor equivalent of the verbal learning serial anticipation method, in which the subject has to predict the next stimulus item. The stimulus item itself provides both knowledge of results of the preceding response and another learning opportunity. The second task, which occurs only on trials 5 and 10 (what a pity it was not done at the very beginning of practice to establish a level of a priori expectancy), requires the subject to generate a track "just like" those which have been experienced. This is a straightforward free-recall paradigm, and its role in memory research is rather different and tells us more about retention and coding, in contrast to serial anticipation, which is useful for charting the progress and efficiency of learning but at the cost of constraining the subjects' learning strategy.

A key question about Harvey's experiment is whether the performance differences he finds can be legitimately interpreted as differences in the internal memory model or whether they are artifacts of the two recall methods. First it must be said that serial anticipation is about the worst possible way of learning a motor sequence (see von Wright, 1957) probably because there are two sets of events to be remembered, first the actual response made and second whether it was right or wrong. Von Wright found errorless following of the correct movement pattern much more efficient than trial-and-error and, I suspect, so would Harvey's subjects. But all subjects carry out both tasks so it can be argued this should not affect the question of what kind of internal model they form of the task. However the two tasks do have quite different demand characteristics. The phrase "just like" in the generation task could imply similarity in any or all of a number of different dimensions such as reversal frequency, mean excursion amplitude and so on. In the serial anticipation task the subject is specifically required to locate the next target. Harvey's results seem to indicate that in the serial anticipation task subjects are responding to distance rather than direction. It is always possible that under different learning conditions, for instance error-free practice, other features of the track might become prominent. The same could be true for different amounts of practice, as in the classic study of the acquisition of a tracking skill by Fuchs (1962), subjects only became sensitive to the acceleration component of the track after a great deal of practice.

Papers by Frohlich (7) and Swinnen and Walter (8) are concerned with dual task learning and both have something interesting to say about the development of coordination between two limbs based on detailed examination of changes in response patterns over practice. Similar actions carried out simultaneously tend to become entrained, that is temporally coupled. The mastery of a dual task skill may require that the two responses be uncoupled and Swinnen and Walter propose that this becomes possible by a process of temporal staggering in which one action is made to temporarily inhibit the initiation of another. Empirically, the more subjects delayed the initiation of one of the two rather similar arm movements the more the two limbs became uncoupled. The authors are unnecessarily apologetic about introducing an inhibitory deus ex machina. There are plenty of precedents in recent work on serial skills of the necessity for an inhibitory principle, such as Rumelhart and Norman's computer simulation of typing skill (Rumelhart & Norman, 1982) and Mackay's theory of speech generation (MacKay, 1982, 1986). In all these cases it is the timing of the inhibitory process which is critical to fluent performance and so we are left with the problem of how timing is learned.

Frohlich (7) identifies effector function knowledge, knowledge of the correspondence between a movement and its effect on the world, as a significant factor in learning to coordinate the two hands in a bimanual control task. He finds that there are substantial individual differences and it seems that subjects may learn different things as a result of variations in their initial response strategies. I recall once being given an informal lesson in controlling a system with complex dynamics. After some experience with the apparently highly unstable system my tutor suggested I simply "jiggle" the joystick. Not only did my performance improve dramatically but the task looked and felt quite different as I realised, albeit intuitively, that this particular system was sensitive to the acceleration component of the input.

Frohlich argues that specific strategies, for example making alternate left- and right-hand movements in the dual control task, can emerge incidentally as a function of the particular experience of the individual. If this is indeed so it provides a useful insight to the persistence of individual differences in the performance of skilled motor tasks to which Seashore drew attention (Seashore, 1951). With practice performance improves, but not always in the same way for every subject and the performance of individuals tends to become more idiosyncratic rather than uniform with experience.

What, then, does this collection of papers tell us about the issues now facing research on motor control? It has been clear for some time that a classic psychophysical account of movement control (even one which substitutes speed and accuracy for conscious content in the equation) does not work in any straightforward way. There is no simple psychophysical law, even of the more sophisticated "information processing" variety which will hold for a comprehensive range of tasks and subjects. The function of the brain in controlling motor output is not like that of a transmitter with a radio-controlled model plane, or even of a sophisticated autopilot. There are two reasons why variations on the information-processing models of the past 30 years are now seen to be unsatisfactory. The first is that movement information processing is distributed. The second, which is almost certainly a consequence of the first, is that the motor system as a whole is adaptive, changing its operating characteristics as a function of experience and the changing demands of the environment.

The distributed nature of motor control has been well argued and well documented in a number of places but Pew's succinct statement (Pew, 1984) is particularly helpful in respect to the implications of distributed processing for the motor program concept. He argues that it is not always necessary to postulate a central program if the "programmed" characteristics of the motor output can be accounted for by simple biomechanical constraints or relatively local computational processes. If this is the case then great care is needed in drawing conclusions about hypothetical control mechanisms from speed/

accuracy data and about response programming from reaction time experiments. Some of the analyses presented in this symposium, and indeed elsewhere, do not convince me that a satisfactory separation has always been made. We need more discussion of these issues and even closer attention to the justification of particular experimental designs.

I am not arguing that fast aiming and tracking responses are necessarily "non-cognitive", but rather that cognitive processes, including especially learning, may well determine which control processes the subject actually employs. We have begun too slowly to appreciate that practice can invalidate most of the classic generalisations in the motor skills field. The failure of Hick's law after extended practice is the best known example. As Frohlich shows, different strategies may arise from individual experience but instruction and coaching may encourage behaviour which makes certain kinds of learning possible and in this way lead to the adoption of new and effective strategies.

Students of motor control are now facing a new agenda which departs radically from the classical psychophysical and information processing approaches. The very adaptability of motor performance requires a renewed interest in the effects of practice and individual differences on the way in which tasks are performed. Hypothesis-forming research and the use of detailed kinematic analyses will enhance our understanding of programming and control processes more than the search for a unifying psychophysical law.

Note

Numbers in brackets following an author's name in the text denote the chapter number in this volume.

References

Annett, J. (1969). Payoff and the refractory period. Attention and Performance II. (W.G. Koster, Ed.), Acta Psychologica, 30, 65-74.

Annett, J., Annett, M.E., Hudson, P.T.W., & Turner, A. (1979). The control of movement in the preferred and non-preferred hands. Quarterly Journal of Experimental Psychology, 31, 641-652.

Annett, J., Golby, C.W., & Kay, H. (1958). The measurement of elements in an assembly task - the information output of the human motor system. Quarterly Journal of Experimental Psychology, 10, 1-11.

Crossman, E.R.F.W. & Goodeve, P.J. (1963). Feedback control of movement and Fitts' Law. Paper presented to the Experimental Psychology Society, Oxford, July 1963. Published in Quarterly Journal of Experimental Psychology, 1983, 35A, 251-278.

Fitts, P.M. (1954). The information capacity of the human motor system in controlling the amplitude of movement. Journal of Experimental Psychology, 47, 381-391.

Fitts, P.M. & Peterson, J.R. (1964). Information capacity of discrete motor responses. Journal of Experimental Psychology, 67, 103-112.

Fuchs, A.H. (1962). The progression-regression hypothesis in perceptual-motor skill learning. Journal of Experimental Psychology, 63, 177-182.

Henry, F.M. & Rogers, E.E. (1960). Increased response latency for complicated movements and a "memory drum" theory of neuro-motor reaction. Research Quarterly of the American Association for Health, Physical Education and Recreation, 31, 448-458.

Lashley, K.S. (1917). The accuracy of movement in the absence of excitation from the moving organ. American Journal of Physiology, 43, 169-194.

Laszlo, J.I. (1966). The performance of a simple motor task with kinaesthetic sense loss. Quarterly Journal of Experimental Psychology, 18, 1-8.

MacKay, D.G. (1982). The problem of flexibility, fluency and speed-accuracy trade-off in skilled behavior. Psychological Review, 89, 483-506.

MacKay, D.G. (1986). Self inhibition and the disruptive effects of internal and external feedback in skilled behavior. In H. Heuer & C. Fromm (Eds.), Generation and modulation of action patterns. Experimental Brain Research Series 15. Berlin: Springer-Verlag.

Pew, R.W. (1984). A distributed processing view of human motor control. In W. Prinz & A.F. Sanders (Eds.), Cognition and motor processes. Berlin: Springer-Verlag.

Rabbitt, P.M.A. (1981). Sequential reactions. In D.H. Holding (Ed.), Human skills. Chichester: Wiley.

Rumelhart, D.E. & Norman, D.A. (1982). Simulating a skilled typist: a study of skilled cognitive-motor performance. Cognitive Science, 6, 1-36.

Schmidt, R.A., Zelaznik, H.H., Hawkins, B., Frank, J.S., & Quinn, J.T. Jr. (1979). Motor output variability: a theory for the accuracy of rapid motor acts. Psychological Review, 86, 425-451.

Seashore, R.H. (1951). Work and motor performance. In S.S. Stevens (Ed.), Handbook of Experimental Psychology. New York: Wiley.

Sternberg, S., Monsell, S., Knoll, R., & Wright, C. (1978). The latency and duration of rapid movement sequences: comparison of speech and typewriting. In G.E. Stelmach (Ed.), Information processing in motor control and learning. New York: Academic Press.

Taub, E. & Berman, A.J. (1968). Movement and learning in the absence of sensory feedback. In S.J. Freedman (Ed.), The neuropsychology of spatially oriented behavior. Homewood, Illinois: Dorsey Press.

Von Wright, J.M. (1957). A note on the role of guidance in learning. British Journal of Psychology, 48, 133-137.

Wright, C.E. & Meyer, D.E. (1983). Conditions for a linear speed-accuracy trade-off in aimed movements. Quarterly Journal of Experimental Psychology, 35A, 279-296.

Woodworth, R.S. (1899). The accuracy of voluntary movement. Psychological Review Monograph Supplement, 3, (3).

Part II

MOTOR SYSTEMS AND ACTION SYSTEMS APPROACHES TO MOTOR CONTROL

Cognition and Action in Skilled Behaviour
A.M. Colley and J.R. Beech (Editors)

MOVEMENT METAPHORS

Martin R. Sheridan
University of Hull

The motor systems approach and action systems approach are compared. The exclusive prescription for research offered by action theorists, and criticisms directed at a restricted understanding of motor systems concepts, are rejected. The divergence between motor and action systems is considered in terms of, i) The Cartesian Reflex, and ii) The Cartesian Doctrine of Corporeal Ideas. In relation to the reflex, two arguments are advanced. First, that the attack made by action theorists on the reflex, is an attack on the simple Cartesian conception. This ignores a considerable body of early work which radically modified this view, and which has been incorporated into motor systems thinking. Second, that the implicit analogy drawn by action theorists between reflex and motor program in terms of the "release" of a response, has the effect of grossly oversimplifying the concept of motor programming. The implications of the Cartesian Doctrine of Corporeal Ideas are discussed, and finally, a number of arguments and sources of evidence pertinent to the controversy are considered. While favouring the motor systems approach, it is concluded that both approaches have positive contributions to make to our understanding of movement.

> "It is the theory which decides what we can find."
> Albert Einstein

I should say at the beginning of this debate that I adopt an eclectic approach to scientific advance, and that I believe that both the motor systems approach and the action systems approach have positive contributions to make to our understanding of movement. This may cause some raised eyebrows, particularly when one considers Michaels and Carello's (1981) statement concerning the "direct" approach to perception (which equates with the action systems position) compared to the "indirect" or traditional approach (which equates with the motor systems position). They argue that:

> The two approaches ask wholly different questions. Indeed, there is so little common ground that arguments between proponents of each approach are often exercises

> in futility or, at best, exercises in frustration. Answers cannot be compared because the questions are different. Questions cannot be compared because the underlying metatheories are different. (p.17)

I hope that the discussion will not be one of total futility or frustration, even though I am going to oppose the exclusive prescription for research offered by action theorists, and the criticisms directed at a restricted understanding of concepts such as "motor program". It seems perplexing that to accept Reed's (1982) assertions concerning "tenable procedures" of experimentation, would exclude most of the contributions to the recent International Conference on Skilled Behaviour, on which the present volume is based. Moreover, action theorists / direct perceptionists (e.g. Michaels & Carello, 1981; Reed, 1982, 1984) extend their line of argument to reject the approaches of psychophysiology, cognitive psychology, in fact all of traditional psychology, so no one need feel left out!

The Concise Oxford Dictionary defines a metaphor as, "Application of name or descriptive term to an object to which it is not literally applicable". The title of the paper was chosen because throughout history we have described human movement and action using terms and concepts at the current forefront of technical or intellectual development, but which are not literally applicable to human behaviour. The value of metaphors and analogical argument, lies not in any exact description or explanation of the movement system thus provided, rather, it lies in aiding the organization of our thinking and the assimilation of observations into a coherent framework. Note, however, that coherent does not necessarily imply "correct". There is no reason to suppose that current metaphors exactly reflect some discoverable "reality". If such were the case we would be at the end of our scientific quest.

An Historical Perspective

Around 387 B.C. Plato proposed that the brain was the "seat of the soul". He derived this insight not by experimentation but by reasoning. The perfect geometrical shape, he argued, is a sphere, where else could the rational soul be, but in the spherical head, the summit of the body? Physicians of the Hippocratic School four hundred years before Christ also believed that the Sacred Disease of epilepsy, and madness itself, were disturbances of the brain. In contrast, Aristotle, whose gift to science was the method of observation, considered that the seat of the soul was the heart. The soul was seen as a mover, an animator, and what is more necessary for movement and life than the free flow of blood through the body?

Such ideas were incorporated into the hydraulic model which saw its most complete expression by Descartes in the seventeenth century. According to Descartes sensory stimulation produced a flux of the "animal spirits" contained in the heart and arteries. The heart then pushed the spirits into the cerebral ventricles, much as the pumps of an organ push air into its pipes. The animal spirits inflated the cavities and pulled on little tubes which were attached to them, just as the wind can, "fill up the sails of a ship, and pull all the lines attached to them under tension" (Descartes, 1664). Pores were opened in the ventricles and animal spirits flowed down hollow tubes in the centres of the nerves to inflate the muscle, which then moved the limb. The analogies of the pump of a pipe organ or the inflated sail, and the conception of cavities and tubes, served to support the notion that neural information was transmitted via circulatory fluid in the nerves. It was not until Galvani's discovery of "animal electricity" in 1791 that electrical propagation of nervous activity began to supplant animal spirits, although it took until 1850 to become firmly established. The Cartesian conception of cerebral function presents a rigidly structured view of simple automatic reflexes.

The divergence between action and motor systems will, for present purposes, be considered to start with Descartes (circa 1664). There are two main points of departure:-

i) The Cartesian Reflex.
ii) The Cartesian Doctrine of Corporeal Ideas.

The Cartesian Reflex

In this section I shall argue two things. First, that the attack made by action theorists on the reflex, is an attack on the simple Cartesian conception. This ignores a considerable body of early work which radically modified this view, and which has been incorporated into motor systems thinking. Second, there has been implicit analogy drawn by action theorists between reflex and motor program in terms of the "release" of a response. This has the effect of grossly oversimplifying the concept of motor programming. A motor program is thus seen as, "a central command pattern for generating a given pattern of movement" (Reed, 1982, p.102). Keele's (1968) narrow interpretation of a motor program as, "a set of muscle commands that are structured before a movement sequence begins, and that allows the entire sequence to be carried out uninfluenced by peripheral feedback" (p.387) has thus been, almost exclusively, the target for criticism. Even here, Keele's conception was not intended as an exhaustive definition of how a motor program is structured and executed, and in a later paper (Keele, 1981) he modified his view to consider a general central representation of movement.

The Reflex Concept

In attacking the motor program concept, action theorists point to experimental work from the 1970s and 1980s indicating that reflexes are not based on, "unmodifiable input-output connections" (Reed, 1982, p.102). Evidence is provided that the simple reflex movements involved in stepping (Forssberg, Grillner & Rossignol, 1977), looking (Gonshor & Melville-Jones, 1976) and chewing (Lund & Rossignol, 1981) are attuned to the current situation of the movement. In spinal preparations both temporal adjustments to context (Ghez & Shinoda, 1978) and spatially adaptive modulations are discussed (Fukson, Berkenblit & Feldman, 1980). For example, Fukson et al. (1980) have shown that in the spinal frog, hindlimb movements based on the wiping reflex will alter their trajectory to compensate for movement of an irritated limb. But this is not evidence illustrating a new principle, and requiring a new theory of movement. Such adaptive responses have been known for many years.

In 1877 Pfluger noted that if a drop of acid was placed on the side of a decapitated frog, then while flexing its limb it was able to rub the irritated area with its foot. If one then amputated the foot, after several unsuccessful attempts with its mutilated limb, the frog eventually achieved the same end result by using the other, still intact foot. A rather dramatic early demonstration of an adaptive reflex. It is clear that the spinal animal produces no voluntary movements and remains immobile if not stimulated, but that it can react in an adaptive manner when stimulated. In the 1880s Goltz demonstrated this not only in the spinal frog, but in a series of long-term experiments with dogs. He destroyed the brain with a pressurized jet of water injected through a hole in the skull. One such animal was able to live for eight months. Unstimulated, the dog without a cerebrum seemed to sleep. A loud noise "woke" it up, a painful stimulus made it growl, and it would swallow food put at the back of its mouth. Placed on its legs it would even walk, a response requiring considerable coordination of activity.

Sherrington (1906) was quite clear that the simple reflex,

> ... is probably a purely abstract conception, because all parts of the nervous system are connected together, and no part is probably ever capable of reaction without affecting and being affected by various other parts. (p.8)

The simple reflex was thus seen as always being integrated into an action which exceeded it, and which included it as a constituent element. Furthermore, it has been clear for some time that reflexive activity interacts with learning. It is evident that an organism's response to pain has considerable evolutionary significance. However, in his work on conditioned reflexes Pavlov was able to transform overt pain to apparent pleasure, by combining an electric shock with the appearance of food. At first the dog reacted violently to each shock and its appetite was considerably reduced, but later there was no sign of pain, and when the shock came the dog salivated, wagged its tail and turned expectantly to its bowl. More remarkable are some experiments reported by Melzack (1973) on the social context of reflexes. When dogs reared in total isolation were released, they seemed to have little or no sense of pain. They would return repeatedly to sniff at a burning match, and were apparently unable to learn the danger of it.

The Motor Program Concept

Let us return to the concept of a motor program as a structured set of muscle commands, since this seems to be a major point of confusion and the object of action theorists' criticism. Since Flourens' work in the 1820s it has been clear that any higher level motor program would not contain specific instructions for particular muscles. Flourens transposed the nerves normally responsible for raising and lowering the wing in a chicken. According to Flourens, the animal could fly as well as before the experiment. The same type of experiment was subsequently performed in numerous species by different researchers. The general opinion was that the new innervation fulfilled, without fail, its new function (Jeannerod, 1985). Goldstein in the 1930s (Goldstein, 1934) was greatly influenced by this work, and by the "theory of resonance" conceived by Paul Weiss. This type of intervention was thus used in humans paralyzed by trauma or illness such as poliomyelitis. Movements such as extension of the hand or elevation of the foot are essential for the preservation of prehension or normal gait. If an extensor muscle responsible for these postures is paralyzed, it can be replaced by transposition of another, less important muscle, on to its tendon. The muscle was transposed complete with its original innervation, and although the muscle may have had a completely different function, such as flexion, the patients were able to achieve appropriate use of their extremity when they concentrated on the task.

It is no wonder that Requin and his colleagues at the C.N.R.S. (e.g. Requin, Semjen & Bonnet, 1984) despair of attacks made on a motor program conceived of as a rigid set of commands. The early work, together with concepts such as, "kinetic formula" (Liepmann, 1900), "motor scheme" (Head, 1920), "schema" (Bartlett, 1932), "scheme of action" (Del Bianco, 1947) and "action plan" (Miller, Galanter & Pribram, 1960), are all variants of the general idea that a central representation of action contributes to the structuring of the outputs responsible for movement. This is quite different from arguing that the final form of the movement is specified centrally. The kinematic shape of movement unfolds as the result of the interplay of many factors in the hierarchical system. It is this idea which is developed in modern theories of motor programming. Indeed, Bernstein (1967) proposed broadly conceived motor programs or "engrams". The notion of hierarchical motor organization is not new (Bryan & Harter, 1897; Woodworth, 1899). More recently, others (Turvey, Shaw & Mace, 1978) have, along with Bernstein (1967), argued that there cannot be a direct correspondence between the representation of action and the detailed form of the movement. Higher levels are thus argued to have fewer degrees of freedom in determining specific movement details than lower levels. Conversely, higher levels clearly have more freedom in determining the overall action. The context in which the movement occurs, the task demands, the desired outcome, the expectations of the performer, all affect the final detailed specification of the response. The hierarchical view does not mean, however, that higher levels necessarily control lower levels. Lashley (1951) discussed the integration of levels and the transfer of control between them. The concept of transfer of control is important because, as Broadbent (1977) points out, it avoids a rigid view of levels and hierarchies. For, rather than higher levels necessarily incorporating and controlling lower levels it becomes necessary to understand the influence of one level on another, and to recognize that control can shift between levels, or even appear to reside at several levels of complexity simultaneously, with processes occurring in parallel at different levels. Thus, Jeannerod (1985) writes:

> The conceptual level has no order to give to the operational level: the hierarchy of levels we are discussing should be thought of only in terms of the

> information they contain. What the conceptual level transmits to the operational levels concerns the goal to be attained, the general climate in which the action will take place, the nature of the programs to be constructed. In return, the operational level informs the conceptual level of the degree of execution of the action: it is by this constant flux of information, circulating in both directions, that a level can know its own state and influence the state of other levels. (p.123)

The control of movement can be seen as being distributed vertically and horizontally in the nervous system. Such a conception has sometimes been referred to as a heterarchy. We should be quite clear that this concept owes nothing to the hierarchies of association or connection alluded to by action theorists. There is no difficulty in reconciling this view with concepts such as synergy (Bernstein, 1967; Ferrier, 1886), functional synergy (Kelso, Putnam & Goodman, 1983), co-ordinative structures (Easton, 1972; Michaels & Carello, 1981), and the equations of constraint discussed by Turvey and his colleagues (Turvey, Fitch & Tuller, 1982). Underlying such discussion is the idea that much of the co-ordination and control of movement can take place at a relatively low level in the system, and the motor systems approach would add, thereby reducing the amount of movement control that needs to be computed at higher levels. Runeson and Frykholm (1983) have elegantly stated the basic rationale for this view:

> We must not think of our anatomy as arbitrarily concatenated. Rather, our geometrical proportions, the distribution of mass, the intricate connections of muscles and tendons across joints, and the elasticity and damping of the tissues have been delicately tuned through evolution to provide adequate constraints. In the dynamic system thus established the options for motion have been reduced substantially toward those conducive to adaptive action. (p.593)

In a similar vein, the "peripheral"/"central" dichotomy claimed by Reed (1982) also needs to be rejected. There is no border between the perceptual domain and the motor domain in our representation of the outside world. For years we have talked about perceptual-motor skills, meaning just that. One can consider so-called "mixed" theories of motor control in which the central and peripheral origin of motor command are closely integrated. It is known that control processes occur during responses (Ostry, 1980) and that feedforward control, based on perceptual knowledge, is used in addition to sensory feedback (Arbib, 1981, 1984; Poulton, 1952). Thus, there are conceptions in which feedback and feedforward mechanisms are the source of the adaptive flexibility of control exerted by different levels in the hierarchy (Brooks, 1979). The program concept has, moreover, been extended to include postural adjustments accompanying and/or anticipating movements (Gahery & Massion, 1981). Mixed approaches to motor control have been widely advocated (e.g. Bizzi, 1980; Kelso, 1978) and Reed (1982) acknowledges that they "have much to offer", but rejects them because he perceives confusions and conceptual difficulties.

Direct versus Mediated Action

This brings us to the main point at issue, the rejection by proponents of action systems and direct perception of not just the motor systems approach, but of all "traditional" psychology. This involves the rejection of all cognitive or epistemic mediators including representations, schemas, programs, models, organizing principles, meanings, concepts and the like (Turvey & Kugler, 1984).

To support their position, action systems theorists frequently cite the work of Bernstein and Gibson. Differences of interpretation clearly exist, however, concerning the work of these authors. Such differences, in their extreme, are exemplified by the writing of American based scientists such as Turvey, Shaw, Mace, Kugler, Michaels, Carello, Reed, etc., compared to the position of French scientists such as Requin, Bonnet, Semjen, Jeannerod, etc.. To be sure, there are numerous points of contact and agreement, particularly in relation to Bernstein's work, and much of his thinking has influenced modern motor systems approaches. More contentious are the interpretations and implications of Gibson's position (e.g. Gibson, 1950, 1966, 1979). Interestingly, Jeannerod (1985) describes Gibson as a behaviourist, a description which I imagine would mortify his supporters, with its vision of stimulus-response cycles. And yet, while rejecting behaviourism and reaffirming the mediated nature of perception and action, Jeannerod is quite comfortable with the Gibsonian concept of "affordance". Similarly, Neisser (1976) uses the concept of affordance to argue that perception informs us about things as more than "mere objects", geographically and physically defined. Thus, he writes:

> In the normal environment most perceptible objects and events are <u>meaningful</u>. They afford various possibilities for action, carry implications about what has happened or what will happen, belong coherently to a larger context, possess an identity that transcends their simple physical properties. These meanings can be, and are, perceived. (pp.70-71)

Despite this, Neisser's work is rejected by direct perceptionists and action theorists (e.g. Michaels & Carello, 1981). Where does the divergence arise? Followers of Gibson's approach believe that knowledge of the world is obtained directly unaided by inference, memories, or representations. Perception is seen simply as the detection of information, and information is structure that specifies an environment to an animal. Information is structure generated in a lawful way by environmental structure (e.g. surface layout), and by movements of the animal. Thus, a perceiver is said to directly perceive its environment and no elaboration is needed. In contrast, the indirect approach argues that knowledge of the environment is a derivative of information processing and that perception involves the intervention of memories, representations, etc.. Cognitive psychologists thus consider that an affordance is derived, Gibson considers that it is perceived directly.

The Cartesian Doctrine of Corporeal Ideas

To find the point of departure we need to return to Descartes. Descartes, like Plato, doubted the reliability of his senses. Simply stated, his doctrine proposed that all knowledge is knowledge about states of the mind. The generic use of the term "body" included the brain and nervous system, which he distinguished from the soul or mind. The problem then posed is, how one can know and act upon the environment, when the ideas one has about such things are based on awarenesses simply of brain states. Descartes proposed rules, inferences, and judgements, to obtain "indirect" evidence about activity and environment from "directly" given brain states. According to this principle human perception and action are not direct, but mediated, that is, we actively construct our perception and knowledge of the world. In current terminology, the mediators are such things as programs, schemas, models, concepts, representations, etc., which are at the heart of traditional psychology. Turvey and Kugler (1984) argue, however, that:

> ... there is nothing in this explanation to guarantee that the proposed inferential operations performed on the brain states will yield conclusions that are objective and accurate rather than fatuous. (p.379)

I oppose this assertion for a number of reasons, although I do not have the space to develop the argument fully. Turvey and Kugler derive the need for objectivity and accuracy, from Bernstein's (1967) arguments concerning the need for accurate awareness of the objective facts of the environment and of one's actions, for meaningful and reliable control of adaptive activity. What might "accurate" and "objective" mean? One can consider this at both a conceptual and operational level. At a conceptual level we can, and do, hold many beliefs or hypotheses about the world that may be inaccurate, and yet still act reasonably successfully within the world. Did it affect the survival of early man whether or not he believes that sacrificing to the gods would produce a good harvest? Such a belief may be both inaccurate and lack objectivity, but it need not affect survival, although it clearly would affect behaviour. Hypotheses that we hold can affect our perceptions and actions, and can even influence our tests of those hypotheses. In early microscopy, scientists saw and drew tiny proto-people within sperm cells. What they saw was, in part, constructed from and constrained by what they expected to see. If invariant properties of the optic array specify structure directly, why do people not see the same thing when they look down a microscope? There are many examples of this type in psychology.

According to Einstein's relativity principle, "objective" would simply mean agreement between observers. At a conceptual or operational level, for a particular factor, the greater the intervention of evolutionary pressure, the greater the likelihood of agreement between conspecific observers. Thus, I see shapes, textures, etc. the same way as other humans. One could not say, however, that my perception was more accurate or objective than lower animals. Another example is our adaptation to distorted vision. Our perception of the world here is both "subjective" and "inaccurate", nevertheless, we can adapt relatively successfully to the distortion, where it is consistent. This idea of consistency is important, because it relates to the tests of our inferences. As I understand it, Descartes does not deny a "real" and consistent world, only our ability to know it directly. I have not got the space available for a full philosophical discourse, but I believe that the Gordian knot of regressive inference Turvey outlines (e.g. Turvey & Kugler, 1984) can be cut. The inferences and tests of the inferences derive from association, experience / societal evolution ("memes" etc.), and genetic evolution, depending on the level of analysis. "Objectivity" and "accuracy" are tested at the conceptual and operational levels through agreement between conspecific observers, framed by lawful physical relationships where these bear on the issue. Thus, for example, evolution has intervened such that, "infants are born with biodynamic structures that embody a certain 'knowledge' or functional readiness for experience of objects" (Trevarthen, 1984, p.252), as evidenced by orienting and pre-reaching behaviours.

Arguments and Evidence

In this section a number of sources of evidence pertinent to the motor systems / action systems controversy are considered. Ullman (1980) has outlined a number of arguments against direct perception which pose a problem for action theorists, but these will not be discussed in detail here. For further consideration of some of the theoretical issues, the reader is referred to Fodor and Pylyshyn (1981) and to the reply by Turvey, Shaw, Reed and Mace (1981).

i) There is now a considerable body of work on the use of the time-to-contact variable (T(t)) in adaptive behaviour (e.g. Lee, 1976 1980). I can see no overriding reason for the motor systems approach to dispute the significance of this work, particularly when one considers locomotor activity. Whether such information is perceived directly, or computed at a low level in a hierarchical system, seems largely a matter of perspective, as does whether one talks of catching a ball in terms of T(t) (Lee, 1980) or feedforward and feedback processes (Arbib, 1984). Those advocating direct perception and ecological realism, do not deny mediation in the sense that, "perceptual systems modulate information" (Michaels & Carello, 1981, p.182), that is, brain structure operates to "detect" information not "manufacture" it. It seems strange to argue that although evolution may have (via invariant optical structure) designed a perceptual computer, it does not compute. Similarly, whether an affordance is seen as being perceived directly or indirectly is again a matter of philosophical perspective. For infants, a visual drop in the visual cliff experiments does not afford support, and so is avoided. If the invariant optical structure specifies an affordance for a particular animal-environment interaction, then infants at a particular stage of development ought to respond similarly to the visual cliff. There is, however, evidence from research on locomotion artificially assisted by means of wheeled "crawlers" or "walkers" before unaided crawling or walking is possible, that infants show variation in sensitivity to a visual drop (Rader, Bausano & Richards, 1980). Avoidance of the deep side of a visual cliff may occur for crawling before it does for walking, however, it should be remembered that in both cases the infant would fall.

ii) In support of the action systems position Turvey (Turvey & Kugler, 1984) and Reed (1982) refer to Lishman and Lee's (1973) study indicating that humans walking forward will report they are moving backwards when given global optical information generated by backward locomotion. Turvey, however, suggests that they report walking backwards. This is clearly not the same thing, and the reafferent information discussed by Held (1965) would certainly make any such report odd. Reed only suggests that subjects report moving backwards. The situation is analogous to walking slowly the wrong way on a moving walkway; are we surprised at our ability to say that we are travelling backwards? Many of Lee's experiments demonstrate the dominance of vision when compared with other sources of information. The reason seems clear. Vision provides, amongst other things, feedforward information, the ability to predict what will happen in the future, thus allowing anticipation.

iii) Accounting for the adaptation to distorting prisms can be argued to be a problem for the action systems approach. While adaptation has been reported with passive movement, adaptation is quicker and more complete with active movement (Pick & Hay, 1965; Welch, 1978). Thus, with two people wearing prisms, one walking and pushing the other in a wheelchair, the active subject adapts better. Held's ideas and data oppose Gibson point for point. Gibson's supporters try to account for adaptation by a process of "normalization". That is, some axes are argued to be omnipresent (through gravity, the vertical). Subjects can indeed "normalize" to a room tilted a few degrees, but the subjects have been free to move their head and eyes, as has been the case in many studies of passive adaptation.

iv) Reed (1982) has cited Darwin's (1881) observations of earthworms, in support of the action systems position. Worms are argued to perceive that leaves have an affordance for plugging burrows. The behaviour of worms in plugging burrows is not a fixed action pattern, but is adaptive to conditions. Thus if the weather is too cold or dry, worms plug the burrows more effectively. Precision of behaviour is increased as the problem becomes more acute. Rather than recourse to perception of an affordance, such behaviour could be explained by a variant of Miller, Galanter and Pribram's (1960) TOTE. This, coupled with the likelihood that "pulling leaves the best way to plug burrows" has been selected by evolution, could account for the observed behaviour.

v) The work of von Hofsten (1979, 1980) on infants' reaching behaviour is also cited by action theorists as supporting their position. As with Darwin's worms, the infants increased precision when the motor problem became more acute. However, this observation is perfectly compatible with the motor systems approach. It is the simplified notion of programming that leads action theorists to believe that these data support only their position. In any event, von Hofsten (1983) explains the performance by assuming that the infant makes a direct internal representation of the various vectors of displacement.

vi) Action theorists argue that responses are not "released" and that actions are not "triggered". Reed (1982) goes so far as to assert that, "under almost all environmental circumstances this never occurs" (p.109). There are, in fact, many examples of released action patterns in the animal literature. For example, Bolles and Woods (1964) observed an adult scratching pattern in the neonate rat, and even though no contact was actually made with the skin, the animal proceeded to clean its paw after the pseudo-scratching sequence. More importantly, Trevarthen (1984), when observing the pre-reaching grasp to objects in newborn human infants, concluded that, "although the form of movement was pre-adapted to grasp an object, its evocation was not dependent upon perception of a target" (p.238). That is, it could be triggered without the infant seeing a target to grasp. Such reaching and grasping are, moreover, observed before birth (Humphrey, 1969).

vii) Shepard's experiments in the early 1970s on mentally rotating 3-D objects (e.g. Shepard & Metzler, 1971) would seem to present a problem for the action systems approach. One had to say whether two tachistoscopically presented objects, having different angles of rotation, were the same or different. The time taken to decide depended on the difference in the angle of rotation, with the implication that subjects were mentally rotating the objects. Similarly, if you ask someone to travel a route in their mind, the longer one waits, the further along the route they are. Proponents of Gibson's direct perception attempt to counter such criticisms by arguing that perception need not be direct in time, but can occur over a period of time. In fact, proponents of direct perception deny a past-present-future trichotomy, thus denying memory-perception-expectation. There is acceptance that perceivers have experiences of "nowness" but they suggest that it is illusory.

viii) It is difficult to see how the ecological approach can account for experiential dimensions of a hedonic tone (humour, pleasure etc.) that appear to have no physical stimulus referents. The answer provided by action theorists, that they must be very high-order, seems rather weak. Does the optical information contained in looking at a watch directly specify the time? Furthermore, regarding higher- and lower-order invariants, what rule specifies "the ordering of abstract properties all of which, one would think, are equally abstract in their description" (Kolers, 1978)? Action theorists have, as yet, provided no answer.

ix) Visual agnosia (e.g. Humphreys & Riddoch, 1987) would seem to present a real problem for direct perception. Here, the visual information is available but there is no understanding, the conceptual level is absent.

x) Lastly, and probably most seriously, learning does not fit easily into the action theorist's position. They attempt to account for learning by arguing that events can change the structures upon which direct perception depends, although the explanatory power of this notion would seem limited.

Having presented some problems with the action systems approach, what does it add to our understanding of motor behaviour? First, a perspective on the richness of optic information (optic flow field, time-to-contact etc.) and the degree to which movement is controlled at a low level in the system. This complements the motor systems approach and is a significant addition, particularly when considering locomotion. Second, an emphasis on the importance of the interaction between animal and environment, which has the spin-off of cautioning us against the over-free use of cognitive theorizing and model building.

In a speech delivered in 1872, du Bois-Reymond concluded that there are absolute limits to our knowledge of nature: "Ignoramus, ignorabimus". I think that we may approach an understanding, but only by attacking it from different perspectives and at different levels of analysis. As quoted at the start of this paper, it was Einstein who argued that, "It is the theory which decides what we can find". Attempting to restrict research options constrains our ability to gather and assimilate information, since there is a tendency for humans to operate as "confirmatory hypothesis-testers" (Snyder, 1981). In the spirit of rhetorical argument (Billig, 1987; Shotter, 1986), I trust that I have confirmed my hypothesis!

References

Arbib, M.A. (1981). Perceptual structures and distributed motor control. In V.B. Brooks (Ed.), Handbook of physiology, Section 1, The nervous system, Vol.II, Part 2, Motor control. Bethesda, Md.: American Physiological Society.

Arbib, M.A. (1984). From synergies and embryos to motor schemas. In H.T.A. Whiting (Ed.), Human motor actions: Bernstein reassessed. Amsterdam: North-Holland.

Bartlett, F.C. (1932). Remembering. Cambridge: Cambridge University Press.

Bernstein, N.A. (1967). The coordination and regulation of movement. London: Pergamon Press.

Billig, M. (1987). Arguing and thinking: A rhetorical approach to social psychology. Cambridge: Cambridge University Press.

Bizzi, E. (1980). Central and peripheral mechanisms in motor control. In G.E. Stelmach & J. Requin (Eds.), Tutorials in motor behavior. Amsterdam: North-Holland.

Bolles, R.C. & Woods, P.J. (1964). The ontogeny of behaviour in the albino rat. Animal Behaviour, 12, 427-441.

Broadbent, D.E. (1977). Levels, hierarchies and locus of control. Quarterly Journal of Experimental Psychology, 29, 181-201.

Brooks, V.B. (1979). Motor programs revisited. In R.E. Talbott & D.R. Humphrey (Eds.), Posture and movement. New York: Raven Press.

Bryan, W.L. & Harter, N. (1897). Studies in the physiology and psychology of the telegraphic language. Psychological Review 4, 27-53.

Darwin, C. (1881). The formation of vegetable mould through the action of worms, with observations on their habits. London: J. Murray.

Del Bianco. (1947). Cited in H.T.A. Whiting (Ed.), Human motor actions: Bernstein reassessed. Amsterdam: North Holland, 1984, p.479.

Descartes, R. (1664). Traite de l'homme. Leiden. Reproduced in F. Alquie (Ed.), Descartes, R. Oeuvres philosophiques. Paris: Garnier, 1963.

du Bois-Reymond, E. (1872). Uber die grenzen des naturkennens. Leipzig. Cited by M. Jeannerod, The brain machine. Cambridge, Ma.: Harvard University Press, 1985.

Easton, T.A. (1972). On the normal use of reflexes. American Scientist, 60, 591-599.

Ferrier, D. (1886). The functions of the brain. London: Smith, Elder.

Flourens, P. (1824). Recherches experimentales sur les proprietes et les fonctions du systeme nerveux dans les animaux vertebres. Paris: Crevot; 2nd expanded ed., Paris: Bailliere, 1842.

Fodor, J.A. & Pylyshyn, J.W. (1981). How direct is visual perception? : Some reflections on Gibson's "Ecological Approach". Cognition, 9, 139-196.

Forssberg, H., Grillner, S., & Rossignol, S. (1977). Phasic gain control of reflexes from the dorsum of the paw during spinal locomotion. Brain Research, 132, 121-139.

Fukson, O.I., Berkenblit, M.B., & Feldman, A.G. (1980). The spinal frog takes into account the scheme of its body during the wiping reflex. Science, 209, 1261-1263.

Gahery, Y. & Massion, J. (1981). Co-ordination between posture and movement. Trends in Neurosciences, 1981, 4, 199-202.

Ghez, C. & Shinoda, Y. (1978). Spinal mechanisms of the functional stretch reflex. Experimental Brain Research, 32, 55-68.

Gibson, J.J. (1950). The perception of the visual world. Boston: Houghton-Mifflin.

Gibson, J.J. (1966). The senses considered as perceptual systems. Boston: Houghton-Mifflin.

Gibson, J.J. (1979). The ecological approach to visual perception. Boston: Houghton-Mifflin.

Goldstein, K. (1934). Der aufbau des organismus. The Hague: Nijhoff.

Goltz, F.L. (1880). Cited in Jeannerod, M. The brain machine. Cambridge, M.A.: Harvard University Press, 1985, p.32.

Gonshor, A. & Melville-Jones, G. (1976). Short term adaptive changes in the human vestibulo-ocular reflex arc. Journal of Physiology, 256, 361-379.

Head, H. (1920). Studies in neurology 2. London: Frowde, Hodder & Stoughton.

Held, R. (1965). Plasticity in the sensory motor system. Scientific American, 213, 84-94.

Humphrey, T. (1969). Postnatal repetitions of human prenatal activity sequences with some suggestions of their neuroanatomical basis. In R.J. Robinson (Ed.), Brain and early behaviour. London: Academic Press.

Humphreys, G.W. & Riddoch, M.J. (1987). To see but not to see: A case study of visual agnosia. Hillsdale, N.J.: Erlbaum.

Jeannerod, M. (1985). The brain machine. Cambridge, M.A.: Harvard University Press.

Keele, S.W. (1968). Movement control in skilled motor performance. Psychological Bulletin, 70, 387-402.

Keele, S.W. (1981). Behavioural analysis of motor control. In V.B. Brooks (Ed.), Handbook of Physiology, Section 1, The nervous system, Vol.II, Part 2, motor control. Bethesda, Md.: Amer-

ican Physiology Society.
Kelso, J.A.S. (1978). Joint receptors do not provide a satisfactory basis for motor timing and positioning. Psychological Review, 85, 474-481.
Kelso, J.A.S., Putnam, C.A., & Goodman, D. (1983). On the space-time structure of human interlimb co-ordination. Quarterly Journal of Experimental Psychology, 35A, 347-375.
Kolers, P.A. (1978). Light waves. Contemporary Psychology, 23, 227-228.
Lashley, K.S. (1951). The problem of serial order in behavior. In L.A. Jeffress (Ed.), Cerebral mechanisms in behavior. New York: Wiley.
Lee, D.N. (1976). A theory of visual control of braking based on information about time-to-collision. Perception, 5, 437-459.
Lee, D.N. (1980). Visuo-motor coordination in space-time. In G.E. Stelmach & J. Requin (Eds.), Tutorials in motor behavior. Amsterdam: North-Holland.
Liepmann, V. (1900). Das krankheitsbild der apraxia ("motorischen asymbolie") auf grund eines falles von einseitiger apraxie. Monatschrift fur Psychiatrie und Neurologie, 8, 15-44, 102-132, 188-197.
Lishman, J. & Lee, D.N. (1973). The autonomy of visual kinaesthesis. Perception, 2, 287-294.
Lund, J. & Rossignol, S. (1981). Modulation of the amplitude of the digastric jaw opening reflex during the masticatory cycle. Neuroscience, 6, 95-98.
Melzack, R. (1973). The puzzle of pain. Harmondsworth: Penguin Books.
Michaels, C.F. & Carello, C. (1981). Direct perception. Englewood Cliffs, N.J.: Prentice-Hall.
Miller, G.A., Galanter, E., & Pribram, K.H. (1960). Plans and the structure of behavior. New York: Holt, Rinehart & Winston.
Neisser, U. (1976). Cognition and reality. San Francisco: Freeman.
Ostry, D.J. (1980). Execution-time movement control. In G.E. Stelmach & J. Requin (Eds.), Tutorials in motor behavior. Amsterdam: North-Holland.
Pfluger (1877). Cited in Jeannerod, M. The brain machine. Cambridge, M.A.: Harvard University Press, 1985, p.31.
Pick, Jr., H.L. & Hay, J.C. (1965). A passive test of the Held reafference hypothesis. Perceptual and Motor Skills, 20, 1070-1072.
Poulton, E.C. (1952). Perceptual anticipation in tracking with two-pointer and one-pointer displays. British Journal of Psychology, 43, 222-229.
Rader, N., Bausano, M., & Richards, J.E. (1980). On the nature of visual-cliff-avoidance response in human infants. Child Development, 51, 61-68.
Reed, E.S. (1982). An outline of a theory of action systems. Journal of Motor Behavior, 14, 98-134.
Reed, E.S. (1984). From action Gestalts to direct action. In H.T.A. Whiting (Ed.), Human motor actions: Bernstein reassessed. Amsterdam: North-Holland.
Requin, J., Semjen, a., & Bonnet, M. (1984). Bernstein's purposeful brain. In H.T.A. Whiting (Ed.), Human motor actions: Bernstein reassessed. Amsterdam: North-Holland.
Runeson, S. & Frykholm, G. (1983). Kinematic specification of dynamics as an informational basis for person-and-action

perception: expectation, gender, recognition, and deceptive intention. Journal of Experimental Psychology: General, 112, 585-615.

Shepard, R.N. & Metzler, J. (1971). Mental rotation of three-dimensional objects. Science, 171, 701-703.

Sherrington, C.S. (1906). The integrative action of the nervous system. New Haven: Yale University Press.

Shotter, J. (1986). The rhetoric of theory in psychology. In J.F.H. van Rappard, A.W. Staarts, & M.E. Hyland (Eds.), Proceedings of the Founding Conference of the International Society for Theoretical Psychology. Amsterdam: North-Holland.

Snyder, M. (1981). Seek and ye shall find: Testing hypotheses about other people. In E.T. Higgins, C.P. Herman, & M.P. Zanna (Eds.), Social cognition: The Ontario symposium (Vol. 1). Hillsdale, N.J.: Erlbaum.

Trevarthen, C. (1984). How control of movement develops. In H.T.A. Whiting (Ed.), Human motor actions: Bernstein reassessed. Amsterdam: North-Holland.

Turvey, M.T., Fitch, H.L., & Tuller, B. (1982). The Bernstein perspective. I. The problems of degrees of freedom and context-conditioned variability. In J.A.S. Kelso (Ed.), Human motor behavior: An introduction. Hillsdale, N.J.: Erlbaum.

Turvey, M.T. & Kugler, P.N. (1984). An ecological approach to perception and action. In H.T.A. Whiting (Ed.), Human motor actions: Bernstein reassessed. Amsterdam: North-Holland.

Turvey, M.T., Shaw, R.E., & Mace, W. (1978). Issues in the theory of action: degrees of freedom, coordinative structures and coalitions. In J. Requin (Ed.), Attention and performance VII. Hillsdale, N.J.: Erlbaum.

Turvey, M.T., Shaw, R.E., Reed, E.S., & Mace, W.M. (1981). Ecological laws of perceiving and acting: In reply to Fodor and Pylyshyn (1981). Cognition, 9, 237-304.

Ullman, S. (1980). Against direct perception. Behavioral and Brain Sciences, 3, 373-415.

von Hofsten, C. (1979). Development of visually directed reaching: The approach phase. Journal of Human Movement Studies, 5, 160-178.

von Hofsten, C. (1980). Predictive reaching for moving objects by human infants. Journal of Experimental Child Psychology, 30, 369-382.

von Hofsten, C. (1983). Catching skills in infancy. Journal of Experimental Psychology: Human Perception and Performance, 9, 75-85.

Welch, R.B. (1978). Perceptual modification: Adapting to altered sensory environments. New York: Academic Press.

Woodworth, R.S. (1899). The accuracy of voluntary movement. Psychological Review Monograph Supplements, 3, No.3.

Cognition and Action in Skilled Behaviour
A.M. Colley and J.R. Beech (Editors)

REPRESENTATIONAL AND PHYSICAL ACCOUNTS OF MOTOR CONTROL AND LEARNING: CAN THEY ACCOUNT FOR THE DATA?

R.G. Marteniuk, C.L. Mackenzie
University of Waterloo, Canada

J.L. Leavitt
University of Windsor, Canada

The purpose of this paper is to evaluate the effectiveness of two different theories of motor control to explain the results of a series of studies completed by us and our colleagues. In so doing we wish to draw attention to potential strengths and weaknesses in these theories for explaining the results and, in the discussion section, present a view of motor control and learning that is consistent with our data.

Recently, much has been written on the distinction between Motor and Action Theories of motor control (for reviews see Beek & Meijer, 1988; and Schmidt, 1988). For the purposes of this paper a brief account of the pertinent distinctions follows.

Motor Theory

This approach to understanding motor control is based on information processing theory as typified by the Fitts and Posner (1967) book that attempted to break down skilled behavior into its component parts (e.g. perception, decision, and action). Inherent in this approach are the constructs of memory and representations, feedback, feedforward, motor program, and closed-loop control. Early information processing accounts of skilled behavior used the term "information" in the communications theory sense, i.e. the reduction of uncertainty. More recent accounts of information processing in motor skills have used information as synonymous with "knowledge" and interest has centred on the role that this cognitive information plays in motor control and learning. Regardless of the exact definition of the term "information", a main thesis of Motor Theory is that the performer must act on or process information received through the various senses in order that it can be used to control movement. This, in turn, implies the existence of smart mechanisms within the CNS that allow for the "embellishment" or interpretation of information received through the senses.

Action Theory

Central to this position is the interaction between the performer and the environment termed the performer-environment synergy (see Turvey, 1977; Turvey & Carello, 1986; Turvey & Kugler, 1984). This view rejects the motor theorists' reliance on mechanisms within the performer's central nervous system. Moreover, action theorists maintain that perception and action cannot be logically separated and should not be studied independently in that perceptual information is so much a part of the performer-environment interaction that it is inseparable from movement. As such, the concept of information is different from that used in Motor Theory and is synonymous with the concept of "affordance" (Gibson, 1966). Finally, the most important tenet of Action Theory, in terms of the purpose of the present paper, is the denial of any form of representation within the CNS. To these theorists no special brain processes that make the right inferences are necessary to understand the "information" from the environment. On the other hand, those action theorists who admit central representations relegate these ideas to a current unimportant level of investigation so that no theoretical development of these ideas has taken place within the framework of action theory. Overall, then, this non-representational view has, in general, led to an emphasis on physical principles to explain movement control, with a special reliance on non-equilibrium thermodynamics (e.g. the reliance on limit cycle oscillators as a basic mechanism of motor control).

The Issues

The first issue for this paper is whether there is evidence to support some form of internal (central) representation that acts to constrain human movement control and learning. We believe our data speak in favour of this viewpoint and thus offers difficulty to Action theorists who relegate this issue to a current low level of priority.

The second issue we wish to address with our experimental data concerns the Motor Theory issue of central motor programs in terms of what kind and how much information they contain for purposes of motor control. Specifically, we will address the question of whether a motor program concept can explain the control and learning of prehension and other types of arm movements.

Studies in Motor Control

1. Movement trajectories in aiming: Implications for control.

The organization and control of movement have been investigated by observing the characteristics of movement trajectories over a variety of different tasks (Atkeson & Hollerbach, 1985; Flash & Hogan, 1985; Hollerbach & Atkeson, 1987; Munhall, Ostry, & Parush, 1985; Soechting, 1984). Trajectory formation refers to the planning and control of the kinematics of movement and, more specifically, is concerned with the path the movement describes in space and with the speed of movement from the initial to the final position in space.

If the characteristics of trajectory profiles remain invariant over various task demands, support is gained for a movement organization and production mechanism (i.e. an internal representation) that is both general and abstract (Keele, 1981; Schmidt, 1975). Thus a wide variety of trajectories might be produced by selecting appropriate temporal and spatial parameters. The idea is that for movements of different speed, distance, or load, the movement trajectories, as represented by the velocity profile, could be scaled along one or both axes to show that they all belong to a scalar family of curves. In fact there is considerable evidence to support the idea that trajectory planning might occur in this fashion (Atkeson & Hollerbach, 1985; Flash & Hogan, 1985; Hollerbach & Flash, 1982; Munhall et al., 1985; Soechting, 1984). One consistent finding reported is that movements have bell-shaped velocity-time profiles that can be scaled in both the amplitude and time domains.

A general research strategy that we have pursued is to see how the above findings relate to a wide variety of tasks. We have been examining the effects on movement trajectories of varying the number and extent of potential movement constraints. A movement constraint is defined as a variable that limits the way in which movement can be organized and controlled (MacKenzie & Marteniuk, 1985a; Marteniuk, MacKenzie, Jeannerod, Athenes, & Dugas, in press). Marteniuk et al. (in press) suggested that various potential movement constraints might include: target size; conditions of speed and accuracy; specific task characteristics; the structure inherent in communicated information (e.g. music structure); anatomical structure; neurological structure; and, experience and intentions (goals) of the performer.

In an attempt to determine whether target size and movement amplitude were constraints on the planning and control of movement trajectories, MacKenzie, Marteniuk, Dugas, Liske and Eickmeier (in press) examined three-dimensional movement trajectories over a broad range of movement difficulty, as measured by Fitts' index of difficulty (Fitts & Peterson, 1964). Pilot data indicated that it was not index of difficulty (ID) per se that determined the nature of the movement trajectory, but rather the unique combination of amplitude and target width giving rise to ID. So our results could be compared directly with those of Fitts and Peterson (1964) we used the same ID conditions they did. This allowed us to evaluate the separate effects of amplitude and target width since there were six different levels of ID.

The movement time results of this study replicated Fitts' Law in that the line of best fit between ID and movement time accounted for 96% of the variance. The three-dimensional motion analyses consisted of analyzing the movement trajectory of the stylus for the various aiming movements. The kinematic variable selected to form the trajectory was the resultant velocity (a combination of the tangential velocities from each of the three planes of the movement) of the movement throughout its duration. Our analysis of the salient trajectory characteristics showed that for a given ID, trajectories changed dramatically (even though movement time remained almost identical). In an attempt to understand this result we normalized the resultant velocity profiles and found that the profiles scaled to a common profile when dealing with trajectories to a specific target size over the different amplitudes. With respect to target size the profiles differed by the proportion of time spent prior to and after peak resultant velocity. Smaller targets showed skewed velocity profiles with longer right hand tails or deceleration phases. Thus target size determined the shape of the trajectory in terms of relative time spent in acceleration and deceleration.

What do the above results suggest for the idea of an abstract, generalized representation or program for movement in the type of movement we studied? Our data is suggestive of a representation of a movement trajectory but it is not simply scalable in the time domain as has been frequently suggested (Schmidt, 1982; Terzuolo & Viviani, 1980). Remember, our logic in examining the normalized resultant velocity profile was to look for scalability as a function of movement amplitude or target size. The results showed that for a given target size, the resultant speed was scaled as a function of amplitude. However, movements could not be scaled over different target sizes. Thus, since invariance in relative time suggests a program with a scalable parameter, for the conditions of this experiment one might say that a base trajectory (program) exists for a given target width and this trajectory is scaled or parameterized according to the movement amplitude.

These data could be interpreted differently by an action theorist since the target size and movement amplitude are given by the environment and its relation to the individual. However, we next show that for the same index of difficulty movements change according to mechanisms which must operate in the CNS.

2. Reaching and grasping objects of different types for different purposes: The role for planning, context and intent in motor control.

Advocates of the strong version of Action Theory stress that the environment contains all the information necessary to guide movement, given that the performer has a purpose for moving. For example, to a thirsty individual, a glass full of water conveys information at an ecological level that constrains movements of the individual in a way that the glass can be reached for, grasped, and taken to the mouth for drinking purposes.

Motor Theory, on the other hand, might argue that movements have a central nervous system representation which is involved in organizing and controlling the movement in light of past experience and the context in which the movement is performed. Arbib (1981; 1985), for example, suggests that movement is organized and controlled by knowledge of the environment that is far greater than is possible through sensory stimulation. Abbs and his colleagues (Abbs, Gracco, & Cole, 1984; Cole & Abbs, 1986) hold a similar view in that skilled movement is postulated to be dependent on sensorimotor knowledge acquired through experience.

In the above descriptions, both theoretical views would predict functionally specific movements being generated to solve the movement problem. That is, unlike some versions of Motor Programming theory, these views hold that movements are generated by the specific demands of the task and as a result every movement is relatively unique in terms of its kinematic or kinetic expression. Recent work by Marteniuk et al. (in press) and Proteau, Marteniuk, Girouard and Dugas (1987) goes into more detail on the functional specificity hypothesis and presents some results relevant to the present paper.

One goal of the Marteniuk et al. (in press) study was to investigate whether past experience could influence the form of movement resulting from reaching and grasping tasks. To do this, the actual physical size and shapes of the to-be-grasped objects were kept as similar as possible so that the only variable affecting the reach and grasp was the past experience the subject had with the specific objects. In the first experiment, subjects were required to reach and grasp either a tennis ball or the round end of a light bulb. Both objects had a diameter of approximately 6 cm and were placed on a table top 30 cm in front of the seated subject. No instructions as to speed of the reach and grasp was given.

Data analyses were done through the use of a three-dimensional movement recorder which allowed reconstruction of the arm movement trajectories during the reach and grasp. The results showed that movement trajectories to the two objects differed. In particular, movement to the light bulb took longer and the trajectory reached peak velocity sooner. When the trajectories were normalized in the time domain to equate them for this time difference, it was shown that peak velocity for reaching and grasping a light bulb still occurred sooner than for the tennis ball condition. This meant that subjects spent proportionately more of the time involved in reaching for the light bulb in a limb deceleration phase. This is similar to the precision effect noted in the Fitts' data presented above, under conditions where target size became smaller. Here the ID of the to-be-grasped object was constant. Presumably the precision effect occurred for the light bulb condition as a result of the subject making sure the hand was travelling slow enough, when contact was made with the light bulb, in order to avoid breaking it. No such caution was needed for grasping the tennis ball so subjects could spend more time in accelerating their limb to the object and proportionately less in decelerating. One interpretation of these results is that since the objects were approximately the same size and shape, the deciding difference between the two conditions was the prior experience that subjects had with these objects. It was this prior experience, probably acquired early in their movement experiences, that exerted its influence on the movement planning and control processes involved in the reach and grasp.

In a second experiment from the above paper, we tried to structure the task in order to determine the effect of a person's intent on the movement planning and control processes. Here, subjects were asked to reach for an grasp a wooden disk (1 cm thick and 4 cm in diameter) placed 30 cm in front of them. Two movement conditions were employed differing only in what the subject was asked to do after the disk had been grasped. In one, the disk was to be placed in a tight fitting well (4.1 cm in diameter) situated close to where the disk initially lay. In the other condition, the disk was to be thrown into a 20x40x15 cm cardboard box positioned 15 cm to the left of where the disk lay.

Results of this experiment showed that the movement trajectory of the wrist in picking up the disk was influenced by what the subject was going to do with the disk once it had been picked up. Working with time normalized trajectories it was shown that proportionately more time was spent in the deceleration phase of the trajectory when subjects were planning to place the disk in the well. It was as if the precision required in placing the disk in the tight fitting well exerted an influence back in time on the movement planning and control processes. It is likely, however, that it was the planning before the reach and grasp portion of the task that resulted in the movements being specifically designed for the unique demands of the two conditions.

The results of these two experiments show that object properties (softness and fragility) and movement intent (to throw or carefully place an object) influence the way in which movement is controlled. While one might argue that object softness or fragility represent ecological properties that constrain movement in an Action Theory sense, one might ask why these properties are not apparent to young children whose parents go to great lengths to keep fragile objects out of their grasps! One conclusion is that it is direct experience with objects that results in object knowledge being acquired and, in turn, these representations are used when the appropriate context is present.

In terms of the intent of object usage, the second experiment was clear in showing that this variable influenced the grasping of identical objects. Here, the environmental information for reaching and grasping the disk is the same and one might expect Action Theory to predict that no difference should exist in the movement trajectory concerned with grasping the disk. The fact that differences were found speaks to the presence of a relatively high (cognitive/intentional) process exerting its influence on the movement planning and control processes.

3. Reaching and grasping objects of varying size: Inferring movement control processes by a search for invariant kinematic trajectories.

In another study, (Marteniuk, Leavitt, & MacKenzie, in preparation) we asked the question how people planned and executed movements when they were asked to reach and grasp objects of varying sizes. Here we wanted to look at the resulting movement trajectories and attempt to infer what planning and control processes underlie this type of movement, much like in the logic we applied to understand the kinematic basis for Fitts' Law (as described earlier).

Of course, in terms of the purpose of the present paper, since Action Theory does not postulate any internal representations, advocates of this theory would predict that movement trajectories would be functionally specific to the ecological information afforded by the to-be-grasped object. Thus, the trajectories for grasping different sized objects would not have invariant characteristics but rather each trajectory would be rather unique in terms of its kinematic pattern.

The study by Marteniuk, Leavitt, and MacKenzie (in preparation) required subjects to reach for and grasp ten different sized disks (from 1 to 10 cm in diameter, and all were 1 cm thick) that were placed on a table top 30 cm in front of them. The instructions to subjects were to reach as quickly as possible but without so much speed that would result in fumbling the object during the grasp.

Results showed that the mean movement time (from the start of the subjects' reach to point of contact with the disk) decreased as disk diameter increased. While this might be predicted from Fitts' Law, the actual strength of the relationship between movement time and disk size was not as strong as has been reported in the past for other types of tasks described by Fitts' Law. However, movement time did decrease significantly over the ten disk sizes which indicated the size of the disk did influence the trajectory kinematics.

To determine how the trajectory kinematics were affected by increases in disk size, the resultant velocity function was calculated from the three-dimensional coordinates of the wrist as the subject reached and grasped the objects. These velocity profiles were normalized in time and tested to see if they could be scaled to a base trajectory. This test was negative because the profiles were not symmetrical and bell shaped as has been reported about arm velocity profiles in the past (Atkeson & Hollerbach, 1985). Rather, the acceleration portion of the velocity profile (from the start of the movement to zero acceleration at peak velocity) was constant while the deceleration portion of the movement became shorter with increases in disk size. In essence, the smaller the disk, the more time the subject took in decelerating the limb before contact with the disk. This "precision" effect on deceleration was very similar to the effect noted above and very consistent with the results of the experiment on Fitts' Law (MacKenzie et al., in press) where the index of difficulty correlated to a greater degree with time of the acceleration phase than with total movement time. In terms of theoretical significance, these results indicate that the planning and control processes are task specific in that each disk size resulted in a relatively unique movement trajectory being produced by the subject.

Other results from this study were concerned with describing the hand aperture as the hand approached the disk. The aperture was defined as the distance between the index finger and thumb markers, calculated directly from the three-dimensional data. The first analysis showed that the maximum grasp aperture (achieved in time approximately three-quarters of the way to the disk) correlated with the size of the disk, $r=.998$. While all subjects' maximum aperture was larger than the disk to be grasped, the time based profile of the aperture was always the same. That is, during the first three-quarters of the movement the aperture opened to its maximum and then during the final quarter of the movement duration, it closed down to the size of the disk until contact with the disk was made. The fact that the above correlation was so high indicates that there is a highly integrated relationship between the physical demands of this task and the resulting fine motor control in response to those demands.

Results from both the wrist (arm) trajectory and the grasp aperture indicate functionally specific responses of the motor system to task demands. Without other data one might conclude strong support for Action Theory accounts of motor control in that it appears that properties of the person-environment interaction (affordances) are resulting in movements that are specifically tailored to solve the movement problem. Thus, while the results from the ten disk size study would be supportive of Action Theory, the results of the Fitts' Law study, the study that manipulated object properties of softness and fragility, and the study that manipulated the intent of what a subject was going to do with a to-be-grasped object would speak more in favour of a theory that incorporated some form of representation into its constructs.

Collectively, the above studies argue for a view of motor control that is dependent on a knowledge base (not necessarily conscious) that is acquired and represents knowledge about past movements and their consequences in specific situations. As MacKenzie and Marteniuk (1985a,b) have argued, this type of knowledge is possible if one invokes the idea that movements are produced through integrated stores of sensorimotor information. Before discussing a theory of motor behavior based on the principle of sensorimotor integration, further evidence for the influence that past experience has on motor control will be presented.

Studies in Motor Learning

One of the corner stones of Action Theory is the tenet that information for motor control is derived directly from the environment. To account for increases in skill proficiency these theorists (Michaels & Carello, 1981) maintain that information from different levels of abstraction from the environment is used by the performer. However, no representations or memory develop within the performer as increases in skill level occur. Given this, one prediction of Action Theory would be that motor learning should not only be specific to the task but also experience on one task should not influence the level of skill attainment on another task. In essence, skill level on one task should be independent from the level of performance on another related task. If performance on one task influences performance on another task, then this would indicate that some change within the performer's central nervous system, caused by experience with the first task, influenced (either negatively or positively) the performance of the second task. One could argue, from an Action Theory viewpoint, that affordances from the first task influence the level of the affordance of the second task. However, how this could occur without the subject "transporting" the bias from task to task cannot be explained without recourse to some form of change within the CNS.

The two following sections offer evidence for the effects that experience on one task has on another task. The results show that there are carry-over or transfer effects between tasks which are very difficult to explain by current versions of Action Theory. Also, why the transfer occurs is not at all apparent. One option for explanation resides in considering the formation of a cognitive representation for one task which influences the performance of the second task. A second option (not necessarily independent of the first) would be that learning a movement skill results in some reorganization of the CNS in terms of feedback, feedforward, and other motor control processes, both cognitive and non-cognitive. These will be discussed in the final section of the paper.

The functional specificity of motor learning.

Proteau, Marteniuk, Girouard, and Dugas (1987) have shown the functional specificity of motor learning and have attempted to provide a theoretical framework for understanding this phenomenon. They studied the learning of an aiming task where subjects were required to use their left (non-preferred) arm in an underswinging movement to attempt to hit a small target with a hand held stylus. The basic objective of the subjects in this task was to move the hand (there was a straight line distance of 90 cm between the starting position of the hand and the target) in 550 ms with as much accuracy as possible. After each attempt the experimenter gave feedback to the subject by orally giving the movement time and the spatial accuracy in the two axes of the target.

There were four different groups of five subjects each. Two groups were given 200 trials of practice while the other two were given 2,000 trials. One group from each level of practice practiced the task in normal laboratory conditions while the other two groups practiced in total darkness. Thus, for the latter two groups, only the small target was visible to them; they could see neither the moving arm nor the hand as it hit the plate containing the target. After the last training trial all subjects were transferred to a condition which involved the same conditions as the groups who practiced in total darkness, except that feedback for movement time and spatial accuracy was not given. Twenty trials of transfer performance were given. This meant that subjects initially practicing under normal conditions were now in a condition where no visual information about the task or their movements were available.

The results indicated that all subjects improved their performance (both movement time and spatial error) over practice. Furthermore, subjects who practiced with only the target visible were constantly worse than those groups who had the normal conditions. The interesting results were what happened to performance during the transfer condition. After 200 trials of practice, both the normal and vision of target only groups showed a small increase in spatial errors due to the transfer task conditions. Statistically, the difference between the two groups at the end of the 200 trials of practice was maintained during the transfer condition except that both groups' performance here was worse than at the end of the regular practice.

After 2,000 trials of practice the transfer task conditions produced a different set of results. The target only group maintained their pre-transfer level of performance. The normal group, deprived of vision of everything except the target, showed a large increase in spatial error in their transfer performance. In fact, the spatial error of this group was about 400 times larger than their spatial error at the beginning of practice. Obviously taking away vision after 2,000 trials of practice was devastating to their ability to perform the task.

The above results support the idea that learning a movement results in some change within the central nervous system that probably results in the performer becoming more skilled at the task, and, at the same time (at least for the conditions of the present study), interferes with performance of a task that has different feedback conditions. Here, the inference is that some kind of internal structure develops that allows for efficient planning, execution, and movement correction processes necessary for skilled movement. Since this structure is rather specific to the task and the types of information received about the task-performer interaction, when relevant feedback channels are eliminated (as in the transfer condition of the normal practice group of the present study) performance declines dramatically, especially if the performer is skilled.

The above conclusion, of course, goes contrary to Action Theory. However, given the conditions of the present study, it seems difficult if not impossible for this theory to explain the transfer performance of the normal vision group. Remember, their transfer performance after 2,000 trials of practice was 400% worse than their initial performance level. Action Theory might predict that transfer performance would be worse because the task afforded a different type of information not as relevant as in normal vision. However, this viewpoint has difficulty explaining the large amount of negative transfer that occurred. At present we believe that the only inference that can be made is that some kind of internal structure resulted from learning the normal task and this structure interfered with performing the same task but under different planning and feedback conditions.

The case of asymmetrical transfer

In a recent paper (Bamford & Marteniuk, in press) we studied the learning of two versions of the same task and asked what would happen when subjects were switched to the other version. The logic of the design was similar to the above study, in that our hypothesis was that when people learn a movement task, internal structures are developed to efficiently represent and process information about the task. We reasoned that one way of uncovering the nature of the internal structure was to have subjects learn two versions of the same task where the versions differed either by the type of information available for movement execution or by some other type of manipulation relevant to motor control and learning processes. In the present case we manipulated the information display-movement compatibility. We used an elbow rotation task where the subject was seated next to a horizontal arm rest that pivoted around one end. The arm of the subject was placed on the manipulandum so the elbow was directly over the point of rotation and the subject's hand held a handle attached at the other end. By flexing or extending the elbow the subjects could move the manipulandum in the horizontal plane. At the base of the manipulandum was a potentiometer that was used to record the amount of elbow rotation. This potentiometer was interfaced with a computer that performed an analog to digital conversion and then put this signal out to a graphics terminal. The result was a display on the graphics terminal in the form of a continuous line, the amplitude of which was proportional to the amount of elbow rotation.

Subjects were required to learn a series of elbow rotations that were defined by a criterion wave form generated by the experimenter. This criterion "movement" (identical to the one used by Marteniuk & Romanow, 1983) was used to define the required movement to the subjects. The subjects then attempted to produce the criterion by moving the manipulandum in a manner that would produce a wave form identical to that of the criterion. After each attempt, the experimenter displayed the subject's waveform on the graphics terminal and then superimposed the criterion on it. The subject could then see the discrepancy between what was produced and what was required.

There were two groups of subjects that attempted to learn the criterion movement. One was the compatible group where the criterion and subject produced wave form moved in the same direction as the subject's arm. That is, when the subject extended the elbow (movement to the right) the line, coming down from the top of the graphics terminal, would move to the right. Similarly a movement to the left by the subject resulted in the line moving to the left. Thus the movement was described by the terminal in a compatible manner with the subject's movement. The orthogonal condition had the line coming from the left side of the terminal and when the subject's arm moved left the line would go down. Movements to the right caused the line to go up. Thus, the wave form was orthogonal to the movements of the arm.

Both groups of subjects had 90 learning trials where their produced wave form and the criterion were displayed after every trial. Discrepancies between these two wave forms was measured by Root Mean Square Error. Results showed that both groups of subjects reduced error over the 90 trials and they had identical performance at the end of practice. After this learning, the two groups were switched to the other condition for 20 trials. These results proved interesting. The orthogonal group, now performing under the compatible condition, showed a decrement in their performance of about 30% of their pre-switch level. The compatible group, now under the orthogonal condition, showed a much greater decrement (about 70% of the pre-switch level) in their performance. In fact, this group's mean performance for the first five switch trials was at the same level as the mean of their first five trials under the compatible condition. In essence there was no transfer when switching from the compatible to the orthogonal condition.

These results indicated that the orthogonal group learned something that transferred to the compatible condition. On the other hand, the compatible group's initial switch performance indicated no transfer or benefit from their previous experience. These findings are of interest to the purpose of the present paper in that they show asymmetrical transfer which we believe is very difficult for Action Theory to account for. We interpret the orthogonal group as learning something about their interaction with the task that aids them when they attempt the compatible version of the same task. As we (Bamford & Marteniuk, in press) explain, this group has perhaps developed an information processing stage that deals with transforming the information from the display to body centred coordinates within a visual-spatial map. The compatible group was not concerned with this transformation since information from the display was already directly compatible with limb movement. When the two groups were switched to the opposite condition, transfer occurred for the group switched from the orthogonal condition because of the similarity of the two tasks. The other group, however, lacked the ability to transform display information into useable body information and as a result no transfer occurred.

The foregoing is another example of how experience, acquired through interacting with the environment, can affect the way in which a task is performed. To us this implies some kind of relatively persistent structure being developed through learning that influences the way in which a subsequent task is performed. This kind of finding is difficult to explain without invoking concepts related to a representational account of motor control and learning.

Discussions and Implications

Action Theory

Overall, we believe the results from the above studies speak strongly in favour of some form of internal representation being needed to account for skilled movement behavior. The most striking features of the results for this conclusion come from the experiments that showed that object characteristics of softness and fragility influenced the kinematic characteristics of prehension as did movement intent and object size. The results of the second set of two studies on learning also give Action Theory problems in terms of attempting to explain the findings without postulating the existence of changes occurring within the CNS. Specifically, these latter studies point to the relatively persistent effects that past experience has on motor control. It is difficult to see how Action Theory would account for these findings without incorporating concepts more closely aligned with Motor Theory. Here, we are referring to concepts like memory, sensorimotor integration, feedback, and feedforward.

In terms of the studies on prehension which showed that the arm and grasp aperture were tightly coupled to the exact demands of the task, Action Theorists might argue that it was the affordances of the to-be-grasped objects that led to this coupling. However, we do not see it this way in that prehension might be interpreted as depending on internal representations if one argues that prehension is partly the product of development and learning. In other words, learning is necessary if prehension is to be specifically tailored to meet the exacting demands of the multitudinous objects one interacts with in daily life. To determine if learning is necessary for precise prehension, one could ask what would happen if the experiment on grasping a light bulb vs a tennis ball were repeated with infants that could reach and grasp relatively proficiently? Without doing the experiment we believe the infant would demonstrate similar arm trajectories to the two objects. This is because the infant has yet to appreciate the distinction between glass and rubber and what this means in terms of potential injury to the hand. The objects thus afford grasping but without the knowledge of object properties the infant is not yet fully skilled in prehension. In this case it is knowledge derived through experience that will lead to the highly tuned prehension skill that is characteristic of adults.

Consistent with the above, we also wish to make the point that strong versions of Action Theory cannot unambiguously account for human motor behavior. We say this because of the current absence in Action Theory accounts of learning functionally effective movements. Related to this issue is the issue of how the human changes as a function of learning: whether in the development of representations or other types of CNS changes. These changes are not acknowledged in present versions of Action Theory. Our logic for this position is based on the data we presented above and for the conclusion we drew with regard to the role that experience (knowledge) plays in making prehension movements so specifically suited to task demands. If our interpretation is correct we are demonstrating the combined influences of biophysical properties and learning on human movement capabilities. Thus, when one studies movement trajectories as we have, it is important to realize these trajectories have been produced from a very complex system with several levels of control all interacting to make the movement responsive to the exact demands of the human's movement goal as well as to the properties of the environment. Teasing apart the contribution of these different levels will be very difficult and hence the experimental paradigms used for this purpose must be carefully chosen in light of the knowledge of this complexity. Furthermore a neglect of "higher" levels and their influence on "lower" levels will result in an accumulation of movement data that may be misinterpreted in terms of explaining how they were produced. In this regard we think Action Theorists who take the extreme position of there being no internal representation may produce erroneous conclusions as to the nature of their data. One side comment: our use of the terms "higher" and "lower" should not be interpreted as a fixed hierarchy of control. Rather, in any complex system with different levels of control, no one level always has control over any other level. What we stress from a theoretical development viewpoint is a cooperative levels or distributed control systems approach to motor control problems.

Motor Theory (Motor Programs)

As we have mentioned above, we feel our results support the existence of internal representations. However, one purpose of the present paper was to evaluate the concept of the motor program as an internal representation of movement for explaining the data we presented. Here we wish to restrict our comments to the idea of the motor program made popular by the works of Keele (1981) and Schmidt (1975, 1976, 1982, 1988). A generalized motor program was defined by Schmidt (1982) as an internal prototypical representation of a motor act capable of changes in scale which preserve the basic form of the movement. Inherent in this definition is the notion that one could take three-dimensional arm trajectories (as in the data presented above) for different versions of the same task and when linearly scaled in both the time and amplitude domains, the trajectories would literally superimpose upon one another.

For the three-dimensional results we presented (the first three studies), only one aspect of one of the studies comes out in favour for the existence of a generalized motor program. This occurred in the Fitts' aiming experiment where for different movement amplitude requirements to the same target, the resulting resultant velocity profiles scaled to a base trajectory. As soon as the target size was changed, however, unique trajectories resulted. Similar precision effects were shown in the other two studies on reaching and grasping objects where trajectories were unique to the objects being grasped or to the intent of the use of the object. In this regard our overall results agree with those studies reviewed by Gentner (1987) which show only limited support for the idea of the generalized motor program.

Given the foregoing, what is the viability of the generalized motor program concept? Zelaznik, Schmidt, and Gielen (1986), after showing no support for this type of control in aimed hand movements, comment that while the evidence is damaging for a linear account of a general motor program, it may be that more complicated, nonlinear models will be more successful in showing support for the idea of time rescalability. This view is partly based on the observation that the motor system has known nonlinear properties and therefore one should not expect a simple linear scaling of time to be an adequate model.

Our current view of motor program theory is that movement is the result of several interacting levels of the central nervous system. To the extent that central commands are part of this complex system and that there is evidence to show that movement plans, developed through previous experience, have an effect on the control of movement (as shown above), then motor programs probably exist. However, as to how prestructured these commands are (do they prestructure the whole movement or only part of it?) and how much they extend into the evolving movement, we prefer to leave such issues to future research. Until then, we feel that the best explanation that can be advanced for the production of movement comes from theories that stress the cooperation of the various parts of the central nervous system to produce movement that is specifically tailored to meet the exact demands of the performer's goals and of the environment that the performer must interact with. Our account of one version of such a theory follows.

Sensorimotor integration

We (MacKenzie & Marteniuk, 1985a,b) have argued that at the base of all coordinated movement is an integrated store of sensory and motor information that defines relations among body parts for the achievement of movement goals. The actual expression of coordinated movement, however, is modified by an interplay of motor and sensory information that fine tunes movement to the specific context of the situation. We have borrowed the term multimovement coordination from Abbs, Gracco, and Cole (1984) to describe this kind of coordination.

An example of multimovement coordination can be found in insect flight. Altman (1982) has discussed the relationship between the concepts of the central pattern generator and sensory inputs in terms of their contributions to insect flight. Evidence shows that phasic sensory inputs play a crucial role in regulating the output of the central pattern generator. These sensory inputs come not only from wing receptors but also from the head, tail, and, perhaps, the entire body surface. More importantly, the inputs from the central pattern generator and sensory receptors during flight summate to produce a stable yet flexible motor output. In fact, Altman raises the possibility that there may be no such thing as a central pattern generator but rather a flying insect might be more properly thought of as a combination of components, mechanical, sensory, and central neurons, all oscillating in resonance at flight frequency.

Analogous examples to the above can be found in human motor behavior. The work of Abbs and his colleagues, summarized in Abbs and Gracco (1983) shows that coordination of multiple speech movements is not entirely preprogrammed but is subject to refinement through sensorimotor feedforward adjustments. Evidence for this comes from data showing that during speech, when the lower lip is perturbed, compensations occur in synergistic movements of the upper lip. This is significant since the lower and upper lips are controlled independently, thus ruling out a closed-loop process. It is believed that the basis for this open-loop adjustment is a sensorimotor translation, established through prior experience, between the lower-lip afferent signals and upper-lip motor actions. Abbs and Gracco call this sensorimotor translation a predictive or feedforward process.

Feedforward processes have also been implicated in the interaction of postural muscles with muscles involved in rapid arm movements. Work (Nashner & Cordo, 1981) has shown that leg stabilizers produce EMG responses about 50 ms prior to EMG appearance in an arm that must be rapidly moved. Data like these implicate a feedforward anticipation of the kinematic consequences of the muscular contractions in the prime mover.

The nature of feedforward processes is such that a movement is generated to cancel a previously generated error before that error can cause a functional disturbance in the motor output (Ito, 1975). Houk and Rymer (1981) postulate that in multimovement coordination the feedforward controller consists of a neural model of the motor system that translates a predicted error in one component of the movement to an adjustment in a synergistic movement, which cancels the effect of the error on the functional output of the multicomponent movement.

Abbs, Gracco, and Cole (1984) and MacKenzie and Marteniuk (1985) have commented on how such a system might be acquired. Prediction in such a system is derived from past experience where the relationship between afferent signals from muscles comprising the system are related to efferent signals of the same muscles. In other words, sensory events are coded in efferent terms. The establishment of this representation (the neural model) is specific for each learned task. Abbs, Gracco, and Cole (1984) point out that to implement the interdependent actions that make up a compound motor gesture, a motor program is constructed which results in the establishment of pertinent sensorimotor contingencies which ensure coordination of the multiple movement to one common goal. When executed the movement is dependent on the exact demands of the environment in that the program only sets up the correct patterns of interaction among the components of the movement. Hence, it is the result of the initial planning and the resulting interaction among the components of the multimovement that determine the exact nature of the motor output. In this way, it makes sense to not build conceptually too much into the motor program since feedback and feedforward processes can efficiently and rapidly guide movement to accomplish the performer's goal.

References

Abbs, J.H. & Gracco, V.L. (1983). Sensorimotor actions in the control of multimovement speech gestures. Trends in Neuroscience, 6, 391-395.

Abbs, J.H., Gracco, V.L., & Cole, K.J. (1984). Control of multimovement coordination: sensorimotor mechanisms in speech motor programming. Journal of Motor Behavior, 16, 195-231.

Altman, J. (1982). The role of sensory inputs in insect flight motor pattern generation. Trends in Neuroscience, 5, 257-260.

Arbib, M.A. (1981). Perceptual structures and distributed motor control. In V.B. Brooks (Ed.), Handbook of Physiology: Vol.2 Motor control. Bethesda, Maryland: American Physiological Society.

Arbib, M.A. (1985). Schemas for the temporal organization of behavior. Human Neurobiology, 4, 63-72.

Atkeson, C.G. & Hollerbach, J.L. (1985). Kinematic features of unrestrained vertical arm movements. Journal of Neuroscience, 5, 2318-2330.

Bamford, R.B. & Marteniuk, R.G. (in press). Spatial ability and the early learning of a complex arm action. Human Movement Science.

Beek, P.G. & Meijer, O.G. (1988). On the nature of "the" motor-action controversy. In O.G. Meijer & K. Roth (Eds.), Complex movement behaviour: "The" motor-action controversy. Amsterdam: North Holland.

Cole, K.J. & Abbs, J.H. (1986). Coordination of three-joint digit movements for rapid finger-thumb grasp. Journal of Neuroscience, 55, 1407-1423.

Fitts, P.M. & Peterson, J.R. (1964). Information capacity of discrete motor responses. Journal of Experimental Psychology, 46, 199-210.

Fitts, P.M. & Posner, M.I. (1967). Human performance. Belmont, C.A.: Brooks/Cole.

Flash, T. & Hogan, N. (1985). The coordination of arm movements: an experimentally confirmed mathematical model. Journal of Neuroscience, 5, 1688-1703.

Gibson, J.J. (1966). The senses considered as perceptual systems. Boston: Houghton-Mifflin.

Gentner, D.R. (1987). Timing of skilled motor performance: Tests of the proportional duration model. Psychological Review, 94, 255-276.

Hollerbach, J.M. & Atkeson, C.G. (1987). Deducing planning variables from experimental arm trajectories: Pitfalls and possibilities. Biological Cybernetics, 56, 279-292.

Hollerbach, J.M. & Flash, T. (1982). Dynamic interactions between limb segments during planar arm movement. Biological Cybernetics, 44, 67-77.

Houk, J.C. & Rymer, W.Z. (1981). Neural control of muscle length and tension. In V.B. Brooks (Ed.), Handbook of Physiology, Vol.2. Motor control. Bethesda, Md.: American Physiological Society.

Ito, M. (1975). The control of mechanisms of cerebellar motor systems. In E.V. Evarts (Ed.), Central processing of sensory input leading to motor output. Cambridge, Mass.: MIT Press.

Keele, S.W. (1981). Behavioral analysis of motor control. In V.B. Brooks (Ed.), Handbook of Physiology. Section 1: The nervous system. Vol.II, Part 2: Motor control. Bethesda, Md.: American Physiological Society.

MacKenzie, C.L. & Marteniuk, R.G. (1985a). Motor skill: Feedback, knowledge, and structural issues. Canadian Journal of Psychology, 39, 313-337.

MacKenzie, C.L. & Marteniuk, R.G. (1985b). Bimanual coordination. In E.A. Roy (Ed.), Neuropsychological studies of Apraxia and related disorders. Amsterdam: North-Holland.

MacKenzie, C.L., Marteniuk, R.G., Dugas, C., Liske, D., & Eickmeier, B. (in press). Three dimensional movement trajectories in Fitts' task: Implications for control. Quarterly Journal of Experimental Psychology. Human Experimental Psychology.

Marteniuk, R.G., Leavitt, J.L., & MacKenzie, C.L. (in preparation). Prehension characteristics related to different sized objects.

Marteniuk, R.G., MacKenzie, C.L., Jeannerod, M., Athenes, S., & Dugas, C. (in press). Constraints on human arm movement trajectories. Canadian Journal of Psychology.

Marteniuk, R.G. & Romanow, S.K.E. (1983). Human movement organization and learning as revealed by variability of movement, use of kinematic information and Fourier analysis. In K. Magill (Ed.), Memory and control of action. Amsterdam: North Holland.

Michaels, C.F. & Carello, C. (1981). Direct perception. New York: Prentice-Hall.

Munhall, K.G., Ostry, D.J., & Parush, A. (1985). Characteristics of velocity profiles of speech movements. Journal of Experimental Psychology: Human Perception and Performance, 11, 457-474.

Nashner, L.M. & Cordo, P.J. (1981). Relation of automatic postural responses and reaction-time voluntary movements of human leg muscles. Experimental Brain Research, 43, 395-405.

Proteau, L., Marteniuk, R.G., Girouard, Y., & Dugas, C. (1987). On the type of information used to control and learn an aiming movement after moderate and extensive training. Canadian Journal of Psychology, 6, 181-199.

Schmidt, R.A. (1975). A schema theory of discrete motor skill learning. Psychological Review, 82, 225-260.

Schmidt, R.A. (1976). Control processes in motor skills. Exercise and Sport Sciences Reviews, 4, 229-261.

Schmidt, R.A. (1982). Motor control and learning: A behavioral emphasis. Champaign, Ill.: Human Kinetics.

Schmidt, R.A. (1988). Motor and action perspectives on motor behavior. In O.G. Meijer & K. Roth (Eds.), Complex movement behavior: "The" motor-action controversy. Amsterdam: North Holland.

Soechting, J.F. (1984). Effect of target size on spatial and temporal characteristics of a pointing movement in man. Experimental Brain Research, 54, 121-132.

Terzuolo, C.A. & Viviani, P. (1980). Determinants and characteristics of motor patterns used for typing. Neuroscience, 5, 1085-1103.

Turvey, M.T. (1977). Preliminaries to a theory of action with reference to vision. In R. Shaw & J. Bransford (Eds.), Perceiving acting and knowing: Toward an ecological psychology. Hillsdale, N.J.: Erlbaum.

Turvey, M.T. & Carello, C. (1986). The ecological approach to perceiving-acting: A pictoral essay. Acta Psychologica, 63, 133-155.

Turvey, M.T. & Kugler, P.N. (1984). An ecological approach to perception and action. In H.T.A. Whiting (Ed.), Human motor actions: Bernstein reassessed. Amsterdam: North-Holland.

Zelaznik, H.N., Schmidt, R.A., & Gielen, S.C.A.M. (1986). Kinematic properties of rapid aimed hand movements. Journal of Motor Behavior, 18, 353-372.

Cognition and Action in Skilled Behaviour
A.M. Colley and J.R. Beech (Editors)

EXPLORING A LAW-BASED, ECOLOGICAL APPROACH TO SKILLED ACTION[§]

M.T. Turvey[†] and Claudia Carello
Center for the Ecological Study of Perception and Action
University of Connecticut

With respect to skilled behavior, competence refers to the conditions that must hold for humans and other animals to coordinate their acts with objects and events, and performance refers to how those conditions are exploited. An argument is made for a theory of competence expressed in terms of the lawful regularities of the ecological scale rather than in the conventional terms of the computational capability of the nervous system. The principal assumption is that where there is fluent behavior, it must be lawfully grounded. A number of different analyses and experiments are presented identifying the kinds of action-relevant lawful regularities and principles available at the coarse scale of animals and their environments. The analyses and experiments express collectively what might be termed an ecological approach to skilled behavior and the competence that underlies it.

Animals (including humans) are active explorers of their environments. They perceive environmental properties that enable them to guide their actions effectively with respect to those properties. James J. Gibson (e.g. 1961, 1966, 1979) argued that understanding perceiving and acting requires that the environment to be perceived and the activities that animals need to perform be described in a mutually compatible fashion. The relevant descriptions, therefore, are to be found at the level of ecology rather than the level of physics or physiology. His ecological approach is directed explicitly at problems of "looking around and getting around" (1979, p.2) and at uncovering the laws at the ecological scale that permit those activities. Our concern will be skilled activities (e.g. soccer, baseball, tennis, and so on) that involve large movements of the limbs relative to the body and relative to the surroundings. Following Gibson's lead, it is assumed that these activities will be understood primarily in terms of lawful regularities at the ecological scale. This general perspective will be elaborated first and then contrasted with a computational perspective that takes complex information processing

---

[§] The writing of this paper was supported in part by a James McKeen Cattell Fellowship awarded to the first author.

[†] Also at Haskins Laboratories.

systems as the object of understanding. Then we will turn to specific examples of how the law-based, ecological approach is applied to particular action problems.

Gibson's ecological approach to perception

"There are almost certainly laws by which some variables in the optic array specify some environmental facts" (Gibson, 1961/1982, p.69). This statement is as radical today as it was over twenty-five years ago (cf. Fodor & Pylyshyn, 1981). To argue that there are ecological laws of perceiving and acting means that perceiving and acting are underwritten by lawful relations among properties. The lawfulness is revealed, however, only if the problems to be understood are described at the appropriate scale. Traditionally, the scale deemed appropriate for vision has been set by sensations, which are fashioned as much by the anatomy and physiology of the eyeball as by the physical features of objects in the environment. Physical features are presumed to be things such as the orientation or length of lines; anatomical distortions include the flatness and inversion of the retinal image. This starting point, Gibson argued, guarantees that lawfulness remains hidden and that extra-perceptual knowledge structures become the focus of theories of perception. Physical features such as lines and angles have little to do with activity. Moreover, a substantial proportion of organisms that "look around and get around" do not have the kind of eyeball that produces retinal images. This led Gibson to try a new starting point —— a thoroughgoing description of the patternings of light distributions that provide information relevant to getting around regardless of the type of occular apparatus that might detect them.

In Gibson's perceptual theory, the term "information" has a precise usage. In the case of vision, it is structured light that specifies the animal-environment circumstances that generated it. The formulation "**A** generates **B**, **B** specifies **A**" is the formulation of a law of ecological optics. As an example, forward locomotion generates a pattern of global expansion in the optic array; global optical expansion specifies that a point of observation is moving forward. The pattern of optical flow distinguishes forward locomotion from the other styles of locomotion such as moving backwards or turning, and from movement of something toward the point of observation. Invariant relations between properties of the foregoing kind make possible the everyday successes of animals in guiding their activities.

Competence and performance

The focus on everyday successes is an important one. The ecological approach is in the business of explaining what allows animals to do what they do. Is information available that is specific to what one has to do to catch a baseball or to tackle a ball carrier or to clear a high jump? The fact that there are occasions when the ball is dropped or the tackle is missed or the bar is hit does not diminish the lawfulness of the informational support for those activities. The conditions that make one lose the ball in the lights or tackle too high or not lift the trailing foot are a separate issue. (For a discussion of what is usually termed "perceptual error", see

Carello & Turvey, 1984; Michaels & Carello, 1981, Chapter 5; Shaw, Turvey, & Mace, 1982.)

This is the distinction that Chomsky drew in natural language between "competence" and "performance". Competence is said to be what the speaker-hearer knows (tacitly) about his or her language that allows it to be used creatively and effectively. Performance refers to how the language is actually used in a given situation (Chomsky, 1965). Performance will be a direct reflection of competence only in the ideal, when the speaker-hearer "... is unaffected by such grammatically irrelevant conditions as memory limitations, distractions, shifts of attention and interest, and errors (random or characteristic) in applying his knowledge of the language in actual performance" (p.3). But understanding competence is not undermined by the vicissitudes of performance. To reiterate, a description of intrinsic competence is a characterization of the knowledge of language that provides the basis for actual use of language by a speaker-hearer; without competence, performance would not even be close. A theory of competence, though, need say nothing about how a speaker might construct a particular sentence in a particular situation; that is the task of a theory of performance.

Marr (1981, 1982), too, enforces this kind of distinction, with respect to solving information processing problems. He includes three levels: (1) the underlying computational theory, (2) the particular algorithms for implementing a computation, and (3) the hardware in which the algorithms must be instantiated. For Marr, the computational theory is the most important because it is concerned with identifying the kinds of problems that have to be solved. These will dictate ultimately what algorithms have to do and why.

> If one believes that the aim of information-processing studies is to formulate and understand particular information-processing problems, then it is the structure of those problems that is central, not the mechanisms through which they are implemented ... The most fruitful source of such problems is operations that we perform well, fluently ... since it is difficult to see how reliability could be achieved if there were no sound underlying method (Marr, 1981, p.139-140).

He suggests that Chomsky's notion of competence is a good example of a computational theory — it takes an undeniably fluent operation and highlights what is being computed and why without worrying about the "gory details of algorithms that must be run to express the competence (i.e. to implement the computation)" (1981, pp.130-131).

This call for investigations of competence is echoed by ecological queries as to what makes the evolution and everyday realization of perceiving-acting possible. Gibson's characterization of the what of perception — identifying its problems — sets his approach and its proponents apart from orthodox perceptual theory. The ecological approach would, of course, deny that those problems are information processing problems. An information processing device is characterized as mapping from one set of formal symbols — equated with "information" — to another, where the abstract properties of this mapping must be defined precisely. But this is a very different use of the term information from that described earlier. For the ecological approach, information ought not be divorced from law even if the appropriate laws have yet to be identified. The ecological assumption is that where there is fluent behavior, it must be lawfully constrained; the ecological strategy is to search for the lawfulness and regularity until it is found. The search most likely will lead beyond the constructs of traditional psychology and to those sciences that treat the behavior of natural systems as central. What we seek are not mechanisms that have the imprimatur of physics but design principles that serve the cause of behavior. What makes perceiving-acting possible?

A physical challenge

This last question is usually posed with more detail with respect to the form of expected answers: What are the laws, scalar constants, symmetry operations, adiabatic invariants, and so on, at the ecological scale that make perceiving-acting possible (Kugler & Turvey, 1987)? What are the deep constraints, the underlying attractors? That is, what states do perceiving-acting systems relax onto or regulate around in the absence of imposed boundary conditions? The form of these questions is designed to reinforce the notion that perceiving-acting systems are natural, physical-biological systems whose behavior is guided by laws just as is the behavior of any natural, physical-biological system. This is not to say that the laws of relevance will be just those laws that have been identified in classical physics. Nor is it to say that the behavior of perceiving-acting systems is determined. The challenge posed by the problems of skilled action is to identify lawful regularities at the ecological scale — the scale of animals and their environments — that provide a reliable basis for the successful conduct of every-day acts. Information is determinate; behavior is nondeterminate (Kugler & Turvey, 1987).

Physically speaking, perceiving-acting is a circularly causal process involving (a) forces giving rise to noninertial flows, forms, and times, and (b) noninertial flows, forms, and times giving rise to forces. Laws of type (a) are found in orthodox physics (particle and statistical mechanics, equilibrium and nonequilibrium thermodynamics). Orthodox physics does not embrace laws of type (b) which are demanded by the problem of perceiving-acting and are revealed at appropriate scales of space and time. The physical challenge for the ecological approach is to identify the physical principles by which noninertial flows, forms, and times give rise to proportionate forces and to uncover the manner in which these lawful regularities are harnessed selectively in skilled action.

The foregoing describes a principled strategy for pursuing an understanding of skilled activity. The remaining sections will be devoted to illustrating how this strategy has been applied in a variety of experimental settings.

Information about action boundaries: Properties of optic flow

Much skilled action involves perceiving behavioral category boundaries. An individual must be able to perceive whether or not a given act is permitted by present (or imminent) conditions. If behavior **Y** is possible, then there must be information specific to that fact, information that can be detected by appropriately attuned perceivers. If behavior **Y** is not possible, then there must be information specific to that fact as well. A theory of competence for behavior **Y**, and for skilled behavior more generally, would identify the particular patternings of the structured energy distribution (say, light) lawfully generated by the conditions of the behavior and, thereby, specify to its criterial properties, such as its boundaries. In strong terms, performing **Y** is possible if and only if information about **Y** is available and perceivers can detect it.

Consider the problem faced by a softball outfielder. If a ball is catchable, then she should move so as to catch it; if a ball is not catchable then she should move so as to cut it off after it bounces. As it turns out, there is a dimensionless, macroscopic optical property available to a point of observation that specifies where a ball will land relative to that point of observation (Todd, 1981). The starting point for the analysis is **Tau**, the inverse of the relative rate of dilation of a closed optical contour generated by the movement of a surface (such as a softball) toward an observation point (such as the eyes of an outfielder) or vice versa. **Tau** was originally shown to specify the time to contact of the observation point with the upcoming surface (e.g. Lee, 1976). The Todd Number is built from a ratio of two **Tau**s, one specifying time to contact with the horizontal plane through the point of observation (the ball's vertical drop) and the other specifying time to contact with the vertical plane through the point of observation (the ball's horizontal traverse). When the Todd Number

$\mathbf{Tau}_{\mathbf{vertical}}/\mathbf{Tau}_{\mathbf{horizontal}} > 1$, the ball will land behind the point of observation. When

$\mathbf{Tau}_{\mathbf{vertical}}/\mathbf{Tau}_{\mathbf{horizontal}} < 1$, the ball will land in front of the point of observation. The Todd Number — precisely, a highly particular patterning of optical structure — specifies what a person must do (e.g. charge in, retreat) in order to intercept a projectile in the person's sagittal plane (it is, therefore, the limiting case of a much more general law statement).

By the arguments pursued here, the existence of the preceding, lawfully generated optical property makes the act of catching a softball (baseball, cricket ball, etc.) possible. In the absence of an optical property specific to the relation between an observation point and the kinetic and kinematic properties of a projectile, successful repeatable acts of catching would be ruled out regardless of nervous system sophistication. The Todd Number underscores an important point we wish to make: The theory of competence for visually guided behavior, so often conceptualized as addressing nervous system computational capability, is conceptualized more profoundly as addressing the order defined over surface layouts, structured energy distributions and the paths of observation points.

Let us consider some other behaviors, those that require one to modulate the force with which a surface or another person is contacted. For example, under certain game conditions, a linebacker in (American) football may need to use just enough force to push a ball carrier out of bounds; under other conditions, it may be desirable to tackle the ball carrier hard enough to make him drop the ball. In physical terms, as a point of observation approaches a substantial surface, the current force structure (that moves the point of observation) may or may not result in a hard collision. Since collisions are indeed controlled (birds alight gently, not violently, on branches and rooftops), we are motivated by our theory of competence to ask whether or not there is an optical property related lawfully to the current forces and the momentum exchanges that they will engender if continued. As observed by Lee (1976, 1980), the first derivative of **Tau**, another dimensionless quantity, is specific to the category of an upcoming collision. When the Lee Number **dTau/dt** $< -.05$, the contact will be hard; when **dTau/dt** $\geq -.05$, the contact will be soft. That is to say, the optical property captured by the Lee Number specifies the collision type given the current kinetic conditions. A person or animal able to detect **dTau/dt** has, therefore, a reliable basis for determining what must be done (e.g. accelerate, maintain current speed) in order to effect a given kind of contact. The existence of this optical property makes controlled collisions possible.

Information about action boundaries: Body-scaled units

Animals routinely perceive the environmental layout in their own scale. While a rabbit would scamper under a fence, a horse would jump over that same fence. But there will be some fences so high that the horse would not attempt to jump them. In order for an animal to perceive that a given layout permits behavior **Y**, then by the theory of competence proposed here, information about that fact must be available. If behavior **Y** is not possible, then there must be information about that fact as well. Our attitude toward the competence that underwrites body-scaled categorical behaviors of the preceding kinds constrains us to believe that optical structure generated lawfully by surface layout at a point of observation must be in the dimensions of the point of observation. The most obvious scale or metric for observation points is elevation above the ground.

Recent investigations have highlighted the ability of people to perceive surface layout in body-scaled terms. Whether or not a given stair is climbable depends on the size of the actor — what is climbable for a tall person might not be for a short person. But Warren (1984) demonstrated that the maximum perceived climbable stair riser height for tall and short people was the same when that riser was scaled by the person's leg length. Moreover, the action boundary riser/leg length = .89 was the same as that predicted from a biomechanical analysis of stairclimbing.

In an important extension of Warren's work, Mark (1987) showed that optical structure in eye heights underwrites the ability to perceive the behavioral category boundary. Subjects who wore 10 cm blocks strapped to their feet (thereby increasing their eyeheight 10 cm) indicated a higher absolute maximum climbable riser even though the blocks did not, in fact, increase the height of stair that could be climbed (because the two legs are used differently in climbing — what is added to the support leg is effectively lost by the climbing leg which must step onto the tread). In eyeheight units, riser/eye height = .46, the value obtained without blocks. Mark also showed that perceived maximum seat height is body-scaled (seat height/leg length = .88, seat height/eye height = .44). The addition of 10 cm blocks does, indeed, increase maximum seat height but it does so by more than would be the case if one were simply 10 cm taller (distributed proportionately throughout the length of the body). In this circumstance, subjects indicated a lower maximum seat height than was possible with their longer legs. Both perceptions — of the limits of sitability and climbability — appear to be based on optical structure scaled to eyeheight; in both riser and seat height, perceived maximums were consistent with the new eyeheight. Interestingly, when Mark permitted his subjects to walk around in between trials (but not look at the blocks), the amount of over- and under-estimation decreased gradually and asymptotically at the appropriate maximum after about ten pairs of (ascending and descending) trials with the new legs. In other words, with postural and ambulatory exploration the individual subject became increasingly aware of the fit between his or her new body dimensions and the surrounding surfaces.

Warren and Whang (1987) have extended the aforementioned style of investigation to perception of the maximum passable aperture. Subjects place this category boundary at 1.2 times shoulder width, presumably including a margin of safety for sway. As it turns out, this, too, is related to eyeheight. The apparatus was arranged so as to introduce a surreptitious manipulation of eyeheight. The aperture to be judged (two vertical surfaces, parallel to the plane of the subjects' shoulders, whose separation was controlled by the experimenter) was on a floor 24 cm higher than the floor on which the subjects stood. Subjects viewed the opening through a peephole and, consequently, could not see the discrepancy in floor heights. This had the effect of lowering their eyeheights and had the expected result on perceived maximum passable aperture: It was narrower than their actual shoulder width but, when scaled in eyeheight units, the ratio was the same as before. Attunement of perceivers to optical structure that is in the scale of the actor seems to underwrite all of these abilities.

Smart perceptual instruments

A baseball fielder who catches a fly ball or a soccer player who heads a ball into the net are performing very special skills. What they do — and what they must know to do it — are quite different from when those same players throw the ball to homeplate or direct a pass across the goal mouth. In each case, information relevant to guiding a particular activity has been detected and the musculature has been organized to perform that activity. In order to perform behavior **W**, optical property **v** must be detected; in order to perform behavior **Y**, optical property **x** must be detected.

The point is that different activities require the detection of different information. A now celebrated example is provided by the gannet.

Diving into a body of water to snare a fish, a gannet initiates the folding of its wings at a particular value of **tau** (Lee & Reddish, 1981). Presumably, when the gannet's goal is to land gently on the water's surface, the initiation of decelerating manoeuvres is at a different value of the same variable. The competence underwriting these skilled behaviors can be formulated as follows: The intention to do **Y** selects or specifies the optical property **x** that must be detected if **Y** is to be achieved. A theory of competence, as we see it, would have to (a) identify the natural basis of the linkage between **x** and **Y**, and (b) provide an account of how intentional states can specify the requisite optical states. Without going into detail, our hunch is that satisfaction of (a) and (b) will require the identification of a gauge (local) symmetry at nature's ecological scale.

Investigations of the hand-related haptic subsystem illustrate the foregoing demands on a theory of competence. Suppose that one is asked to wield a visually occluded rod in order to determine where its tip could reach. Experiments show that the distances reachable with uniformly dense rods are perceived to a high degree of accuracy (Solomon & Turvey, in press). The typical result is that perceived reachable distance relates linearly to actual reachable distance, with a near zero intercept and a slope that does not differ significantly from unity. This linear relation holds for rods of different densities, for rods wielded in, and perpendicular to, the body's sagittal plane, and for rods wielded at different rates. Manipulating the position of an attached weight on an otherwise uniformly dense rod and manipulating where the rod is grasped, reveals that the moment of inertia of the rod about its axes of rotation is the kinetic basis for this haptic distance perception (Solomon & Turvey, in press). In the terms of the preceding paragraph, the intention to perceive the distance reachable (**Y**) with an unseen hand-held rod is realized by detecting a particular kinetic property (**x**), namely, the rod's principal moment(s) of inertia.

Because the motions of a rod during wielding about axes in the wrist are the three-dimensional motions of a rigid body about a fixed center of rotation, the moment of inertia in the rod's motion equations is in the form of the inertia tensor. The six off-diagonal terms in this symmetric tensor are the products of inertia that engender reactive forces at the center of rotation, causing it to wobble. The three diagonal terms are the moments of inertia with respect to the three coordinate axes. There is an operation — namely, the transformation to the principal or symmetry axes of the rigid body — that eliminates the products of inertia and leaves only the principal moments of inertia on the diagonal (Kibble, 1985). The experimental data suggest that the haptic subsystem separates off the principal moments of inertia from the products of inertia. That is, the haptic subsystem behaves in a manner that is functionally equivalent to the principal axis transformation. Moreover, given that the rigid-body motions of a hand-held rod bring about deformable body motions in the tissues comprising the haptic subsystem, the implied functional diagonalization must include the. deformation (stress/strain) tensor that characterizes deformable body motions.

A particularly pertinent experimental result is that subjects can perceive fractional lengths when rods are held at positions intermediate between their ends ("how far could you reach with the portion of the rod extending beyond your grasp?"). As before, this perceptual achievement depends on detecting principal moments of inertia — but now they are the principal moments of the rod fraction (Solomon & Turvey, in press; Solomon, Turvey, & Burton, submitted). Apparently, the haptic subsystem can decompose the inertia tensor for a given axis of wielding into distinct components corresponding to the mass distributions above and below the given axis. For simplicity, let $\mathbf{I}$ be the moment of inertia of the entire rod about a given axis, and let $\mathbf{I_a}$ and $\mathbf{I_b}$ be the moments of inertia of the rod above the axis and the rod below the axis, respectively. Then it can be argued that when the task is to perceive the whole length of a rod (regardless of hand position), the haptic subsystem behaves as a mechanism that registers the dynamics of the whole hand-held object through the principle of superposition or parallel composition ($\mathbf{I} = \mathbf{I_a} + \mathbf{I_b}$). In contrast, when the task is to perceive fractional length, the haptic subsystem behaves as another kind of mechanism, one that filters the dynamic of the requisite portion of the rod through subtraction ($\mathbf{I} - \mathbf{I_b} = \mathbf{I_a}$).

What is significant about the foregoing experimental results and theoretical analyses is that, depending on the person's intention, the haptic subsystem behaved as one or another smart perceptual instrument (Runeson, 1977; Solomon & Turvey, in press). A smart perceptual instrument is a determinate dynamical machine that executes a single-valued function. Given the task of perceiving property **Y** it detects property **x**, a property that maps uniquely to property **Y** and is a special law-based feature of the situation. In the haptic experiments, the law-based property is the inertia tensor. The challenge for a theory of competence is identifying the grounds for the linkage between the two very different properties involved, namely, the inertia tensor (a kinetic property) and the distal tip of a hand-held object (a geometric property).

Physical principles of cooperativity

The movements involved in skilled action are often complex, involving a great many degrees of freedom. Ordinary locomotion involves very many different kinds of units at the grain sizes of limbs, joints, muscles, neurons, blood vessels, and so on. It is a coordinated act that must be able to accommodate — or reorganize to accommodate — its multiple details to variations in speed and terrain. The control requirements for this so-called degrees of freedom problem have long been recognized (Bernstein, 1967; Turvey, 1977): Although the system's dynamic is describable in a state space of very many dimensions, control is effected through a state space of very few dimensions. More simply, any skilled act presupposes an underlying generic ability to unitize or chunk. This unitizing ability can be conferred — and ordinarily is conferred — on the nervous system. Custom regards the nervous system as an efficient cause (in Aristotle's sense). By this custom, the nervous system is responsible for unitizing. Our view of competence, however, places the means for unitizing in natural laws embodied by the nervous system (Kugler & Turvey, 1987). Contrary to custom, we see the nervous system in the capacity of a supportive basis not an efficient cause (see Ben-Zeev, 1985; Turvey & Carello, 1986).

A physical biology has been evolving in recent years that promises to shed light on the formation and control of movement units comprising skilled action. Broadly construed, physical biology is a law-oriented program that attempts to give an account of biological phenomena (such as coordinated movement) that is continuous with physical methodologies (Kelso, Schöner, Scholz, & Haken, 1986; Kugler & Turvey, 1987). A simple but important example in the movement domain follows.

A transition has been observed between two different modes of rhythmic hand movements, namely, between an antiphase motion in which the relative phase of nonhomologous muscles are 180 degrees and an in-phase motion in which the relative phase of homologous muscles is 0 degrees (Kelso, 1984; Kelso, Sholz, & Schöner, 1986). The observation is made in paradigm in which a person is required to oscillate the two index fingers (or the two hands) at the same frequency. Frequency is then varied (e.g. with a metronome that the person tracks). The main features of the transition are as follows: (a) phase relations of 180 and 0 degrees are the only two steady states; (b) starting in antiphase and increasing the frequency of oscillation leads to an abrupt, involuntary bifurcation to in-phase; (c) immediately prior to the transition, there is a significant increase of critical fluctuations in the relative phase relation; (d) immediately prior to the transition there is a critical slowing down: the time taken to return to antiphase, subsequent to a brief perturbation, increases significantly; and (e) the transition is hysteretic: reducing frequency after the transition does not yield a shift back to antiphase, and starting in-phase and increasing frequency does not eventuate in antiphase organization.

The properties just noted are characteristic of the nonequilibrium phase transitions that occur widely in nature and which are governed by a generic physical mechanism of loss of stability. The physical analysis advanced by Haken, Kelso, and Bunz (1985) and Schöner, Haken, and Kelso (1986) is illuminating. First, it identifies the phase relation as an order parameter. In general terms this is a macroscopic quantity, usually composed of very few component quantities, that expresses the extent of order in a system. An order parameter is of low dimensionality yet it provides an efficient, simple description of the discontinuous behavior of a system comprising a very large number of microscopic degrees of freedom. Second, the physical analysis identifies the antiphase and in-phase coordinations as point attractors in a smooth potential defined with respect to the order parameter (ϕ) as the state variable: $\mathbf{V}(\phi) = -\mathbf{a}\cos(\phi) - \mathbf{b}\cos(2\phi)$. Third, it identifies frequency of oscillation as a control parameter, one whose changes result in qualitative changes in the potential. Specifically, the coefficients a and b change as the frequency of oscillation increases; these changes transform the local minima in the smooth potential — located at $\pm$ 180 deg. — into local maxima. Consequently, at a critical frequency the antiphase equilibrium state disappears and the system jumps suddenly into the in-phase equilibrium state. Fourth, it identifies $\phi = 0$ as the global minimum of the potential; reversing the change in the control parameter does not, therefore, produce a sudden jump back to the antiphase state.

Analyzing movement coordination in terms of its major observables and their dynamics steers thinking toward general principles rather than modular, anatomical, or information processing devices. The theory of competence advocated here demands an appreciation of the lawfulness underwriting the assembling, maintenance, and disassembling of skilled patterns of movement.

Coupling of optical properties to properties of the movement system

A good many skilled activities require continuous adjustment to circumstances as they are revealed. Obstacles that were hidden come into view, opponents block paths to the goal, fly balls die in the wind. For circumstances that are revealed visually, information about them is described kinematically; that is, the optic array consists of optical solid angles transforming over time but there are no masses. In contrast, the behavioral adjustments that must be made are described kinetically; that is, masses must be moved over space and time with the appropriate force. In order to perform a behavior **Y** in a particular circumstance, kinematic information specific to that circumstance must specify kinetic properties of **Y**. A theory of competence for behavior **Y** must delimit how kinematic properties of the optics are coupled to kinetic properties of the movement system.

Just such a coupling has been demonstrated in the adjustment of locomotion over uneven terrain. A runner on a path of irregularly spaced stepping stones must adjust stride length in order to hit the stones rather than the spaces in between them. This adjustment appears to be governed by vertical impulse supplied by the support foot such that the impulse is large when the next stone is far and small when the upcoming stone is near. Vertical impulse is modulated by the optical property **Tau** (Warren, Young, & Lee, 1986) and this makes running over uneven terrain possible.

A similar coupling can be found in the link between **Tau** and the opening of the batter's stance in baseball. In baseball batting, the step and swing are coordinated to the pitch as follows: The start of the step is correlated with the release of the pitch, but the speed of opening of the stance (from start to finish of the step) and the start of the swing are linked to the velocity of the pitch (Hubbard & Seng, 1954). This has the effect of leaving the duration of the swing invariant for pitches of various speeds. That is to say, the swing commences a constant amount of time before the ball is hit. Optical information - in the form of **Tau** - is specific to this fact and makes the act of hitting a baseball possible.

Conclusion

In this article we have attempted to provide the reader with a brief overview of a particular strategy for understanding skilled behavior. The strategy is termed ecological and is so called because of its emphasis on discovering the sources of order - both very general and particular - at the scale at which animals and their niches are defined. The guiding intuition of the ecological approach is that the competence that underlies everyday performances comprises lawful relations among properties. In our view, the theory of competence, as expressed in this article, is preliminary to a thoroughgoing theory of skilled behavior.

References

Ben-Zeev, A. (1985). The Kantian revolution in perception. Journal for Theory of Social Behavior, 14, 69-84.

Bernstein, N. (1967). The coordination and regulation of movements. London: Pergamon (originally published in 1917).

Carello, C., & Turvey, M.T. (1984). On vagueness and fictions as cornerstones of a theory of perceiving and acting: A comment on Walter (1983). Cognition and Brain Theory, 7, 247-261.

Chomsky, N. (1965). Aspects of the theory of syntax. Cambridge, M.A.: MIT Press.

Fodor, J.A., & Pylyshyn, Z. (1981). How direct is visual perception? Some reflections on Gibson's "Ecological Approach". Cognition, 9, 139-196.

Gibson, J.J. (1961). Ecological optics. Vision Research, 1, 253-262.

Gibson, J.J. (1966). The senses considered as perceptual systems. Boston: Houghton Mifflin.

Gibson, J.J. (1979). The ecological approach to visual perception. Boston: Houghton Mifflin.

Gibson, J.J. (1982). Ecological optics. In E.S. Reed & R. Jones (Eds.), Reasons for realism. Hillsdale, N.J.: Erlbaum.

Haken, H., Kelso, J.A.S, & Bunz, H. (1985). A theoretical model of phase transitions in human movements. Biological Cybernetics, 51, 347-356.

Hubbard, A.W., & Seng, C.N. (1954). Visual movements of batters. Research Quarterly, 25, 42-57.

Kelso, J.A.S. (1984). Phase transitions and critical behavior in human bimanual coordination. American Journal of Physiology: Regulatory, Integrative and Comparative Physiology, 15, R1000-R1004.

Kelso, J.A.S,. Schöner, G., Scholz, J., & Haken, H. (1987). Phase locked modes, phase transitions, and component oscillators in biological motion. Physica Scripta, 35, 79-87.

Kelso, J.A.S., Scholz, J.P., & Schöner, G. (1986). Nonequilibrium phase transitions in coordinated biological motion: Critical fluctuations. Physics Letters, 118, 279-284.

Kibble, T.W.B. (1985). Classical mechanics. London: Longman.

Kugler, P.N., & Turvey, M.T. (1987). Information, natural law, and the self-assembly of rhythmic movement. Hillsdale, N.J.: Erlbaum.

Lee, D.N. (1976). A theory of visual control of braking based on information about time to collision. Perception, 5, 437-459.

Lee, D.N. (1980). Visuo-motor coordination in space-time. In G.E. Stelmach & J. Requin (Eds.), Tutorials in motor behavior. Amsterdam: North Holland.

Lee, D.N., & Reddish, P.E. (1981). Plummeting gannets. A paradigm of ecological optics. Nature, 293, 293-294.

Mark, L.S. (1987). Eyeheight scaled information about affordances: A study of sitting and stair climbing. Journal of Experimental

Psychology: Human Perception and Performance, 13, 361-370.

Marr, D. (1981). Artificial intelligence: A personal view. In J. Haugeland (Ed.), Mind design. Cambridge, Ma.: MIT Press. (Originally published in Artificial Intelligence, 9, 37-48, 1977).

Marr, D. (1982). Vision. San Francisco: W.H. Freeman.

Michaels, C.F., & Carello, C. (1981). Direct perception. Englewood Cliffs, N.J.: Prentice Hall.

Runeson, S. (1977). On the possibility of "smart" perceptual mechanisms. Scandinavian Journal of Psychology, 18, 172-179.

Schöner, G., Haken, H., & Kelso, J.A.S. (1986). A stochastic theory of phase transitions in human hand movement. Biological Cybernetics, 53, 247-257.

Shaw, R.E., Turvey, M.T., & Mace, W.M. (1982). Ecological psychology: Consequence of a commitment to realism. In W.H. Weimer & D.S. Palermo (Eds.), Cognition and the symbolic processes, Vol.2. Hillsdale, N.J.: Erlbaum.

Solomon, Y., & Turvey, M.T. (in press). Haptically perceiving the distances reachable with hand-held objects. Journal of Experimental Psychology: Human Perception and Performance.

Solomon, Y., Turvey, M.T., & Burton, G. (submitted). Perceiving the partial and total lengths of rods by wielding: Haptic diagonalization and decomposition of the inertia tensor.

Todd, J.T. (1981). Visual information about moving object. Journal of Experimental Psychology: Human Perception and Performance, 7, 795-810.

Turvey, M.T. (1977). Preliminaries to a theory of action with reference to vision. In R.E. Shaw & J. Bransford (Eds.), Perceiving, acting and knowing. Hillsdale, N.J.: Erlbaum.

Turvey, M.T., & Carello, C. (1986). The ecological approach to perceiving-acting: A pictorial essay. Acta Psychologica, 63, 133-155.

Warren, W.H. (1984). Perceiving affordances: Visual guidance of stair climbing. Journal of Experimental Psychology: Human Perception and Performance, 10, 683-703.

Warren, W.H., & Whang, S. (1987). Visual guidance of walking through apertures: Body-scaled information for affordances. Journal of Experimental Psychology: Human Perception and Performance, 13, 371-383.

Warren, W.H., Young, D.S., & Lee, D.N. (1986). Visual control of step length during running over irregular terrain. Journal of Experimental Psychology: Human Perception and Performance, 12, 259-266.

Cognition and Action in Skilled Behaviour
A.M. Colley and J.R. Beech (Editors)

THE KINEMATIC CHAIN AS A MODEL FOR HUMAN ASYMMETRICAL BIMANUAL COOPERATION

Yves Guiard
Centre National de la Recherche Scientifique,
Marseille.

"If movements are classified from the point of view of their biological significance to the organism making them, it is clear that on the first level of significance we have acts which solve one or another particular motor problem which the organism encounters. (...) Meaningful problems which can be solved by motor action arise, as a rule, out of the external environment."

N. Bernstein (1967, p.115; italics in the original.)

This article presents a tentative theoretical framework for the study of asymmetrical bimanual cooperation in man. It is assumed that each hand represents a motor, i.e. a device controlling a variable position (VP) relative to a reference position (RP). Three modes of assembling the two motors to form a bimanual cooperative structure are distinguished: the orthogonal and the parallel assembly modes, which are basically symmetrical, and the serial assembly mode, which is basically asymmetrical. It is suggested that in man the two hands typically cooperate as two motors assembled in series (with the VP of the left hand serving as the RP for the right hand), thus forming a kinematic chain. Four conspicuous principles governing the behaviour of kinematic chains, namely (i) distal-to-proximal reference, (ii) proximal-distal scale differentiation for time and space, (iii) proximal precedence and (iv) terminal dominance, are described. It is then shown that each of these principles, when applied to asymmetrical bimanual cooperation, leads to predictions consistent with preliminary evidence regarding human real-life bimanual activities. A final suggestion is that the kinematic chain model, which lays emphasis on the hierarchical organization of human bimanual gestures, may help in understanding the adaptive advantage of human manual specialization.

In this paper I present a tentative theoretical framework for the study of asymmetrical bimanual cooperation in man. The activities to which we shall mainly refer are those demanding simultaneous involvement of the two hands appointed to different, complementary roles (such as, for example, playing a guitar or swinging a golf club).

Coordinative and cooperative structures

The problem of coordination in space and time arises as soon as two or more motor organs are simultaneously involved in the activity of an organism. In natural situations, the reason several organs have to come into action concurrently is that, generally, the motor problem encountered by the organism cannot be solved at the level of a single organ: an effector system (Saltzman & Kelso, 1987), or cooperative structure, must be mobilized. This notion may be applied to various scales of the biological reality. A muscle is a cooperative structure whose elements are individual contractile fibers: in order for their common action to be effective, the contractions of the muscle components must be tightly coordinated (a condition that is always met, thanks to hardwired mechanisms). At a higher level, there is cooperation between the various links that form a primate's upper limb in a gesture like reaching and grasping. The contribution of proximal elements, in bringing the hand close to the object to be grasped, and that of distal elements, in grasping the object, are both necessary, and again they must be accurately coordinated in order for the overall gesture to be successful (Jeannerod, 1981). At a still higher level, there is cooperation between the two hands of man for more elaborate activities like, say, manual sewing. Such a task demands a contribution of both the left and the right hands (one to manipulate the piece of fabric, one to manipulate the threaded needle), and these two contributions must be coordinated in time and space.

It is apparent that although cooperation and coordination are two closely related concepts, particularly in the sense that a cooperative structure cannot work in the absence of coordination, they must be carefully distinguished. To decide whether two or more motor organs form a cooperative structure in a particular context, one has to consider what must be done in the environment, that is, examine the motor problem. Two or more motor organs simultaneously involved in the activity of an organism can be said to form a cooperative structure to the extent that they contribute to the solution of one and the same motor problem. In contrast, the concept of coordinative structure (Turvey, Shaw, & Mace, 1978) has to do with the actual execution of simultaneous movements by different effectors, irrespective of whether there is cooperation between the effectors. This is why, in principle, coordinative structures can just as well be studied in the context of dual or even multiple tasks, characterized by the mere superimposition of two or more independent motor problems (for example, Kelso, Southard, & Goodman's (1979) double-handed pointing task), as in the context of single integrated tasks (for example, Kelso, Tuller, & Fowler's (1982) study of the coordination that takes place between the various speech articulators cooperating in utterances).

In short, a cooperative structure is a coordinative structure, that is to say, "a functional grouping of many neuromuscular components that are flexibly assembled as a single, functional unit" (Kay, Kelso, Saltzman, & Schöner, 1987, p.179), but one that serves a common action of the organism. In this sense, it is important to acknowledge that, in general, coordinative structures, while they deserve to be studied per se in multiple-task paradigms, have biological significance to the acting organism only to the extent that they display true cooperation.

Differentiated division of labour and human asymmetrical bimanual activities

As cooperation, unlike coordination, implies homogeneity of purpose in the task to be carried out by the organism, this concept is strongly linked to that of division of labour. There is division of labour between the numerous contractile fibers of a working muscle, as well as between the various joints of an arm engaged in the act of grasping, and between the two hands of a person sewing. The same three examples can serve to illustrate a further useful distinction, the distinction between undifferentiated and differentiated division of labour. Basically, all the fibers of a muscle provide similar contributions to the task of the muscle. Although in action some quantitative differences probably exist between the elements of this cooperative structure, each of them pulls on the tendon, so that division of labour can be said to be undifferentiated. There are, in contrast, marked qualitative differences between the contributions of the various joints of an arm used for reaching and grasping an object, and between the contributions of the two hands in sewing. In the second and third examples, unlike the first, there is differentiation in the roles played by the simultaneously involved organs.

Coming now to the specific subject of this paper, there is little doubt that in humans, as opposed to non-human primate species, manual acts typically rely on differentiated bimanual cooperation. Most skilled human gestures (those which demand at least some learning) can be said: (i) to involve both manual effectors; and (ii) to be asymmetric in the sense that the two manual roles differ qualitatively. This fact, surprisingly, has so far been largely overlooked by experimental psychologists. On the one hand, students of human manual lateralization have traditionally conceived of human manual behaviour as if the problem of laterality amounted to a forced choice between the left and the right hands before action (e.g. Annett, 1985 Hécaen, & Ajuriaguerra, 1964; Oldfield, 1971; Porac, & Coren, 1981). In reality, unimanual instances represent rather rare exceptions in the real repertoire of human skilled manual activities (see Guiard (in press) for a full justification of this statement). Quite typically, human manual tasks demand the building of bimanual cooperative structures, and therefore raise the problem of bimanual coordination during action.

On the other hand, students of motor coordination have generally designed bimanual experimental tasks which are (for reasons that need not be discussed here) basically symmetrical, in the sense that they demand the coordination of two manual activities that are *a priori* equivalent (e.g. Fagard, Morioka, & Wolff, 1985; Kay *et al*., 1987; Kelso *et al*., 1979; Marteniuk, MacKenzie, & Baba, 1984; Turvey, Rosenblum, Kugler, & Schmidt, 1986; Yamanishi, Kawato, & Suzuki,

1980; for notable, but isolated counter-examples, see Guiard, 1986, 1987; Ibbotson, & Morton, 1981; Peters, 1981, 1985; and Schonen, 1977).

Thus, with respect to the understanding of human bimanual behaviour, one is placed in an unfavourable position, which may be summarized as follows. Traditionally, the literature on human manual asymmetry has overlooked the problem of bimanual coordination, while the more recent and more theoretically elaborate literature on motor coordination has so far ignored the fact that, in real task contexts, the two hands of man not only cooperate with each other, but do so according to a differentiated division of labour, leading to marked asymmetry. In the rest of this paper, I shall present an attempt to formulate an approach to the study of human bimanual behaviour that recognizes man's fundamental propensity to form, with his two hands, asymmetrical cooperative structures.

The hands of man as motors, and the problem of assembling them in action

The hand as an anatomical versus task entity

The current use of the word "hand" and its various cognates in phrases such as manual behaviour, hand preferences, bimanual coordination, and the like conceals a minor, but interesting logical oddity. Why for example should one refer to a movement like throwing a stone as a "manual movement"? The act of throwing, after all, involves not only the hand but also, undoubtedly, the elbow, the shoulder, and certainly a number of other motor organs whose contributions may be just as necessary to the performed act as is that of the hand itself. There seems to be a two-stage answer to this question. Firstly, the term of hand in the evoked context is clearly used in a metonymic sense (that is to say, the whole is evoked by denoting one of its parts), otherwise the term would be inappropriate. But, secondly, why choose the hand to refer to the whole cooperative structure, rather than any other part of this structure? The reason, one may presume, has to do with the fact that, to use Saltzman and Kelso's (1987, p.85) terminology, the hand represents the "terminal device of an effector system", that is, the element of the system that is "directly related to the goal of a performed action". Other instances can easily be found of effector systems that are referred to by merely designating their terminal devices. Consider, for example, the lower limb metonymically called "foot" in a gesture like kicking, or the complex hydraulic machine globally called a "shovel", and so on.

Nevertheless, the hand concept, indispensable to the student of human movement, is seriously inaccurate from a concrete, anatomical point of view, because the ensemble of cooperating musculoskeletal organs that it designates metonymically cannot be defined absolutely. For a given action, no list can be a priori drawn of the organs to be involved, because, from repetition to repetition of the same act, there is no guarantee that the same set of organs will be recruited (see the principle of motor equivalence, Hebb, 1949). In contrast, the cooperative structure to which the hand belongs can be abstractly, but accurately, defined as the set of organs that contribute to a given action. Therefore, when we consider "bimanual" behaviour below, it is clear that we shall be dealing with the relationships established, not between two anatomically defined entities, but rather between two functional entities, that is to say, two manual sub-actions or roles.

The hand as a motor

Any device, whether artificial or natural, serving the function of creating motion can be termed a motor. Motors can be identified at many levels of analysis in the same organism. For example, an individual muscle fiber is a motor, but the whole set of fibers that form a muscle can just as well be considered as a motor. At a higher level, one may say that the various muscles that cooperate for controlling a given degree of freedom at a joint collectively represent a motor, and, skipping a few steps, that the hand (metonymically standing for a larger cooperative structure) is a motor.

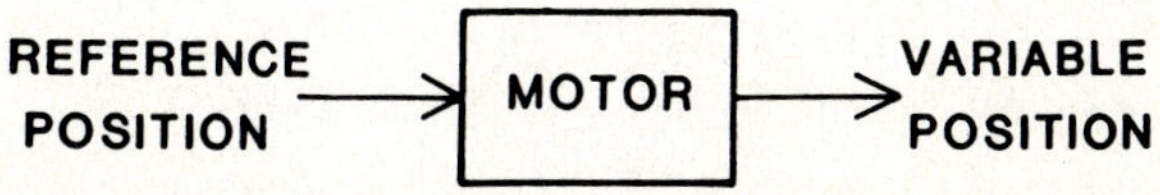

Figure 1. Minimal representation of a motor simply defined as a natural or artificial device whose function is to produce motion. A motor acts upon the difference between a variable position, which it controls, and a reference position, which it receives as an input. This macroscopic representation deliberately ignores both the internal mechanism of the motor (considered as a black box), and the information processing system.

The function of a motor is to create motion, that is to say, to produce a change of position over time. As no position can be conceived of in the absence of another position playing the role of a reference, a motor must be described as a device that controls the difference between two positions, a variable position (VP) which is under its control and a reference position (RP) which it receives passively (see Figure 1). Thus, for example, an engine moving a lift cabin controls the position of the cabin (the VP) relative to the ground (the RP), or the biceps brachii (with the help of other muscles) controls the orientation of the forearm (the VP) relative to that of the upper arm (the RP).

The problem of assembling motors: Orthogonal, parallel and serial assembly modes

Once it has been admitted that the two hands represent two motors, in the abstract sense defined above, the question of bimanual cooperation can be conveniently reduced to that of the cooperation between motors that are assembled in one of several ways. We shall principally consider the case of two-element assemblages, which have the virtue of simultaneously being the simplest and the most relevant to our subject.

There appear to exist basically three ways of assembling two motors to form a cooperative structure (giving rise to another motor at the next level of analysis): the motors can be assembled orthogonally, in parallel, or in series (see Figure 2).

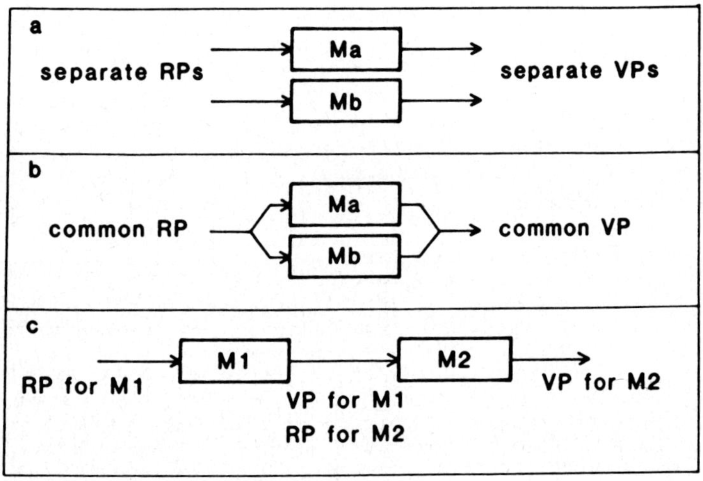

Figure 2. The three conceivable ways of assembling two motors to form a cooperative structure. (a) orthogonal assemblage; (b) parallel assemblage; (c) serial assemblage. Mb, M1, M2 = motors a, b, 1, 2. RP = reference position. VP = variable position. See explanations in text.

An orthogonal assemblage corresponds to the case in which the motors, although they act on the same object, separately control different dimensions of its motion. The basic property of an orthogonal assemblage of motors is mutual independence between the components of motor action, as illustrated diagrammatically in the upper part of Figure 2, in which each of the motors has its own RP and VP. A simple mechanical example is an XY pen recording table, with two servo-motors working along orthogonal axes. The orthogonal assemblage of two motors can also model bimanual cooperation in some instances: for example, consider a milling machine operator manipulating, with the two hands, a pair of cranks that separately control the position of the piece to be wrought along the X and Y axes.

In a parallel assemblage, the motors act upon an object in a synergistic fashion, essentially adding[1] qualitatively non-differentiated contributions to the same action. A parallel assemblage presents the property of mutual dependence, in the sense that the motors have the same RP and control the same VP (see the middle part of Figure 2). Such is the case for example with the left and right engines of an aircraft. As regards bimanual cooperation, the two hands of an athlete lifting a weight, or those of a child skipping rope can be described as motors assembled in parallel.

Finally, in a serial assemblage, the motors are required to act upon the same dimension(s) of the position of an object, with the VP for one motor serving as the RP for the other (see the lower part of Figure 2). A serial assemblage of two motors has the property of asymmetric dependence, in the sense that motion produced by the distal motor (M2 on the figure) is produced relative to the output of its proximal partner (M1), while the inverse is obviously not true. An arm is a familiar instance of a serial assemblage of rotary or torque motors: to consider just two contiguous elements, the set of muscles acting at the elbow forms a motor that is assembled in series with that formed by the set of muscles acting at the wrist. The orientation of the forearm, which represents a VP for the former, simultaneously represents an RP for the latter. Among bimanual cooperative activities, handwriting[2] and sewing can be taken as examples: the left hand manipulates the page relative to the table, while the right manipulates the pen relative to the page (Guiard, & Athènes, 1985; Guiard, & Millerat, 1984); the left hand manipulates the fabric relative to the body, while the right manipulates the needle relative to the fabric.

As shown in the last three paragraphs, each of the three motor assembly modes can serve to model part of the repertoire of bimanual cooperative activities carried out in everyday life. Any homogeneous bimanual activity (that is, any activity describable as solving a single motor problem, rather than several combined motor problems) should, in principle, be classifiable in the language of assembly modes. Thus, the logic of motor assemblages has a taxonomic utility for describing the disheartening variety of human real-life manual gestures.

This is not to say, however, that the orthogonal, parallel and serial modes of assembling are equally useful for modelling human bimanual cooperation. Instances of human gestures that can be modelled in terms of an orthogonal or parallel assemblage of the two manual motors are, in fact, rather hard to find, whereas the serial assemblage seems appropriate for the modelling of quite a large family of human manual activities. The reason for the privileged status of the serial assemblage of two motors with regard to our problem is that this assemblage, contrary to the two others, has the crucial property of asymmetry, due to the fact that such a structure has an orientation, with its elements being qualitatively differentiated by their ranks. Since asymmetry is a prominent characteristic of human manual activities, as already emphasized earlier, the serial motor assemblage is worth examining in greater detail.

The kinematic chain as a model of human asymmetrical bimanual cooperation

A set of serially assembled motors is commonly known as a kinematic chain (e.g. Morasso, 1986). Concretely, a kinematic chain may be composed of torque motors (e.g. a limb), or linear motors, or a mixture of torque and linear motors (e.g. a pneumatic drill mounted at the end of an articulate arm). The view I wish to propose in this section is that there is quite an instructive isomorphism between the way in which two contiguous elements of a kinematic chain and the two hands of man cooperate with each other, considering bimanual cooperation in general. I shall first describe some notable properties of the relationships between the elements of a kinematic chain, and then attempt to show that analogous principles apply quite interestingly to between-hand cooperation in humans placed in a variety of task contexts.

Some principles governing cooperation and coordination between the elements of a kinematic chain

Distal-to-proximal reference

The first principle one must note is true by construction: If a set of motors are assembled in series, then the VP for any motor of rank n represents the RP for the contiguous distal motor of rank n+1 (ranking from the proximal to the distal). Worded differently, the output from any motor of rank n is the input to its distal neighbour of rank n+1.

Proximal-distal scale differentiation for time and space

A second principle is that, both for time and space, a kinematic chain forms a hierarchical structure in which resolution of motion varies as a positive function of the rank. The more distal a motor in a chain, the finer the scale of its contribution to the action of the whole chain. Consequently, if one considers any pair of elements, the one occupying the more distal rank will contribute to the chain's action at a micrometric scale, relative to the other.

As regards time the proximal-distal metric gradient presumably has its origin in the fact that any motor of rank n is carried by the motor of rank n-1, cumulatively true from the periphery to the most proximal motor of the chain (if M3 is carried by M2 and M2 is carried by M1, then M1 carries M2 + M3). Hence there exists a monotonic inertial gradient along the chain[(3)], with the effect that the more proximal a motor, the lower the temporal frequency spectrum of its contribution. Assuming a Weber law for the production of periods (that is to say, the variability of movement time, or period, varies as a positive function of mean movement time, as shown by Stevens, 1886 [cited by Wing, 1986] and confirmed, among others, by Schmidt, Zelaznik, Hawkins, Frank, & Quinn, 1979), one is led to expect that the more proximal a motor, the greater the temporal variability of its activity. Thus, motors occupying different ranks in a chain will differ by the temporal metrics, or scale of their contributions, with the contribution of a more proximal motor being characterized simultaneously by longer time periods and a lower temporal resolution.

Much the same analysis can be made with respect to the spatial scale of the various elements of a kinematic chain. Taking an extended arm as an example, it is obvious that a rotation of, say, 10° about the shoulder will have a much larger effect on the position of the tip of the pointed index finger than the same 10° rotation performed about the metacarpo-phalangeal joint of the index finger. Thus, keeping in mind the amplitude of motion that can be produced at the chain's endpoint by the various motors, it seems clear that, as a rule, the more proximal a motor, the lower its spatial frequency spectrum of activity. Again, with the help of a Weber law argument (that is, the spatial variability of movement varies as a positive function of movement amplitude, as shown by Schmidt et al., 1979) one is allowed to conclude that a more proximal motor will tend to contribute to the chain's action on a different, relatively macrometric spatial scale, characterized by larger amplitudes (larger spatial periods) and, accordingly, a lower spatial resolution.

Proximal precedence

A third principle governing the functional relationship between elements of a kinematic chain is that the more proximal a motor, the earlier it is likely to come into action in a given mobilization of the chain. Thus, for example, in a simple movement of the upper limb to touch a point located at some distance with the tip of the forefinger, it is clear that the macrometric proximal organs of the limb will be crucially involved in the initial phase of the movement, for moving the hand to the vicinity of the target point, whereas the participation of the micrometric distal organs of the limb will take place towards the end of the movement, to ensure an accurate final positioning (for clear-cut illustrations of this principle in the cat reaching food with the forelimb, see Hoffmann, Illert, & Wiedemann, 1986, and Kably, Armand, Buisseret, & Moulin, in press).

As suggested by the very formulation of what precedes, the principle of proximal precedence (which pertains to the actual performance of action rather than division of function and, in this sense, is a principle of coordination rather than cooperation) seems to derive logically enough from the hierarchical nature of kinematic chains. There appears to exist a general constraint that once division of labour has been made within a set of organs according to a hierarchical principle, the macrometric organs will intervene earlier than the micrometric ones in the realization of an action (a prototypic instance is the sequential and forcibly-ordered utilization of the two knobs of an optic microscope serving to set the distance from the lenses to the histological section first macrometrically, then micrometrically).

Terminal "dominance"

Reasoning implicitly on the case of effector systems composed of serially assembled organs, Saltzman and Kelso (1987) pointed out that the terminal device of an effector system is "directly related to the goal of the performed action" (p.85). In terms of our motor assembly model, this characteristic of the terminal device can be interpreted as follows: the VP controlled by the last motor of a kinematic chain relative to the output of the penultimate motor also represents the VP of the whole chain, now with reference to the input to the first motor (see Figure 3). Thus, for example, in the act of pointing in a direction "with the index finger", the orientation of the index finger simultaneously represents the output of the muscles acting at the finger joints (relative to the orientation of the metacarpals) and the global output of the whole cooperative structure (the involved limb, but perhaps also other parts of the body, such as the trunk and legs) relative to the environment.

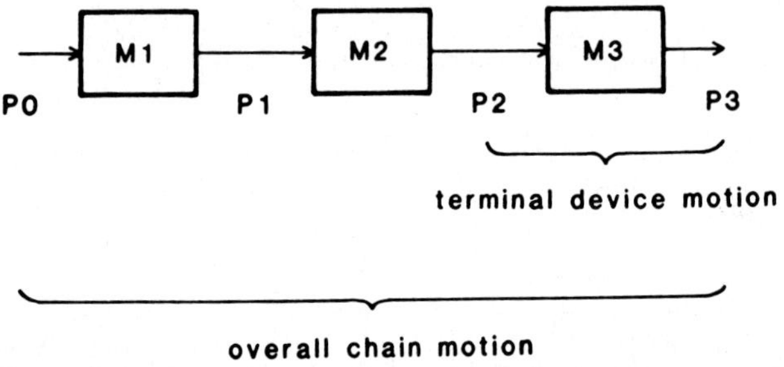

Figure 3. Illustration of the principle of terminal motor "dominance" in a three-element kinematic chain. M1, M2, M3 = motors 1, 2, 3. P0, P1, P2, P3 = positions 0, 1, 2, 3, with P0 standing for a fixed reference in the environment, and P3 standing for the position of the chain's endpoint. A conspicuous characteristic of P3 is that its changes represent action of M3 (relative to P2), while at the same time representing action of the whole chain (relative to P0).

This characteristic of the terminal part of a kinematic chain seems quite clearly to account for the fact that, in the verbal description of motor behaviour, the hand (or even the index finger, as in the example of pointing evoked in the last paragraph) is commonly taken as the representative for a complex chain of motor organs. But another, probably more important, consequence of the special status of the terminal element of a chain is that the acting organism itself is liable to selectively attend to what happens at the extremity of the chain to the detriment of what happens at more proximal levels, for the simple reason that usually the only relevant relationships, from the point of view of motor action, are those established between the chain's endpoint and the environment (an interesting exception in this respect is dancing: see Camurri, Morasso, Tagliasco, & Zaccaria, 1986). Thus, to summarize our fourth principle, we may say that the terminal organ of a kinematic chain is dominant in the sense that its privileged contribution tends to be identified with the global action of the chain, whether by an observer or by the organism responsible for the movement.

The two hands as a kinematic chain

Having described some important high-order principles governing the relationships between elements of a kinematic chain, our task is now to evaluate to what extent these principles apply to the flexible cooperative structure formed by the two hands in the wide variety of everyday asymmetrical tasks. The gist of this section is as follows: not only do humans display a marked propensity to divide labour between their two hands in accordance with the kinematic chain scheme (which represents a regularity in the task domain), but they also (in the ordinary case of right-handedness, which we shall only consider) quite consistently appoint their left and right manual effectors to functions that can be likened to those of the proximal and distal elements, respectively, of a pair of contiguous components of a kinematic chain (a regularity that pertains to the performance domain, and points to the concept of permanent manual specialization).

I shall not try here to formally demonstrate the views that have just been presented (because the realm of human bimanual movements is of a bewildering diversity, and because this paper must have a limited length). My purpose, rather, will be to suggest the feasibility and the interest of treating human asymmetric bimanual cooperative structures as flexible kinematic chains. In practice, I shall examine the applicability of each of the four principles described in the preceding sub-section to two well contrasted classes of bimanual movements: (i) those which can be said, in usual terms, to associate a postural and a manipulative role, as is the case in hammering a nail, peeling a fruit, threading a needle etc. (a very large class indeed); and (ii) those which demand of both the left and right hands a truly dynamic motor contribution, thereby failing to display any qualitative postural-manipulative differentiation of function (more specifically, we shall consider hitting movements performed with bimanually held implements).

Right-to-left reference

Considering bimanual movements in which the left manual role can be deemed as postural, there is no doubt that this role consists not only of providing stability to the object acted upon by the right hand, but also of defining spatial positions that the right hand will necessarily have to take into account for its action to be effective. A postural organ, unlike a clamp or any inert fixation device, remains a motor, that is, a device whose vacation is to change positions.

As suggested by MacNeilage, Studdert-Kennedy and Lindblom (1984), the left, postural hand can be said to offer "frames" into which right hand activity inserts "contents". Along these lines, it is tempting to say that whenever the left hand is appointed to an activity consisting of periodically revising the orientation and/or the position of an object submitted to right-hand action, motion of the right hand organizes itself relative to the orientation and/or position provided.

A clear illustration may be found in handwriting. Naive subjects were asked to produce a complete page of writing on dictation. They used an ordinary A4 sheet of paper but the writing took place on a specially designed desk blotter that hid a sheet of carbon paper. Thus, two writing traces were simultaneously recorded: one was the intended page of writing, corresponding to motion of the pen tip relative to the sheet of paper; the other was the unintended trace formed, through the desk blotter, on the surface of the writing table, and thus corresponding to motion of the pen tip relative to the environment. Quite typically, the two recordings were found to differ markedly, with the latter occupying a much smaller area than the former, due to many line superimpositions (Guiard, in press). The interpretation of this finding is straightforward: as writing proceeds through the page, most skilled handwriters periodically reposition their sheet of paper or notebook, using the left hand, so as to limit the vertical — and, to a lesser extent, horizontal — amplitude of right hand moves relative to the writing table, and thus avoid compromising their overall body posture (Athènes, 1984; Guiard, & Athènes, 1985; Guiard, & Millerat, 1984). The fact that, in such an experiment, the sheet of paper, and not the table surface, bears the appropriately laid out writing when the page has been completed testifies that, in handwriting, right hand (pen) motion is organized relative to left hand (page) temporary positions, and not permanent positions of the environment.

In principle, the notion of right-to-left spatial reference should generally hold for innumerable human bimanual movements characterized by cooperation between a postural and a manipulative roles (the analysis presented above can readily be applied to activities like hammering a nail or a piece of metal, striking a match, sewing, peeling a vegetable, opening a jar, playing the guitar or the violin[4], and so forth). The question of whether the principle of right-to-left reference still applies to cases in which neither hand assumes a postural function, that is, where neither hand defines easily recognizable static positions with respect to the environment, seems more tricky at first glance. It must be recalled, however, that immobility and motion are relative concepts: there is no logical inconsistency in asking oneself whether, given two hands that move simultaneously, one moves relative to the other.

The case of hitting movements performed with bimanually held implements such as the golf club is interesting in this respect, as both hands, which occupy different positions on the implement and therefore are forced to play mechanically differentiated roles, must contribute in a truly dynamic fashion to the acceleration of the distal extremity of the implement. Cochran and Stobbs' (1968) classic analysis of the golf swing has convincingly shown that the structure formed by the golfers' arms and the club can be likened to the serial assemblage of two levers. The left hand, which holds the end of the handle, is the master in controlling the rotation of the upper (proximal) lever, while the right hand, posted below the left, has the responsibility of controlling the rotation of the lower (distal) lever, represented by the club, relative to the (obviously variable) angular position of the upper lever.

Thus, Cochran and Stobbs' (1968) conclusion is plainly consistent with the extension of the principle of right-to-left spatial reference to movements not characterized by distinct postural and manipulative roles. In fact, there is already evidence that the between-hand division of labour governing the golfer's swing holds for the whole family of movements consisting of using a rigid bimanually held implement to hit in rotation (in old martial language, to cut, as opposed to thrusting). Arguing that the double lever model of Cochran and Stobbs (1968) is basically valid for describing the entire repertoire of these movements (including, among other sports implements, the use of the golf club, the cricket and the baseball bats, the lawn hockey stick and the kendo sabre, as well as, among other tools, the use of the pickaxe and the sledgehammer), Guiard (1987) has recently shown that in all cases examined, the preferred order of the two hands on the handle (governed either by institutional prescription or by spontaneous preferences) was the same as in the golfer's grip, with the left hand occupying the higher position on the handle, thus opening the bimanual kinematic chain. In other words, the way in which the two hands cooperate in the golfer's swing, and more generally in the class of mechanically similar rotatory hitting gestures, represents, quite interestingly, a virtually literal application of the kinematic chain model.

Left-right scale differentiation for time and space

As motion and stability are relative concepts, a motor in principle may find its vital spatial references in the positions assumed by any object, whether the latter is immobile or mobile with respect to the environment. There is a limit, however, to this relativity, in the sense that, in practice, a movement can hardly be referred to a body whose motion takes place on a finer temporal-spatial scale.

Let us take handwriting again as an example of postural manipulative bimanual activities. It is clear that a writer's two hands operate in altogether different frequence bands[(5)]. As regards time, the right hand behaves as a quite rapid oscillator (3 to 7 Hz, as shown by Michel, & Laviron, 1972, among others) compared to the left hand, whose cycle of activity, from one move of the sheet of paper to the next, might possibly last tens of seconds. In the spatial domain, a similar contrast can be observed, with the right hand producing small amplitude, high resolution motion at the pen tip by comparison with the large amplitude, low resolution motion periodically imparted to the page by the left, postural hand. Such a marked between-hand difference for the temporal-spatial scale of activity in handwriting is strongly linked to the principle of right-to-left reference evoked above. Generalizing somewhat, one may consider that a postural frame would make no sense, were it defined on a finer scale than the movement content it must incorporate.

Let us return to the other relevant class of human bimanual movements, those consisting of hitting with long implements in rotation. Starting from Cochran and Stobbs' (1968) thorough analysis of the swing of professional golfers, it is easy to show that the left and right hands here contribute to the task on different scales, macrometric and micrometric respectively. For the sake of simplicity, we shall only consider the executory portion of the swing, the so-called downswing. As regards time, the two manual contributions differ considerably in duration, as the acceleration of the upper lever, due to left hand action, is a slow process (high inertia), whereas that of the lower lever, due to right hand action upon the rotation of the club itself, takes the form of a comparatively very short impulse (Cochran, & Stobbs, 1968; see also Connelly, 1984, and Nicklaus, 1983). As regards space, what must be noted is that rotation of the upper lever about the left shoulder has a much larger effect on the position of the clubhead than rotation of the club about the end of its handle, leading us to conclude that the right hand is a motor that ensures a relatively micrometric, high resolution control of the position of the clubhead (as already pointed out earlier, the validity of the double lever model extends to the whole class of bimanual rotatory hitting movements).

In sum, there are clear indications that, as predicted by the kinematic chain model, activities of the two hands simultaneously involved in asymmetric cooperation differ in terms of their spatial-temporal metrics, a fairly general phenomenon, observable both in the context of postural-manipulative action and that of bilateral dynamic action.

Left-hand precedence

The principle of left-hand precedence in the mobilization of the human bimanual cooperative structure also appears to hold in general, as may be suggested by examining successively what happens in the implementation of postural-manipulative and bilaterally dynamic manual actions.

In activities such as handwriting, sewing, hammering a nail, and the like, the left hand obviously must have completed its postural adjfustments before the manipulation proper starts for the right hand, which implies that in any such task the mobilization of the two hands tends to be ordered in time. This fact is readily interpretable in terms of the phenomenon classically known as postural precedence (Belen'kii, Gurfinkel', & Pal'tsev, 1967; Gahery, & Massion, 1985; Nashner, & McCollum, 1985): to the extent that the left hand role is postural, it stands to reason that it must intervene first in time.

In contrast, our second class of bimanual activities, those which are bilaterally dynamic, raises an interesting problem in this respect. For lack of any observable stability during action (with respect to the environment) for either of the two hands involved, the concept of posture is inapplicable, and therefore the postural-precedence principle irrelevant. This is clearly the case, for example, in the golf swing, where we must assume, following Cochran and Stobbs (1968), that although the left hand "carries" the dynamically behaving right hand, it is also acting itself dynamically (a situation analogous to that of, say, the elbow musculature with respect to the wrist musculature in a gesture like hammering).

As a matter of fact, Cochran and Stobbs (1968) have provided data which show that in the golfer's downswing, the principle of left-hand precedence does apply: the acceleration of the proximal lever, corresponding to left-hand action, takes place during approximately the first two thirds of the downswing, followed by a deceleration contemporaneous with the sudden acceleration of the distal lever (the club) controlled by right-hand action(6). In other words, the relatively long-lasting action of the left hand in the golf swing precedes the relatively brief action of the right, in keeping with the model.

Why is it the case that, in human asymmetrical bimanual cooperation, the mobilization of the left hand consistently tends to precede that of the right, regardless of whether the former contributes statically or dynamically to the overall action? The logic of the kinematic chain seems to offer a satisfactory interpretation (see the earlier section on proximal precedence): the left hand tends to be mobilized first, it is suggested, not simply because its role is postural (otherwise the left-right temporal ordering would probably be specific to postural-manipulative bimanual tasks, which it is not), but basically because its contribution represents a relatively macrometric, global component of an action that can be later refined, thanks to the micrometric contribution of the right hand. This interpretation calls upon the principle of global precedence, familiar to students of visual perception (see, for example, Navon, 1977), but conceivably applicable to a wider range of human actions, whether perceptual, intellectual, or motor in nature.

Right-hand dominance

Of course no discussion is needed to admit the existence of the phenomenon of right-hand dominance in man. Nearly ninety per cent of humans are right-handed, and the hand dominance phenomenon has been extensively described by psychologists, in its two aspects: one is hand preference, which can be simply assessed with questionnaires evoking tasks that require a forced choice between the two hands: the other aspect is hand superiority, which can be assessed by experimentally comparing the subjects' ability to perform standard unimanual motor tasks with the left or the right hand (for reviews, see Annett, 1985; Hécaen, & Ajuriaguerra, 1964; Porac, & Coren, 1981).

What is open to discussion, in contrast, is the significance of this familiar, but poorly understood phenomenon. The prevailing conception, it seems, in the current literature on manual motor asymmetry, is that the appearance, in the evolution of the human primate, of special motor skills in a single hand (leading both to hand superiority and hand preference) has represented, per se, a crucial positive evolutionary step (see Calvin, 1982, for an explicit formulation of this view). Such a conception might be criticized, firstly on logical grounds: it seems unclear in what sense the emergence of a left-hand discrepancy for manual motor ability (with one hand becoming skilled and the other remaining unskilled) may have been optimal from an evolutionary point of view. Secondly, and more importantly, this conception is incompatible with the fact that virtually all skilled human manual actions rely on the simultaneous and differentiated participation of the two hands (see the earlier section on the differentiated division of labour).

Beyond the question of whether the dominant right hand is, on the whole, individually superior to its non-dominant partner (a question which might well elicit different answers depending on the criteria used for defining motor ability[7]), it is interesting to examine the right-hand preference phenomenon in the light of the kinematic chain model. The suggestion of the model is two-fold: firstly, our understanding manual skills, in comparison with those of other primates, would rest, not in the special motor abilities of our preferred hand, but rather in our species-specific ability to form asymmetric, differentiated cooperative structures with our two hands to efficiently solve most of the encountered motor problems; secondly, the right-hand preference phenomenon would reflect, not necessarily a real superiority of the right hand over the left, but rather the fact that the right hand, which as a rule ends the bimanual chain, typically shoulders a more conspicuous responsibility[8]. To interpret right-hand preference by analogy with the principle of terminal dominance evoked above, one may say that the concept of right (distal) hand, so to speak, designates the whole bimanual structure, by a metonymical process so effective, albeit unconscious, that the contribution of the (more proximal) left hand is, in many a case, ignored. Such favouritism for the right hand, however, has an air of legitimacy, as the contribution of this hand, unlike that of the other, logically tends to represent the action of the whole chain (see the section on terminal dominance, and Figure 3).

Symmetry, asymmetry and dissymmetry in two-motor assemblies

It has already been pointed out that a serial assemblage of motors, by definition, has the property of asymmetry. An important question in this regard is whether asymmetry is specific to the serial case. I wish to argue that the answer — which hinges on the distinction between asymmetry and dissymmetry, concepts that I shall try to define below — is definitely yes.

Let us consider two instances of bimanual tasks, one orthogonal and one parallel, in which, in some sense, symmetry seems to be broken, thus raising an apparent objection to our position. Frohlich and Elliott (1984) and Fagard et al. (1985) had subjects rotate a pair of knobs (or cranks) in order to steer a cursor along tilted tracks displayed on a screen. Clearly, division of labour between the hands in such tasks was orthogonal, and yet the task demanded, for all track inclinations but one (0° in Frohlich, & Elliott's task, 45° in Fagard et al.'s), that the two control devices be rotated at different angular velocities. As for the parallel instance, think of an athlete rowing with a single oar rotating about a fixed axis. The two hands add their efforts, but as they must operate at different distances from the axis of rotation of the oar, the reactive force and the amplitude of movements will differ between the left and the right components of the task.

It seems tempting to categorize such tasks as "asymmetric", on the simple grounds that there are measurable differences between the two manual activities. This would be, however, inappropriate. The argument, taking place at the level of the logic of division of labour between a pair of motors (to the exclusion of any quantitative aspects), is that any orthogonal or parallel assemblage is a symmetrical structure, as unequivocally illustrated in Figures 2a and 2b. The two examples given in the preceding paragraph are not exceptions: in Frohlich and Elliott's (1984) and Fagard et al.'s (1985) orthogonal tasks, the two dimensions of motion of the cursor are logically equivalent; in rowing with a single oar, the two hands play logically equivalent roles, both consisting of rotating the oar relative to the boat (same VP, same RP). What these examples quite interestingly show, in the final analysis, is that a symmetrical logic of division of labour may suffer a number of quantitative differences arising at the stage of its implementation. This idea may be conveyed by the term of dis-symmetry, denoting a defect in symmetry.

Thus, an orthogonal or a parallel assembly of two manual sub-actions may give rise either to symmetrical activity (e.g. skipping rope) or to dissymetrical activity (e.g. rowing with a single oar), but the term of a-symmetry, which denotes non-validity of the symmetry hypothesis, does not apply. In contrast, a serial logic of assembly, which is properly asymmetrical, as shown in Figure 2c, will necessarily give rise to truly asymmetric activity.

Overview and Conclusion

It will be useful to recapitulate the various theoretical assumptions that have been made so far. The main preliminary choices that have served to define our approach can be summarized as follows. First, deliberately ingoring left-handedness, we have based our reasoning on the within-subject logic of the functional relationships established between the two hands of man when coping with a variety of bimanual tasks. Thus, our stance is that of psychologists interested in the basic study of human behaviour, as distinct from that generally adopted by students of handedness, which can be labelled as a differential stance on the grounds that the central handedness concept has to do with between-individuals variability. Second, our approach can be defined as non-reductionist with respect to the central nervous system, in the sense that we seek to account for behavioural phenomena on the scale, and in terms of behaviour. This choice is based on the contention that, in dealing with behavioural asymmetries, psychology can do more than merely treat them as symptoms of the functional specialization of the cerebral hemispheres (this position obviously amounts, not to denigrating the study of brain-behaviour correlations, but rather to questioning a naive causal understanding of these correlations). A third preliminary choice is to seriously take into consideration theoretically relevant facts that lie in the realm of common knowledge, to the extent that this characteristic reflects their obviousness, rather than any collective illusion. While an experimental demonstration can be trivial (by laboriously showing something that is already known to be true), a fact is simply more or less robust. The point being made here is that besides trying to establish, at a high cost, subtle, and often empirically controversial new lateral differences in the laboratory (as has been generally the case in experimental psychology since Kimura's [1961] discovery of the popular right-ear advantage in dichotic listening), the student of human functional laterality might fruitfully consider the various asymmetries that manifest themselves in the most obvious and robust fashion in the real-life behaviour of man, which may represent just as valuable data to the scientist.

Turning to the constituent assumptions of the model outlined in the preceding sections, it has been assumed in the first place that each hand of man represents a motor, defined abstractly, but rigorously as a device whose function is to create motion in the environment, by changing a position (termed as variable position) relative to another position (termed as reference position). Abstraction refers to the fact that, in reality, one is faced by a complex, multi-joint musculoskeletal ensemble whose anatomical borderline cannot be traced with certainty, and which, by default, must be defined comprehensively, in a given task context, in terms of the function collectively served by its component organs.

In the second place, the problem of assembling several (and notably two) motors was examined, and three cases, the orthogonal, the parallel, and the serial modes of assembly, were distinguished. The main observation was that while the three conceivable assemblages of two motors can serve to model human cooperative bimanual activities, only one of them, the serial assemblage (identified with the concept of kinematic chain) presents the particularity of asymmetry, which characterizes the vast majority of skilled bimanual gestures in man.

Finally, an attempt was made to analyse in greater detail the properties of kinematic chains, and to show that each characteristic feature of a kinematic chain has its strict analogue in human asymmetric bimanual cooperation. Four conspicuous principles governing the behaviour of a kinematic chain were described, namely, distal-to-proximal reference, spatial-temporal scale differentiation, proximal precedence, and terminal dominance. It was then shown that provided that one models the left and right hands as the proximal and distal elements, respectively, of a two-element chain, the four above-mentioned principles convert readily into principles of bimanual cooperation and coordination that not only are quite sensible, but also seem consistent with available preliminary evidence regarding human real-life bimanual activities. The final suggestion, consequently, was that the kinematic chain model may serve as a theoretical framework for exploring the domain of human bimanual cooperation.

It may be useful to remark that although the two hands can be conveniently viewed as forming a kinematic chain by themselves, it does not follow that the bimanual system necessarily works in isolation. In fact, it must be realized that in many task contexts the two-handed kinematic chain represents just one part of a larger chain comprising one or several more proximal element(s). An obvious instance is the golf swing, which can be said to articulate the two-lever manual structure on top of the more proximal structures composed of the trunk and the leg musculatures. To describe a golfer in the spirit of Cochran and Stobbs (1968), but in terms of our motors assemblage model, we may say that the golfer schematically represents a four-element chain, whose last two elements are the hands. The legs rotate the pelvis relative to the ground, the trunk musculature rotates the pectoral girdle relative to the pelvis, the left hand rotates the proximal lever relative to the pectoral girdle, and, finally, the right hand rotates the club relative to the proximal lever. This is not all. A further possibility must be kept in mind, namely that the bimanual chain may carry a more distal organ (as seems to be the case for example in an activity like singing while accompanying oneself with a guitar, in which the voice can be compared with the terminal organ of a three-element chain). Thus, to formulate the model of asymmetric bimanual cooperation in accurate terms, our suggestion is to view the left and right hands of man as two contiguous elements of a kinematic chain whose number of elements need not be specified. At the same time, one is led to a more general treatment of the model: after all, man's propensity to build, with his two hands, asymmetrical cooperative structures that have the form of kinematic chains is liable to represent just one particular, albeit privileged, case of a more general human propensity to build kinematic chains on the various scales of motor action, that is, to proceed to solve motor problems in a hierarchical fashion.

To conclude, it may be appropriate to examine the problem of the biological significance of kinematic chains. In what general, but specific, sense are serial assemblages of motor organs advantageous to the acting organism? Perhaps the most important feature of kinematic chains is that they represent hierarchical structures, as already hinted at in the preceding discussion. I wish to argue that hierarchical division of labour between motor organs makes it possible, at the level of the whole chain's action, to overcome the limitations imposed on movement production by Weber's law (Schmidt et al., 1979).

If one has a single motor at one's disposal for creating movement, or a set of motors that can only be assembled orthogonally or in parallel, one will inevitably have to adopt a particular compromise between two contradictory requirements: one is the temporal-spatial magnitude, the other the temporal-spatial resolution of movement. With the Weber law dilemma, one will be condemned, so to speak, to be either far-sighted or near-sighted in motor action. The point is that if, in contrast, one can proceed to assemble motor organs in series, the invaluable facility to concurrently operate on several scales will emerge, so that overall action will reach a disproportionately high temporal spatial resolution, given its duration and amplitude characteristics.

This principle is visibly at work in the functioning of concrete kinematic chains such as an arm, whose more proximal organs allow the gestures to explore a large control space (Turvey et al., 1978) while its more distal organs ensure a complementary fineness of resolution. It seems conceivable that this reasoning might be extended to altogether abstract hierarchical action systems such as language (duality of patterning; e.g. Hockett, 1960) or to the numerical system. Ranked powers of a given base offer the facility to define a quantity without Weber law constraint, in the sense that even when coping with, say, trillions, it remains possible (although presumably absurd) to be accurate to, say, the thousandth. Between such extreme instances, there seems to be room for the concept of a flexible hierarchical assembly of two manual actions, which the kinematic chain model, it is hoped, may help to formulate.

Footnotes

(1) Two motors working as mutual antagonists (e.g. the biceps and the triceps brachii) must be represented as assembled in parallel, simply because they both control one and the same VP relative to one and the same RP (the orientation of the forearm relative to the upper arm, in the example taken above). As to the notion that they add their contributions, it remains true if these contributions are represented by vectors.

(2) Although handwriting has been traditionally held as a unimanual activity, it is easy to show that the non-preferred hand contributes to this task in a modest but significant way, by not only fixing the

sheet of paper (or notebook) to the writing table but also repositioning it upwards periodically as the writing proceeds downwards in the page, so as to limit the amplitude of the right-hand moves. Deliberately disregarding the value judgements that come to the mind about the relative importance of the two manual roles in an activity like handwriting, it seems necessary, in the context of this study, to scrupulously recognize what is actually done by each hand in every task considered.

(3) This inertial gradient may be particularly strong in a chain composed of rotary motors having different axes of rotation, as is the case with an arm: here not only will mass be added from link to link, but also radius of rotation. Hence a strongly accelerated increase of moment of inertia from the most distal to the most proximal element of the chain.

(4) Complex though it may be, the activity of playing a string musical instrument such as the guitar or the violin can be reduced to the following minimal schema: the left hand controls the position of the instrument (which it holds) as well as its states (the length of the strings, that is, positions again) while the right hand, whether or not equipped with an implement like a bowl acts upon it by exciting the strings.

(5) Throughout this paper it is assumed that the temporal and the spatial metrics or scales of movement quite generally bear a positive correlation: as a rule, the larger the amplitude (the spatial period) of a movement, the longer its duration (its temporal period). Evidence for this position has been recently provided by Kay et al. (1987), who have shown that the amplitude of simple rhythmical hand movements spontaneously decreases in a monotonic way as the frequency of oscillation imposed on the movement increases.

(6) Cochran and Stobbs (1968) account for the intriguing deceleration of the rotation of the hands about the trunk that takes place in professionals towards the end of the downswing (before ball impact) as follows: at the beginning of the downswing, rotation of the proximal lever about the central pivot has the effect of imparting motion to the distal lever (the club), as the two levers form a rigid whole (the reason is that the wrists, initially assuming a maximal angle of 90° or so between the extended left arm and the club, temporarily act as a stop). With the acceleration of this proximal component of rotation, the centrifugal force that tends to align the two levers, that is, to accelerate the distal rotation to the detriment of the proximal rotation, becomes substantial. Low handicap golfers take advantage of this kinetic phenomenon, which represents a transfer of angular momentum from the proximal to the distal lever.

(7) Since the origins of the experimental study of human manual skills (e.g. Woodworth, 1899), investigators seem to have placed much emphasis on relatively high resolution movements, characterized by short durations and amplitudes, typical of those which the right hand is currently required to perform in everyday bimanual movements (Craik, 1947; Fitts, 1954; Schmidt et al., 1979; Meyer, Smith, & Wright, 1982). Consequently, the finding that the right hand performs these kind of tasks better than the left (e.g. Flowers, 1975; Todor, & Cisneros, 1985) is not that surprising. The question of whether

inverse hand superiority can be demonstrated in lower resolution movements remains open. For example, Guiard, Diaz, & Beaubaton's (1983) finding that in a relatively large amplitude (42 cm) open loop aimed movement, the left hand of right-handers displayed a smaller spatial constant error than the right, despite a larger variable error, may be interesting in this regard.

(8) This interpretation of the right-hand dominance phenomenon quite interestingly converges with Peters' (1985) attentional interpretation of the asymmetry that emerges in bimanual rhythmical movements. In a task consisting of tapping a steady beat with one hand and a simple rhythm with the other, it has been observed that right-handed non-musicians perform better if the beat is assigned to the left, and the rhythm to the right hand rather than vice versa (Ibbotson, & Morton, 1981; Peters, 1985). To account for this and other similar results, Peters (1985, p.172) suggested that "in the control of naturally occurring bimanual movement, there is normally a division of the component tasks in terms of one activity that demands and receives focal attention, and one that is capable of being guided by indirect attention".

Acknowledgements

The author wishes to thank Peter Boisvert, David Frohlich and Michel Treisman for helpful comments on the first version of this article, and Alain Durey, Onno Meijer, Sylvan Kornblum and Michael Peters for valuable discussions concerning several of the topics therein.

References

Annett, M. (1985). Left, right, hand and brain: The right shift theory. Hillsdale, N.J.: Erlbaum.

Athènes, S. (1984). Adaptabilité et développement de la posture manuelle dans l'écriture: étude comparative du droitier et du gaucher. Unpublished memorandum. University of Aix-Marseille II.

Belen'kii, J. Ye., Gurfinkel', V.S., & Pal'tsev, Ye. (1967). I. Elements of control of voluntary movements. Biophysics, 12, 154-161.

Bernstein, N. (1967). The co-ordination and regulation of movements. Oxford: Pergamon.

Calvin, W.H. (1982). Did throwing stones shape hominid brain evolution? Ethology and Sociobiology, 3, 115-124.

Camurri, A., Morasso, P., Tagliasco, V., & Zaccaria, R. (11980). Dance and movement notation. In P. Morasso, & V. Tagliasco (Eds.), Human movement understanding. Amsterdam: North-Holland.

Connelly, I. (1984). Learn the correct role of your hands and arms. Golf World, 23, 66-68.

Cochran, A., & Stobbs, J. (1968). The search for the perfect swing. London: Morrison & Gibb.

Craik, K.J.W. (1947). Theory of the human operator in control systems. I. The operator as an engineering system. British Journal of Psychology, 38, 56-61.

Fagard, J., Morioka, M., & Wolff, P.H. (1985). Early stages in the acquisition of a bimanual motor skill. Neuropsychologia, 23, 535-543.

Fitts, P.M. (1954). The information capacity of the human motor system in controlling the amplitude of movement. Journal of Experimental Psychology, 47, 381-391.

Flowers, K. (1975). Handedness and controlled movement. British Journal of Psychology, 66, 39-52.

Frohlich, D.M., & Elliott, J.M. (1984). The schematic representation of effector function underlying perceptual-motor skill. Journal of Motor Behavior, 16, 40-60.

Gahéry, Y., & Massion, J. (1985). Co-ordination between posture and movement. In E.V. Evarts, S.P., & D. Bousfield (Eds.), The motor system in neurobiology. Amsterdam: Elsevier Biomedical Press.

Guiard, Y. (1986). Interlimb role differentiation in pointing with a bimanually held implement. Presented at the 27th Annual Meeting of the Psychonomic Society. New Orleans, Lousiana.

Guiard, Y. (1987). The kinematic chain as a model for asymmetric between-hand division of labour in the manipulation of long tools. Presented at the Fourth International Conference on Event Perception and Action. Trieste, Italy.

Guiard, Y. (in press). Asymmetric division of labor in human skilled bimanual action: The kinematic chain as a model. Journal of Motor Behavior.

Guiard, Y., & Athènes, S. (1985). Main droite et main gauche dans l'écriture: la question de la posture "inversée" chez le scripteur gaucher. In UNICEF, (Ed)., Maitrise du geste et pouvoir de la main chez l'enfant. Flammarion.

Guiard, Y., Diaz, G., & Beaubaton, D. (1983). Left-hand advantage in right-handers for spatial constant error: preliminary evidence in a unimanual ballistic aimed movement. Neuropsychologia, 21, 111-115.

Guiard, Y., & Millerat, F. (1984). Writing postures in left-handers: inverters are hand-crossers. Neuropsychologia, 22, 535-538.

Hebb, D.O. (1949). The organization of behaviour. New York: Wiley.

Hécaen, H., & Ajuriaguerra, J. de (1964). Left handedness: Manual superiority and cerebral dominance. New York: Grune and Stratton.

Hockett, C.F. (1960). The origin of speech. Scientific American, 203 88-106.

Hoffmann, P., Illert, M., & Wiedemann, E. (1986). EMG pattern of cat forelimb muscles during target reaching and food taking movements. Neuroscience Letters supplements, 26, S-215.

Ibbotson, N.R., & Morton, J. (1981). Rhythm and dominance. Cognition, 9, 125-138.

Jeannerod, M. (1981). Intersegmental coordination during reaching at natural visual objects. In J. Long, & A. Baddeley (Ed.), Attention and performance, IX. Hillsdale, N.J.: Lawrence Erlbaum.

Kably, B., Armand, J., Buisseret, P., & Moulin, G. (in press). Précission du mouvement des articulations proximales pour atteindre une cible et son rôle compensateur après ablation néonatale unilatérale du cortex sensorimoteur chez le chat. In M. Laurent, & P. Therme (Eds.), Recherches en activités physiques et sportives II. Marseille: Centre de Recherche de l'UEREPS Aix-Marseille II.

Kay, B.A., Kelso, J.A.S., Saltzman, E.L., & Schöner, G. (1987). Space-time behavior of single and bimanual rhythmical movements: Data and limit cycle model. Journal of Experimental Psychology: Human Perception and Performance, 13, 178-192.

Kelso, J.A.S., Southard, D.L., & Goodman, D. (1979). On the coordination of two-handed movements. Journal of Experimental Psychology: Human Perception and Performance, 5, 229-238.

Kelso, J.A.S., Tuller, B., & Fowler, C.A. (1982). The functional specificity of articulatory control and coordination. Journal of the Acoustical Society of America, 72, S103.

Kimura, D. (1961). Cerebral dominance and the perception of verbal stimuli. Canadian Journal of Psychology, 15, 166-171.

MacNeilage, P.F., Studdert-Kennedy, M.G., & Lindblom, B. (1984). Functional precursors to language and its lateralization. American Journal of Physiology (Regulatory, Integrative and Comparative Physiology), 15, R912-R914.

Marteniuk, R.G., McKenzie, C.L., & Baba, D.M. (1984). Bimanual movement control: Information processing and interaction effects. Quarterly Journal of Experimental Psychology, 36A, 335-365.

Meyer, D.E., Smith, J.E.K., & Wright, C.E. (1982). Models for the speed and accuracy of aimed movements. Psychological Review, 89, 449-482.

Michel, F., & Laviron, A. (1972). Analyse fréquentielle de la vitesse du geste graphique. Psychologie Francaise, 1, 145-151.

Morasso, P. (1986). Trajectory formation. In P. Morasso, & V. Tagliasco (Eds.), Human movement understanding. Amsterdam: North Holland.

Nasher, L.M., & McCollum, G. (1985). The organization of human postural movements: A formal basis and experimental synthesis. Behavioral and Brain Sciences, 8, 135-172.

Navon, D. (1977). Forest before trees: The precedence of global features in visual perception. Cognitive Psychology, 9, 353-383.

Nicklaus, J. (1983). Five views of my new swing. Golf World, 22, 42-43.

Oldfield, R.C. (1971). The assessment and analysis of handedness: The Edinburgh inventory. Neuropsychologia, 9, 97-113.

Peters, M. (1981). Attentional asymmetries during concurrent bimanual performance. Quarterly Journal of Experimental Psychology, 33A, 95-103.

Peters, M. (1985). Constraints in the performance of bimanual tasks and their expression in unskilled and skilled subjects. Quarterly Journal of Experimental Psychology, 37A, 171-196.

Porac, C., & Coren, S. (1981). Lateral preference and human behavior. New York: Springer Verlag.

Saltzman, E., & Kelso, J.A.S. (1987). Skilled actions: A task-dynamic approach. Psychological Review, 94, 84-106.

Schmidt, R.A., Zelaznik, H., Hawkins, B., Frank, J.S., & Quinn, J.T.Jr. (1979). Motor output variability: A theory for the accuracy of rapid motor acts. Psychological Review, 86, 415-451.

Schonen, S. de (1977). Functional asymmetries in the development of bimanual coordination in human infants. Journal of Human Movement Studies, 3, 144-156.

Todor, J.I., & Cisneros, J. (1985). Accommodation to increased accuracy demands by the right and left hands. Journal of Motor Behavior, 17, 355-372.

Turvey, M.T., Rosenblum, L.D., Kugler, P.N., & Schmidt, R.C. (1986). Fluctuations and phase symmetry in coordinated rhythmic movements. Journal of Experimental Psychology: Human Perception and Performance, 12, 564-583.

Turvey, M.T., Shaw, R.E., & Mace, W. (1978). Issues in the theory of action: Degrees of freedom, coordinative structures and coalitions. In J. Requin (Ed.), Attention and performance VII. Hillsdale, N.J.: Erlbaum.

Wing, A. (1986). Presented at the 10th Annual Meeting of the European Neurosciences Association. Marseille, France.

Woodworth, R.S. (1899). The accuracy of voluntary movement. Psychological Review, 3, 1-114.

Yamanishi, J., Kawato, M., & Suzuki, R. (1980). Two coupled oscillators as a model for the coordinated finger tapping by both hands. Biological Cybernetics, 37, 219-225.

Cognition and Action in Skilled Behaviour
A.M. Colley and J.R. Beech (Editors)

EXPLORING THE DYNAMICS OF JUGGLING

P.J. Beek
The Free University, Amsterdam

The dynamics of juggling three balls in a figure-of-eight pattern are explored from a natural physical perspective. A pilot experiment is reported in which the juggling task is scaled on rate in order to test hypotheses as to how this effects: (1) the timing relation between two key time components in the motion of the hands, and (2) the relative balance between harmonic and relaxation behaviour of the effector system. In addition, some clues and ideas are provided as to how perception may constrain the act of juggling.

Consider a skilled juggler, juggling three balls, comfortably, in a figure-of-eight pattern. The ongoing action is one of alternately catching a ball with the one hand and tossing it over to the other. The elliptical movements of the hands, resulting primarily from the coordination of cyclical shoulder, elbow, and wrist motions, tightly match the parabolic flight motions of the balls. Furthermore, the movements of the two hands mirror one another, albeit with a certain phase lag. This situation is depicted schematically in Figure 1, which also defines the symbols as they will be used throughout the paper.

The general problem we would like to address is the following: how is such a seemingly complex skill controlled and coordinated? More specifically, how does the skilled juggler meet the rather severe spatial and temporal constraints of the task? What are the relevant perceptual variables used in steering? What kind of minimal dynamical model can account for the observed kinematic data? In short: what are the dynamics of juggling?

The approach we adopt to this problem is largely inspired by the dynamical approach to movement control, championed by workers of the Haskins Laboratories and the University of Connecticut, but it is not, as will become apparent, identical. We share, however, the overall aim to describe action phenomena in terms of low-dimensional equations of motion and to identify the essential collective variables that govern specific perception-action couplings (Kelso, 1981; Kelso & Kay, 1987; Kugler, 1986; Kugler, Kelso, & Turvey, 1980; Saltzman & Kelso, 1987; Turvey, 1977).

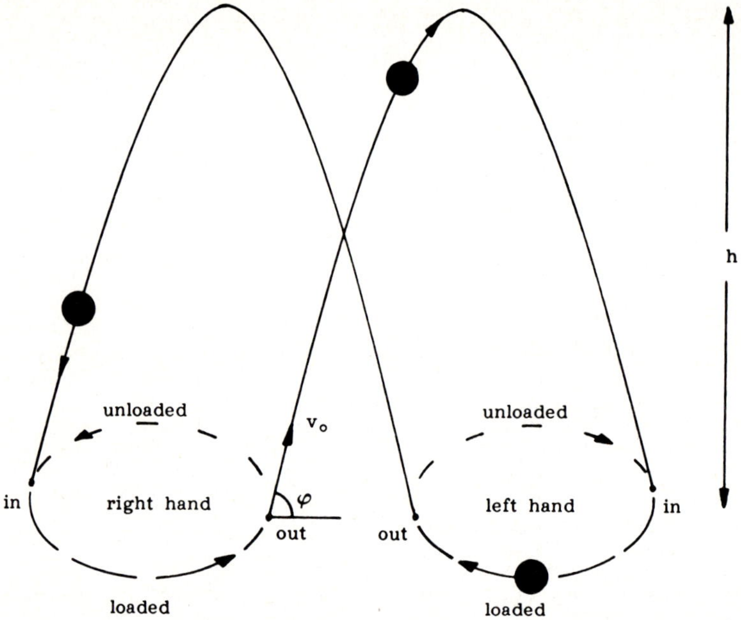

Figure 1. Schematic representation of juggling three balls in a figure-of-eight pattern, momentary situation. φ is the angle of release; v_o is the velocity of the ball at the moment of release; h is the height to which the balls are tossed relative to the point of release.

In the present contribution, our aim is to demonstrate how far a dynamical approach to an advanced skill like juggling with an odd number of balls can contribute to our understanding, how such an approach is to be styled and shaped in order to arrive at the appropriate questions for guiding future research, and to what type of empirical results such an approach may lead. The emphasis is on the development of a theoretically significant research programme rather than, at this stage, on the provision of irrefutable empirical evidence. The data are presented largely as illustration; they are derived from a study involving only one experimental subject.

First, we will develop some theoretical considerations which, in turn, give rise to two experimental hypotheses - one with respect to the delicate timing relations that obtain in juggling three balls, the other with respect to the dynamics of the effector system (Saltzman & Kelso, 1987), i.e. the hand-arm system. Secondly, we will report on a pilot experiment to test these hypotheses. The experimental results are then presented and discussed. The programme pursued for studying action dynamics will also provide us with some clues as to the nature of the relationship between action and perception.

Timing relations and relative timing in juggling three balls

From Figure 1 it is clear that, with an increasing frequency of juggling, the probability of collision of the balls in the air will increase considerably if the flight trajectories of the balls are not precisely controlled. This probability will also increase with the number of balls being juggled, albeit in a different way, since that would change the task itself. In theory, the strategies of the juggler to avoid such mid-air collisions are many. For example, he can ensure:

1) a small, systematic difference in the absolute value of the angle of release of tossed balls between left and right hand (very effective);
2) an alternating change in the height difference between both hand cycles (effective);
3) an alternating change in the horizontal difference between both hand cycles (still effective, but less so);
4) a small forward-backward sway of the body causing the balls to be projected in individual vertical planes (very effective, but difficult to control).

The most effective factor in avoiding collision of balls, however, turns out to be an inherent property of the hand movements proper:

5) the time that a hand is loaded with a ball, t-loaded (tl), is more than twice as long as the time that a hand moves empty, t-unloaded (tu). If N is the number of balls, the mean number of balls in the hand is 2tl/(tl+tu), while the mean number of balls in the air is:

$$\frac{(N-1)2tu + (N-2)(tl-tu)}{tl + tu} = N - \frac{2tl}{tl + tu} . \qquad (1)$$

In the case where tl is equal to tu, the mean number of balls in the hand would be 1 and the mean number of balls in the air would be N-1. For tl greater than tu, however, the mean number of balls in the hand is more than 1, while the mean number of balls in the air is less than 2. Hence, with tl greater than tu a considerably less risky sequence in juggling is promoted than would be the case with tl close to tu.

In order to obtain a smooth performance, a juggler has to match the flight time of the balls (tf), t-loaded and t-unloaded and to keep those times relatively constant. These time elements are, of course, closely related, but how? Irrespective of the exact values of tf, tl and tu, the total flight and loaded time per ball in a complete cycle should equal the total loaded and unloaded time per hand in a complete cycle. In formula form:

$$\frac{(tl + tu)}{H} = \frac{(tl + tf)}{N} , \qquad (2)$$

where H is the number of hands (2) and N is the number of balls (3).

Equation (2) provides a means of gaining some insight into the ratios of the three crucial times involved, if a principle of "phase locking" is assumed which states that the ratios between these characteristic times are simple and pure Pythagorean. We can rewrite Equation (2) as:

$$tf = (\frac{N}{H} - 1)tl + (\frac{N}{H})tu, \tag{3}$$

which is equivalent to

$$1 = \frac{1}{2}\frac{tl}{tf} + \frac{3}{2}\frac{tu}{tf}, \tag{4}$$

for H is 2 and N is 3. The only Pythagorean candidates for this equation are

$$\frac{tl}{tf} = 2, \frac{3}{2}, 1, \frac{1}{2}, \frac{1}{3}, \ldots, \tag{5a}$$

and hence, because of Equation (4)

$$\frac{tu}{tf} = 0, \frac{1}{6}, \frac{1}{3}, \frac{1}{2}, (\frac{5}{9}), \ldots, \tag{5b}$$

From this, it follows that

$$k = \frac{tl}{tl + tu} = 1, (\frac{9}{10}), \frac{3}{4}, \frac{1}{2}, (\frac{3}{8}), \ldots, \tag{6}$$

where the fractions between the brackets are not simply Pythagorean. On the basis of this analysis we can formulate Hypothesis I: In juggling three balls, the relative timing ratio k is a Pythagorean relational invariant independent of angular loop frequency.

The dynamics of the effector system

An exact account of the dynamics of juggling is sought in the theory of oscillators. Functional units of action are thought of as dynamical systems, characterized by a set of time-independent dynamic parameters (e.g. mass or moment of inertia, damping, stiffness) with kinematic variations (e.g. position, velocity, acceleration over time) as a consequence. In the past, for instance, a number of investigators (e.g. Bizzi, Polit, & Morasso, 1976; Kelso & Holt, 1980; Kelso, Holt, Kugler, & Turvey, 1980; Polit & Bizzi, 1978) have hypothesized that such units can be modelled as linearly damped mass-spring systems with the following equation of motion:

$$m\ddot{x} + b\dot{x} + kx = 0, \tag{7}$$

where m is mass, b: damping coefficient, k: stiffness coefficient; and $x, \dot{x}, \ddot{x}$: position, velocity and acceleration. If b is greater than zero, such a system is a point attractor, that is, in the $(x,\dot{x})$-plane (or phase plane) all trajectories settle down to a static equilibrium position, regardless of initial conditions or changes thereof due to perturbation.

In the case of sustained rhythmical movement, however, a different type of dynamical description is required. In principle, there are two ways to transform a linearly damped oscillator into a periodic attractor. One of them is to add a time-dependent forcing function, rendering the equation non-autonomous in a mathematical sense:

$$m\ddot{x} + b\dot{x} + kx = F(t) \quad (8)$$

where all left hand side symbols are as defined in Equation (7), and F(t) is a time-dependent forcing function. An essentially different way is to add a time-independent "forcing" function with a negative damping coefficient, which amounts to inserting energy into the system, and a non-linear dissipative component to balance that energy input. These requirements comprise a non-linear escapement function, rendering the equation of the system (again) autonomous (as in Equation (7)):

$$m\ddot{x} + f(x,\dot{x})\dot{x} + kx = 0, \quad (9)$$

where $f(x,\dot{x})$ is a non-linear escapement function and all other symbols are defined as in Equations (7) and (8).

The oscillators described by Equations (8) and (9) may settle down to an invariant limit cycle trajectory in the phase plane representation, and return to that cycle after perturbation. They differ, however, with respect to their frequency-amplitude relation, phase-locking and phase transitions. Recently, some evidence (e.g. Kay, Kelso, Saltzman, & Schöner, 1987; Kelso & Schöner, in press) has been produced in favour of non-linear autonomous descriptions of rhythmical movement.

An essential feature of oscillators with a non-linear escapement function is that they may exhibit relaxation behaviour. Relaxation oscillations (Van der Pol, 1934, 1939) deviate in some interesting ways from harmonic oscillations. They constitute a periodic repetition of a non-harmonic phenomenon, a discontinuous jump, during which the system is periodically unstable. Typically, their amplitude is fixed, rather than their frequency, while the situation is quite the reverse for harmonic oscillations.

The distinction between harmonic and relaxation behaviour is of particular relevance to an analysis of the dynamics of juggling. Whatever the precise equations of motion for juggling with three balls turn out to be, they will almost certainly be non-linear because the stability of the movements will not be neutral (Kay, Kelso, Saltzman, & Schöner, 1987). Moreover, the spatiotemporal constraints of the task are so severe that the frequency and the amplitude of the hand movements need to be relatively stable.

The relative importance of these two aspects, however, may vary with the rate of juggling. We expect that in the low frequency mode spatial constraints will be more severe than in the high frequency mode. In the low frequency mode, the balls are tossed away more forcefully and even a small deflection in the desired angle of release will have a considerable effect on the locations at which they are to be caught. The juggler, therefore, has to carefully control the amplitude of the hand motion in relation to the velocity vector of the ball. Thus, the relaxation component in the hand motion will be more pronounced than in the high frequency mode. In the high frequency mode, the balls are tossed away less forcefully allowing more variation in the angle of release. Here, temporal constraints are more severe than in the low frequency mode and the overall motion will be more harmonic.

These considerations may be summarized in Hypothesis II: The (non-linear) dynamics of the effector system in juggling allow for dynamic readjustments in the balance of harmonic and relaxation behaviour. When going from high to low pacing, the relaxation component in the behaviour of the effector system will gradually increase relative to the harmonic component.

Hypotheses I and II will be put to the test in the experiment that follows.

Method

Subject

The subject was an experienced professional juggler (age 26). In acknowledgement of his professional commitment, he was paid a small amount of money for his services.

Task

The subject was required to juggle three balls (weight 120 g, diameter 6.7 cm), in his preferred frequency mode, in a figure-of-eight pattern for at least twenty complete cycles (120 consecutive tosses and catches). Subsequently, he was required to slow down or speed up his performance without impairing the smoothness of the operation, thus providing data in low and high frequency modes.

Procedure

Film recordings were made of ten cycles of juggling in each frequency mode (low, preferred, high). The camera (Teledyne), running at a speed of 40 frames per second, was placed directly in front of the subject at a distance of 4 m. For purposes of digital data acquisition, the proximal joint (metacarpophalangeal) of the middle finger of the left and right hand of the juggler were marked with a strip of black tape. The fingers comprise - in the task-dynamic terms of Saltzman and Kelso (1987) - the terminal device of the effector system, i.e. that part of the effector system that is directly related to the goal of that action. Here, we assume that the observed motion of the terminal device reflects sufficiently well the overall system movement.

Data reduction and dependent measures

The films (Kodak 4X Reversal 400 ASA) were projected by means of a NAC (DF-16b) 16mm projector on to an opaque screen. Mounted on the screen was a SAC 14" X-Y tablet, connected to an Apple II micro-computer. Frame by frame analysis of the position of the three balls and fingers allowed the coordinates of these marked points to be read into the computer and stored on floppy disk. For each frequency mode, three out of the ten complete cycles - those that best represented the ongoing rhythmic motion in the sense of being free from minor errors - were digitized. The data were, later, transferred to a much faster Cyber 175-750 mainframe for further processing. The displacement data were filtered with a recursive, second order Butterworth filter with a cut-off frequency of 8 Hz. This procedure was run through twice in order to negate the phase shift (Wood,

1982). Subsequently, the first derivative of the smoothed displacement data was computed by means of a five-point central difference algorithm.

A peak-finding algorithm was used on the velocity data of the balls in order to identify the temporal location of the points of release (positive peak velocity) and the points of catch (negative peak velocity), thus allowing a maximal relative error of 12.5 ms (0.5 frame). The time elements t-loaded and t-unloaded and the relative timing ratio k were computed from these temporal locations. Subsequently, in order to test Hypothesis I, measures of central tendency (means) and variability (standard deviations) for these variables were computed.

In order to test Hypothesis II, a Sine and Cosine Fourier Transform and a Fast Fourier Transform were performed on the filtered displacement data of the first joint of the middle finger of the left and right hand in the x- and y-directions of motion. In addition, the power of the peaks in the power spectra were scaled to the main frequency of the hands (peak a_1) in the preferred mode, which was set to a value of one (hence, arbitrary units).

Results

To obtain a more meaningful impression of the data, reference should be made to Figures 2.1 and 2.2, which exhibit the time plots of the x- and y-coordinates of the hands and the balls in the preferred frequency mode. Essential data points (catches and tosses) and key time elements (t-unloaded, t-loaded, t-flight) are indicated.

Timing relations and relative timing in juggling three balls

The means and variability measures of t-loaded and t-unloaded and their relative timing ratio k for the low, preferred, and high angula loop frequency are presented in Table 1. A one-way analysis of

Table 1

Means and standard deviations of t-loaded, t-unloaded and their relative timing ratio k for the low, preferred and high angular loop frequencies ($\omega_h = 2\pi$ (tl+tu)) of one skilled juggler. Tl and tu are in seconds, k is dimensionless and ω_h is in rad/sec.

frequency	tl	s.d.	tu	s.d.	k	s.d.	ω_h
low	0.63	0.04	0.23	0.03	0.73	0.04	7.30
preferred	0.37	0.02	0.17	0.03	0.69	0.03	11.64
high	0.28	0.02	0.14	0.02	0.68	0.04	14.96

variance was performed on the relative timing ratios k, revealing an effect of angular loop frequency on k, $F(2.44) = 17.00$, $p < .005$.

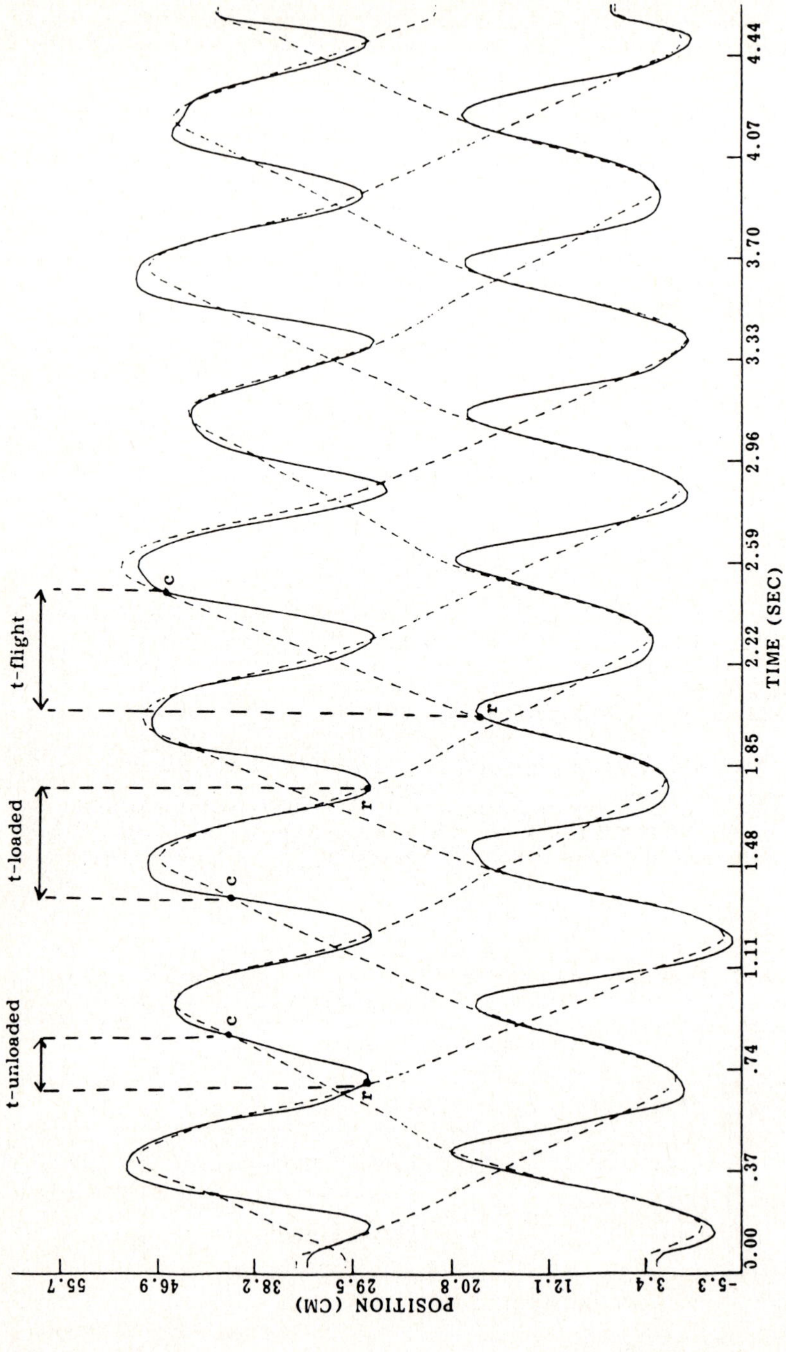

Figure 2.1. The juggling motion of the hands (solid lines) and the displacement of the balls (dotted lines) in the x-direction. Points of catch (c) and points of release (r) are indicated.

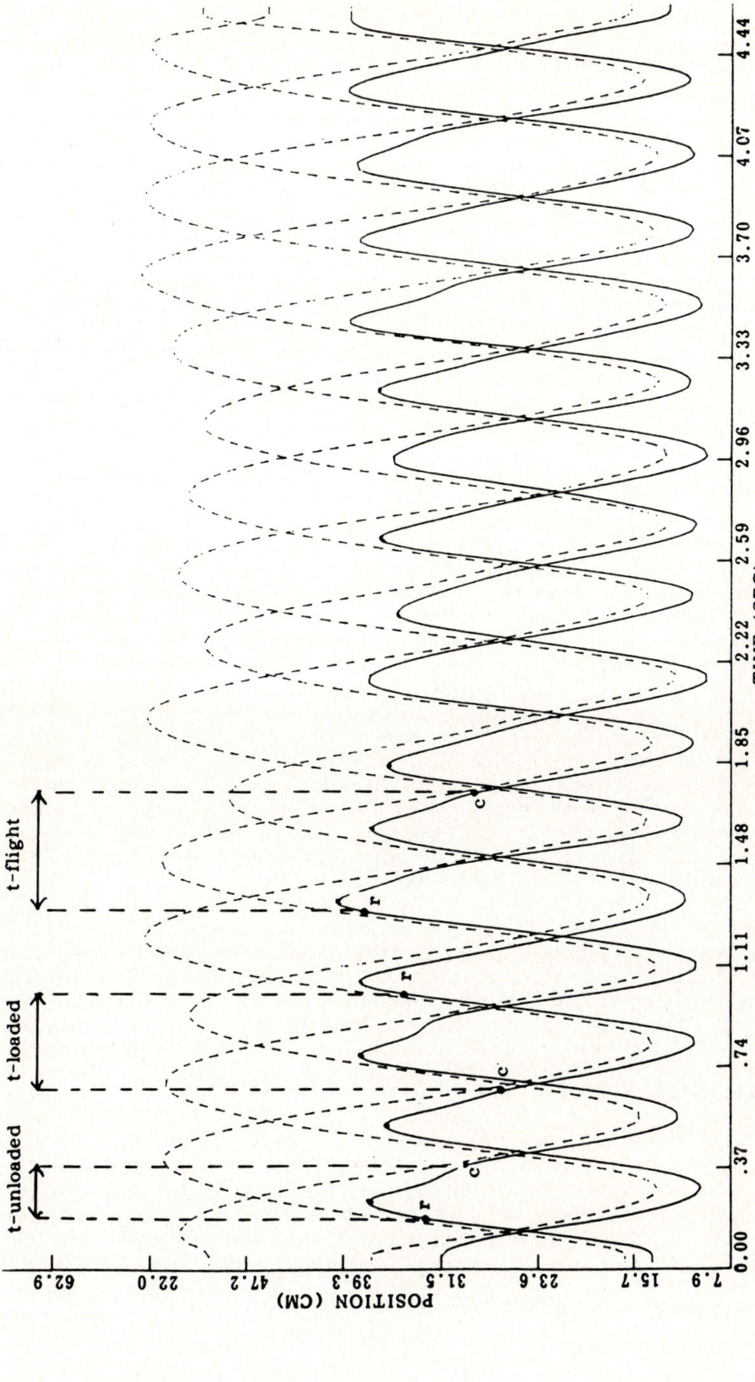

Figure 2.2. The juggling motion of the hands (solid lines) and the displacement of the balls (dotted lines) in the y-direction. Points of catch (c) and points of release (r) are indicated.

The data presented in Table 1 confirm that the above timing analysis, based on simple phase locking (k is a constant Pythagorean ratio), is a reasonable first order approximation: all measured k-values do, in fact, approach the value of 3/4 (0.75). However, the significant result of the one-way ANOVA suggests that there is more to the problem of relative timing than simple, invariant phase locking. Hypothesis I, that the relative timing ratio k in juggling three balls is a Pythagorean relational invariant over different angular loop frequencies, is only true as a first order approximation and should be rejected as a complete description. In the light of this result, we suggest that the dynamics of juggling are such that there are, in fact, several steady k-states, clustered around a Pythagorean ratio, but related to different frequency domains of juggling. To test this new hypothesis, we need to capture the dynamics of juggling such that different dynamical regimes emerge, which then account for the differences in k obtained.

In the present contribution, however, we will refrain from explaining regimes of relational k invariants in terms of the underlying dynamics, but it is a real challenge for the near future to do so. In our opinion, a search for invariance in skilled movement behaviour (Schmidt, 1984) is necessarily a first step in understanding the design of the system, never a final analysis. Once particular invariant features have been traced, a rationalizing of these on principled, physical grounds should be attempted (Kelso, 1981), although there is no guarantee that this in itself will provide a complete answer.

The dynamics of the effector system

The Sine and Cosine Fourier Transform of the y-values of the hands is described by only one harmonic frequency within a noise level of 15%. Its power spectrum in the low frequency mode is displayed in Figure 3.1. This frequency is, when multiplied by 2π, equal to the angular loop frequency of the hands. Apparently, the juggling movements in the y-direction of motion are largely harmonized with the fixed acceleration of the balls due to gravity.

The results of the Sine and Cosine Transform of the x-values of the hands are more complicated. The simple and major part is one sine frequency (again, directly related to the loop frequency of the hands), showing that as a first approximation the hands transverse an elliptical trajectory. The cosine frequencies of the Transform, however, cluster around 0.5, 1.0, and 2.0 times the frequencies of the hands. Figure 3.2 offers an example of this finding, again in the low frequency mode.

Since non-linearity in the dynamics of a system is the only known cause for subharmonics (Van der Pol, 1922, 1934), the lower frequency unequivocally indicates non-linearity in the differential equation(s) of motion of the hands. Physically speaking, the appearance of subharmonics in the power spectrum implies that the movements of the hands are to a certain degree characterized by relaxation behaviour. There is, in other words, a regime of frequencies in juggling at which the hands are spatially, rather than temporally, restricted.

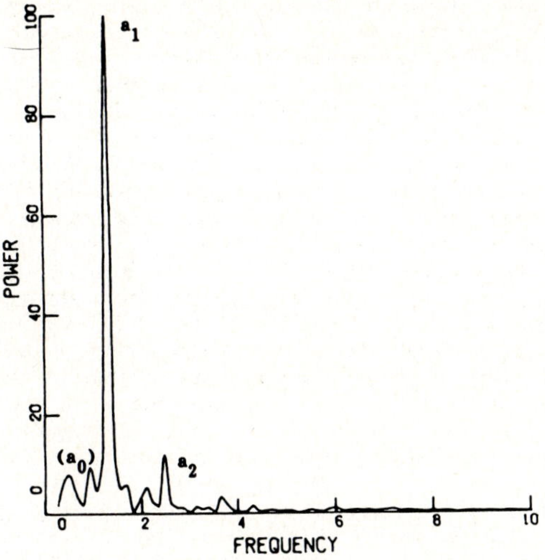

Figure 3.1. The power spectra of the displacement data of the hand in the y-direction. The power is normalized to the absolute power of the largest peak (100%). Low frequency mode of juggling.

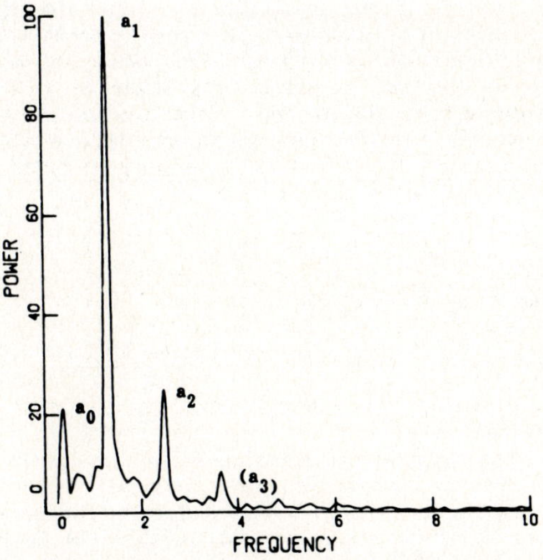

Figure 3.2. The power spectra of the displacement data of the hand in the x-direction. The power is normalized to the absolute power of the largest peak (100%). Low frequency mode of juggling.

The higher or superharmonics may also be ascribed to a non-linear effect in the motion of the effector system, since non-linearity close to frequencies of harmonic behaviour is also known to produce higher harmonics. Although it cannot be ruled out a priori that these higher harmonics are, in fact, due to a persistence of the subfrequencies of the loaded and unloaded parts of the time loop of the hands, the fact that the k-value (see above) is not really an invariant, renders this explanation, at best, incomplete. Thus, we must conclude, that the larger part of the frequency spectrum (sub- and higher harmonics) is accounted for by non-linearities in the equations of motion of the hands. Hence, the system cannot be described by linear equations of the type defined by Equation (8).

Another way to state this result is that the frequency preferred by the juggler is such that a balance is maintained between the frequencies predicted by harmonic and relaxation behaviour. Only then, does he seem to be able to keep the dynamic adjustments of his hands bounded in space and time. For a complete confirmation of Hypothesis II, however, we need to show that the relative balance between harmonic and relaxation behaviour changes with the rate of juggling and, furthermore, that it changes in the predicted direction. Table 2 provides some useful information in this respect. The a-values represent the scaled power of the peaks (a_0, a_1, and a_2) in the power spectrum of the displacement data of the hands in the x-direction of motion.

Table 2

The relative power of the main peaks (a_0, a_1, a_2) in the power spectra of the displacement data of the left hand in the x-direction of motion for the low, preferred and high frequency modes of one skilled juggler. The a-values are based on the scale $a_1 = 1$ for the preferred frequency mode (arbitrary units). The value of $a_0/(a_1 + a_2)$ is a measure for the relaxation component in the overall motion.

	a_0	a_1	a_2	$a_0/(a_1+a_2)$
low	0.55	2.58	0.65	0.17
preferred	0.17	1.00	0.24	0.14
high	0.16	1.09	0.20	0.12

When the juggler is invited to slow down from his preferred frequency mode to a lower one, the relaxation component in the motion of the hands increases slightly, as witnessed by a small, but marked, increase in the ratio $a_0/(a_1 + a_2)$. The relative increase of the relaxation component is limited because the juggler must maintain smoothness of operation (as is supported by the values of a_1 and a_2).

When the juggler speeds up from his preferred frequency mode to a higher one, the relaxation component in the motion of the hands decreases (the value of $a_0/(a_1 + a_2)$ is somewhat lower). Again the effect is limited, since the higher harmonic component of motion (a_2) is also less pronounced. Nevertheless, the overall motion is more harmonic (as is reflected in an increased value of a_1), while non-linear aspects continue to play a role (a_0 and a_2). The juggler still operates in a stable region between harmonic and relaxation behaviour, between temporal and spatial control. (It may be conjectured that non-linear aspects are (also) preserved in the high frequency mode in order that the juggler be prepared for either external or "self-inflicted" perturbations.)

Naturally, the reasoning behind this analysis leads to the question as to how well a juggler controls the angle of release (φ) in the three frequency modes. From the data, the y- and x-velocities of the balls at the moment of release were used to compute φ = arc tg vy_0/vx_0. Table 3 reviews the results.

Table 3

The absolute means of the angles of release (φ) and their standard deviations for the low, preferred and high frequency modes of one skilled juggler. φ is in degrees.

	mean	s.d.
low	82.32	1.84
preferred	70.36	2.35
high	69.09	3.96

On the face of it, the variation in the angle of release does indeed appear to decrease with a decreasing rate of juggling. To test the null hypothesis of equality of variances, the Scheffé (1959, pp.83-87) approximate test for comparison of variances was performed. Since this test is based on the analysis of variance of the logarithms of the sample variances, we had to randomly subdivide each of our three frequency samples into two in order to obtain a variance of variances. The result was such, $F(2,3) = 5.57$, $p<0.10$, that we can only speak of a nearly significant trend here, i.e. that the angle of release is more rigidly controlled, and thus more constant at lower rates of juggling. Nevertheless, it is sufficiently promising to motivate further research in this direction.

All in all, there is sufficient evidence to accept Hypothesis II. The non-linear dynamics of the effector system in juggling do, indeed, allow for dynamic (re)adjustments in the balance of harmonic and relaxation behaviour. When going from high to low pacing, the relaxation component in the overall behaviour of the effector system increases. The qualitative implications of this conclusion should seriously constrain the future mathematical modelling of the dynamics of juggling.

Some considerations on the perceptual information for juggling

Close inspection of Equations (2) and (6) gives an indication of what is involved in skilful juggling as well as in learning to juggle. The "motor problem" of juggling, to use Bernstein's (1984, p.344) apt term, is to a considerable extent a problem of appropriate timing. Hence, part of the problem of motor learning is to master these timing relations. One of the relevant questions in this respect is how perception constrains the relative timing components involved.

Although an extraordinarily skilful juggler might be able to juggle three balls blindfold for a limited period of time, he will normally look at the top part of the trajectory of the ball. To a less experienced juggler the available information at this spot is essential. Austin (1976) demonstrated this with a simple, but crucial experiment. He shielded the eyes of jugglers with a fan-like screen containing a notch that could be gradually closed in such a way that the top part of the ball trajectory could be observed through a smaller and smaller aperture. Failure in performance occurred only when the screen was closed beyond (circa) 10 degrees, which led Austin to the conclusion that it is possible to catch, and with practice, to actually juggle, when as little as one inch of the ball trajectory is visible, as long as that inch is in the top-most part of the flight parabola.

We designed a similar experiment in which a semi-circular screen (radius 25 cms) in the horizontal plane was attached to the nose of the juggler, occluding vision of the hands and the major part of the ball trajectory except for the top. We invited our juggler to reduce the height to which the ball was tossed without elevating the hands. Failure occurred only after less than one third of the ball diameter (circa 2.2 cm) remained in sight. This experimental result, which is in agreement with Austin's study, leads to the conclusion that the observation of an object at the onset of free fall for a period less than 130 ms is sufficient to perform the juggling task without breakdown.

One might be amazed that such a short observation of an object hanging virtually stationary in the air can lead to such an accurate prediction of falling time. How can this be?

In the case of an approaching object, Lee (1976, 1980) and others (e.g. Koenderink & Van Doorn, 1981; Wagner, 1982) have identified the kinematic property of the optic flow field that specifies the time at which the point of observation will make contact with the surface (time-to-contact) of an object approaching along the line of sight. The rate of magnification (dilation) of the object relative to the point of observation, as expressed by the formula (1/s).(ds/dt), is this significant optical property. Wagner (1982) called this variable the relative retinal expansion velocity (RREV), whereas Lee (1976) designated its inverse "tau".

In the case of perceiving a falling ball in juggling, however, there is virtually no retinal expansion. Nevertheless, we hypothesize that the concept of time-to-contact may be still applicable here, albeit in a somewhat different sense. If we assume that the visual system is able to pick up information specifying the height of an object relative to the position of the hands, the computational labour required for obtaining t-fall over that perceived height, i.e. time-to-contact with respect to the hands, is minimal at the top of the toss parabola, since from this position t is simply equal to $\surd(2h/g)$. For all other positions of the ball's trajectory the algorithm required for obtaining t-fall would be much more complicated. Another reason why "the point of singularity" at the top of the toss parabola may be such a potent source of information to the juggler, is the following: At this point the time that elapses between the moment of release of the ball and the moment of zero velocity in the y-direction (t_o) equals the time that will elapse between t_o and the moment of catch, given that the points of catch and release are (more or less) in the same horizontal plane. Thus, the juggler may be able to prospectively control the moment of catch. Of course, it remains to be seen if either of these two possibilities indeed yield the perceptual basis for timing catching.

Returning to Equations (2) and (6), the time element next to t-fall (as a component of t-flight) which ought to be assessed is t-loaded. Active touch promotes discrimination (Dyhre-Poulson, 1978), just as "jiggling" (not juggling!) an object aids discrimination of its mass (Brodie & Ross, 1985). Bingham, Schmidt and Rosenblum (1987), however, have produced evidence that hefting objects for a maximum distance throw provides haptic information specifying, not weight as such, but "throwability" of objects. Presumably, a similar functionally constrained perceptual property is picked up by the haptic system in the case of a fixed height throw, as in juggling. If the height at which the ball is tossed (and thus t-flight) is under control and if t-loaded is perceived, the skilled match of t-unloaded, between tossing one ball and catching the next is, according to our timing relations, the final requirement to meet the timing constraints of juggling.

Conclusions and outlook

In the foregoing, we have explored, from the perspective of natural physics, three aspects of the dynamics of juggling with three balls in a figure-of-eight pattern: (1) the intricate timing relations between the moving hands and balls, (2) the nature of the underlying dynamics of the effector system with respect to the relative mix of harmonic and relaxation behaviour over different rates of juggling, and (3) the way in which perceptual information is used in juggling.

On the basis of our preliminary results, three further hypotheses have been proposed for guiding further investigations into the dynamics of juggling.

1) In the case of juggling three balls, the relative timing component k is not, strictly speaking, a relational invariant. It is a variable that seems to approach the value of 0.75 in the simplest phase locking analysis. There are, probably, different regimes of phase locking with local optima in a region around 0.75.
2) When juggling is scaled on rate, the relative mix between spatial and temporal control changes with the pacing parameter. To adjust this delicate balance to the requirements

of the task, adjustments in the non-linearities of the effector system are exploited.

3) The point of singularity at the top of the ball trajectory is a potent source of visual information, because (1) at this point a very simple algorithm to compute time-to-contact relative to the hands (t-fall), given the perception of relative height, is available, and (2) at this point in time, t-fall equals the time elapsed after release of the ball.

In fact, the experimental and theoretical treatment of these three hypotheses is part of a wider research programme into the dynamics of juggling. To arrive at a more complete understanding of the skill of juggling, we need to describe the dynamics of the effector system so that observed patterns of movement over a larger number of manipulations can be explained. The descriptive levels proposed in the task-dynamic approach of Saltzman and Kelso (1987), i.e. task space, body space, task network and articulator network, may be of help in this respect. In addition to varying the rate of juggling, the number of balls used by the subject needs to be varied as well as their weight and size. When a satisfactory account of these aspects in juggling is reached, the system under study may be so enlarged as to incorporate the motion of the elbow and shoulder, and the posture and sway of the entire body.

The present contribution makes clear, we hope, that our approach is to quantify movement where possible and to offer physical explanations where tractable. The aim, however, is not necessarily to explain human movement exclusively in the language of mathematical physics. There is no reason to believe that this could ever be achieved even at higher levels of abstraction. Our predilection for quantification is based on the maxim that what can be explained in straightforward physical terms should be. Only then can discussions at higher levels of motor control be clarified, such as the relation between perception and task control, the role of intentional action, mnemic influences, personality traits, etc.

To put this into the language of this paper, we are looking for equations of motion of the type:

$$m\ddot{x} + kx + W(x,\dot{x}) = F'(t), \tag{10}$$

where $W(x,\dot{x})$ is an autonomous function that contains all non-linear terms that are necessary to account for the self-organizing features exhibited by a particular effector system and $F'(t)$ is a non-autonomous function that contains all intentional action that can not be accounted for by means of natural physics. In so doing, we hope eventually to achieve a more purposeful discourse on what the intentional act, in terms of $F'(t)$, really means.

Acknowledgements

I am grateful to the following persons for the valuable contributions they made to this paper and/or the work presented in it: Wiero Beek, Reinoud Bootsma, Piet van Wieringen, John Whiting, and two anonymous reviewers. In addition, I would like to express my appreciation to Ann Colley and John Beech for doing such an efficient editing job. Finally, thanks are due to the juggler "Aristotle", whose pseudonym, as far as I have been able to glean from the classic literature, bears no relationship to his motor competencies!

References

Austin, H.A. (1976). A computational theory of physical skill. Unpublished Ph.D. thesis. Department of Electrical Engineering and Computer Science, M.I.T., Boston.

Bernstein, N.A. (1984). Some emergent problems of the regulation of motor acts. In H.T.A. Whiting (Ed.), Human motor actions: Bernstein reassessed. Amsterdam: North-Holland.

Bingham, G.P., Schmidt, R.C., & Rosenblum, L.D. (1987). Smart perceptual mechanisms and the methodological myth of special access: Hefting for a maximum distance throw versus the size-weight illusion. (Submitted for publication.)

Bizzi, E., Polit, A., & Morasso, P. (1976). Mechanisms underlying achievement of final head position. Journal of Neurophysiology, 37, 792-804.

Brodie, E.E. & Ross, H.E. (1985). Jiggling a lifted weight does aid discrimination. The American Journal of Psychology, 98, 469-471.

Dyhre-Poulson, P. (1978). Perception of tactile stimuli before ballistic and during tracking movements. In G. Gordon (Ed.), Active touch. London: Pergamon Press.

Kay, B.A., Kelso, J.A.S., Saltzman, E.L., & Schöner, G. (1987). Space-time behavior of single and bimanual rhythmical movements: Data and limit cycle model. Journal of Experimental Psychology: Human Perception and Performance, 13, 178-192.

Kelso, J.A.S. (1981). Contrasting perspectives on order and regulation in movement. In J. Long & A. Baddeley (Eds.), Attention and performance, Vol.IX. Hillsdale, N.J.: Erlbaum.

Kelso, J.A.S. & Holt, K.G. (1980). Exploring a vibratory systems analysis of human movement production. Journal of Neurophysiology, 43, 1183-1196.

Kelso, J.A.S., Holt, K.G., Kugler, P.N., & Turvey, M.T. (1980). On the concept of coordinative structures as dissipative structures: II. Empirical lines of convergence. In G.E. Stelmach & J. Requin (Eds.), Tutorials in motor behavior, New York: North-Holland.

Kelso, J.A.S. & Kay, B. (1987). Information and control: A macroscopic basis for perception-action coupling. In H. Heuer & A.F. Sanders (Eds.), Tutorials in perception and action. Hillsdale, N.J.: Erlbaum.

Kelso, J.A.S. & Schöner, G. (in press). Self-organization of coordin-

ative movement patterns. Journal of Human Movement Science.
Koenderink, J.J. & Doorn, A.J. van (1981). Exterospecific component of the motion parallax field. Journal of the Optical Society of America, 71, 953-957.
Kugler, P.N. (1986). A morphological perspective on the origin and the evolution of movement patterns. In M.G. Wade & H.T.A. Whiting (Eds.), Skill acquisition in children: Aspects of coordination and control. The Hague: Martinus Nijhoff.
Kugler, P.N., Kelso, J.A.S., & Turvey, M.T. (1980). On the concept of coordinative structures as dissipative structures: 1. Theoretical lines of convergence. In G.E. Stelmach & J. Requin (Eds.), Tutorials in motor behavior. Amsterdam: North-Holland.
Lee, D.N. (1976). A theory of visual control of braking based on information about time-to-collision. Perception, 5, 437-459.
Lee, D.N. (1980). Visuo-motor coordination in space-time. In G.E. Stelmach & J. Requin (Eds.), Tutorials in motor behavior. New York: North-Holland.
Pol, B. van der (1922). On oscillation hysteresis in a triode generator with two degrees of freedom. Philosophical Magazine, 43, 700-719.
Pol. B. van der (1934). The nonlinear theory of oscillations. Proceedings of the Institute of Radio Engineers, 22, 1051-1086.
Pol, B. van der (1939). Paper delivered at the 2th-conference for biological rhythm research, August 25-26, Utrecht (Holland).
Polit, A. & Bizzi, E. (1978). Processes controlling arm movements in monkeys. Science, 201, 1235-1237.
Saltzman, E. & Kelso, J.A.S. (1987). Skilled actions: A task-dynamic approach. Psychological Review, 94, 84-106.
Scheffé, H. (1959). The analysis of variance. New York: John Wiley.
Schmidt, R.A. (1984). The search for invariance in skilled movement behavior. Report No.11/1984, Research Group on Perception and Action at the Center for Interdisciplinary Research (ZiF), University of Bielefeld.
Turvey, M.T. (1977). Preliminaries to a theory of action with reference to vision. In R. Shaw & J. Bransford (Eds.), Perceiving, acting and knowing: Toward an ecological psychology. Hillsdale, N.J.: Erlbaum.
Wagner, H. (1982). Flow-field variables trigger landing in flies. Nature, 87, 255-259.
Wood, G.A. (1982). Data smoothing and differentiation procedures in biomechanics. Exercise and Sport Reviews, 10, 308-362.

Cognition and Action in Skilled Behaviour
A.M. Colley and J.R. Beech (Editors)

DISCUSSION: SELF-ORGANIZATION OR REPRESENTATION? LET'S HAVE BOTH!

P.C.W. van Wieringen
The Free University, Amsterdam

Animals, including man, are part of nature. It is plausible, therefore, that, like other natural systems, they exhibit self-organising qualities. The question being addressed in this short paper is whether a full-fledged account of motor behaviour in terms of self-organisation is possible, an account in which no resort is taken to internal representations in the sense of symbolic knowledge structures specifying prescriptions for action, like plans, schemata, or programmes.

For at least some phenomena in the biological action domain the answer to this question seems to be affirmative. Two very well-known examples are the instantaneous adaptations in gait of the centipede Lithobius demonstrated after successive removal of pairs of legs (Von Holst, 1973/1937) and the abrupt phase transitions in the gait of horses, changing from walking to trotting to galloping when increasing their speed of locomotion (Hoyt & Taylor, 1981). These sudden transitions from one stable spatiotemporal ordering to another, after short periods of instability, are similar to such transitions occurring in non-living systems, like the transition from laminar flow of water to turbulence when increasing the aperture of the water tap. The transition points, marked by instability, are reached when a critical value of some order parameter (Reynold's number in the water example) has been reached.

With respect to the gait of horses, Kelso and Scholz (1986) draw attention to the fact that the changes in locomotory mode are not necessarily hard-wired or deterministic, arguing that horses can trot at speeds at which they normally gallop, although it is metabolically costly to do so. In fact, this phenomenon may be seen during trotting-matches, where the jockeys force their horses in a trotting pattern at speeds where energy demands should lead to galloping. The human counterpart of this example is shown in speed-walking, where the athlete prevents his locomotion pattern from following its "natural" course by repressing the phase transition from walking to running.

Phase transitions in human movement have not yet been studied with respect to locomotion, but data on cyclical finger and hand movements have been presented by Kelso (see Kelso, 1981 and 1984 respectively). Subjects in the latter experiments performed oscillatory movements of either the two hands or two index fingers. They started moving in an out-of-phase, antisymmetrical movement, and were required to gradually speed up movement velocity. It was observed that at some critical frequency the out-of-phase movements gave way to in-phase, symmetrical movements. When this critical frequency was expressed in units of preferred frequency, the resulting ratio was constant (1.33) for all subjects, but one.

The latter, exceptional subject belonged, according to Kelso (1984), to those few subjects who were not naive, and deliberately resisted the transition from occurring, at the cost of extra energy expenditure.

Kelso, Holt, Rubin, and Kugler (1981) stress the fact that in Kelso's phase transition experiments the changed mode of organisation is not due to a priori prescriptions, but emerges as a consequence of the dynamical behaviour of the system itself.

The rhythmic movements of the hands or fingers are conceptualized as limit-cycle oscillations, and these self-oscillations are equated with forced oscillations produced by a force which depends on the nature of the oscillations. The model for such behaviour is found in a clock, the important feature of the clock being "that the periodic tapping of energy to sustain the clock's oscillation (its ticking) depends solely on the position of the pendulum and not on time per se" (Kugler, Kelso, & Turvey, 1980, p.16).

According to this metaphor "timing of impulses does not require a separate device but arises necessarily from the design characteristics - the equations of constraint of the muscle collective" (Kugler, Kelso, & Turvey, 1980, p.18).

The question arising, however, is how to account for the behaviour of Kelso's aforementioned anomalous subject. It seems difficult to deny that the external forcing of the oscillating limbs, which is responsible for the resistance and postponement of the phase transition has something to do with prescriptions, prescriptions reflecting the conscious intention to realize specific characteristics of the movement pattern. It is important to realize that this subject's intention is not only reflected in triggering the movement and allowing them to occur (all of Kelso's subjects, for example, might have decided either to start performing the required movements or to prove their independence by walking out of the lab), but that it is continually involved in the control of them.

In this respect W.J. Beek's (in press) critical remarks with regard to Kugler, Kelso and Turvey's (1980) account of motor behaviour in terms of coordinative structures, deserve to be mentioned: "If non-linear mechanics has primacy and if movement patterns are embedded in the design itself of muscular units, what then gives the signal for the appropriate timing of its design parameters like stiffness and damping? We are then back to questions of movement control and motor programming, be it on the level of a master controlling the autonomous slave of an aggregate of muscles and joints (using the jargon 'master-slave control' from control theory...)."

Recently Saltzman and Kelso (1987) redefined the concept of coordinative structures, speaking about them in terms of abstractly defined action units, which constrain their muscle/joint components to act cooperatively and specifically to the task at hand. They remark that "For different skilled actions, performers transform the limbs temporarily into different special purpose devices, whose functions match the tasks being performed", suggesting that "Thus, an arm can become a retriever, puncher, or polisher; a leg may become a walker or kicker; the body can become a dancer or swimmer; the speech organs may become talkers, singers, chewers, or swallowers, and so on". (p.85)

With regard to autonomy Saltzman and Kelso argue that the "Action units operate relatively autonomously and are, to a large extent, self-regulating. That is, once a given functional organization is established, over a muscle/joint collective, the system achieves its goal with minimal voluntary intervention" (p.85, all underlining mine).

From the latter quote it is clear that the authors discuss the situation in which a specific skill has already been learned ("a given functional organization is established") and that even here they leave room for at least some degree of non-autonomy and voluntary intervention. Saltzman and Kelso illustrate their approach, in describing how task dynamics generates task-specific trajectory shapes in discrete reaching, rhythmic target-to-target, cup-to-mouth, and cranking tasks, indicating the fact that no explicit trajectory planning is called for. The latter consequence of their approach is one of its two major advantages. The second one, immediate compensation, is demonstrated in the case of perturbations occurring during a reaching task.

Saltzman and Kelso's examples refer to relatively simple, overlearned tasks, which certainly are not representative for all of the skills exhibited by human performers. It might be useful here to have a closer look at an example of a more complicated motor skill. It refers to the movement patterns displayed by the actors of Grotowski's famous laboratory theatre from Warsaw, in which postures and movements play an extremely important role. These actors get, next to the rehearsals for the specific play to be performed, three to four hours of basic movement training each day. Some of the exercises have been derived from Hatha-Yoga principles, according to which the movements should be performed very slowly. The actor has to concentrate on so-called "strategic points", i.e. those body parts which are the target of the exercise in question. Only specific muscles have to be contracted, while all the others have to be consciously relaxed. During movements the actors are required to attend to correct performance, to constancy, to relaxation and breathing, to immobility during static phases, as well as to the aforementioned strategic points. The movements have to be initiated in the spinal column and have to be finished by feet, hands and fingers. Training of facial expression is derived from Indian Kathakali; the actor learns to be conscious of each of his facial muscles in order to control them. In this way the actor learns to move facial muscles simultaneously and in different rhythms. Finally the actors are to develop what Grotowski calls "gestic ideograms", till they spontaneously follow from the actor's own images (for further descriptions, see Schwerin von Krosigk, 1986).

Of course this description is in "experiential", and not in scientific terms. It suffices, however, to include the problems one might have in accounting for such skills without taking representations into account. Even if one were to agree with Carello, Turvey, Kugler, and Shaw (1984), that "natural systems do not require explicit instructions in order to perform their natural activities", and that "for natural systems it is largely the free interplay of forces, not a priori prescriptions, that realize stationary and transitory states" (p.231), it seems at least improbable that the movement behaviour of Grotowski's actors, and for that sake, any other actor or dancer, can be accounted for by just "free interplay of forces". Now, supposedly, actors and dancers may be better described as cultural systems performing cultural activities than as natural systems performing natural activities.

According to Thelen (1987) the fundamental disagreement between natural physical and cognitive accounts of motor skills concerns the ultimate source of the information that guides movement. Where the former approach implies that the planning for trajectories of movement and the detection of error and corrections of those movements need not be explicitly stored, the latter approach deems such storage in representations and schemata inevitable. As will be clear by now, it is my opinion that, at least for cultural skills like dancing, such representations, being formed by, for example, instructions, demonstrations, or even reading books, indeed do play an important role.

My view here is compatible with Harvey's (1985) opinion that adherents to the Gibsonian programme may "have difficulty in accounting for performance in artistic and polemical skills, where the goal is not to relate to the environment in a particular way but, via the environment, to affect perception of the audience in a particular way" (p.1592). In this respect it is worthwhile to realise that Turvey's definition of intentionality as "directedness towards objects" (1987, p.153) is too narrow to cover the intentions of, for example, a dancer. Moreover, the information guiding the dancer's action is not restricted to information in the specificational sense, which is Turvey's preferred conceptualisation of information (1987; Carello, Turvey, Kugler, & Shaw, 1984). Questions such as "how is optical structure specific to a place that permits stepping down (...), specific to how the stepping down is to be conducted, and specific to when the stepping down should be initiated" (Carello et al, 1984, p.245), are clearly underconstraining the ways in which a dancer performs his steps. This information is supplemented by information in the indicational sense, which is encoded in, for example, the choreography. The dancer has to represent this code internally, and the symbol strings in question guide the performer in realising his intentions. It seems even not too far-fetched to consider cognitive activity here as being the "main driver of the movements" (Beaubaton, & Pailhous, 1987).

Kinematic trajectories in dancing are often planned in advance, and, as long as the skills are not fully mastered, perturbations are not spontaneously compensated for. What is more, the movements in question may be perturbed by introducing secondary mental tasks (e.g. mental arithmetic), indicating that tapping the symbolic mode interferes with motor performance.

Of course I do realise that there is a wide gap between making the claim that representations and prescriptions play a very important role, and giving a principled account of the way in which such representations constitute "extraordinary boundary conditions on natural laws", to use Turvey's (1986) terminology.

It has to be admitted that terms like representation and other cognitive constructs have unfortunate overtones. Iran-Nejad and Ortony (1984) pointed out that "The problem is that often the essentially metaphorical use of these concepts can give rise to misleading implications. For example, we ordinarily talk about mental representations being stored in memory, searched for, and retrieved. It is easy to see how, if taken literally, such ideas can lead to the conclusion that people's heads are populated with a huge number of pre-packaged permanent structures corresponding to everything they know" (p.173). It remains to be seen if Iran-Nejad and Ortony's account of cognition, in which it is explained in terms of the activity of anatomically distributed constellations of neuronal elements, will bring us nearer to a principled explanation of the way in which cognitions play their part in the learning and control of human skills, or, in terms of Saltzman and Kelso (1987), in the "control regimes (that) serve to convert an effector system into the appropriate task-demanded special purpose device" (p.86).

Maybe the foregoing discussion led to the impression that a sharp distinction should be drawn between natural and cultural, or phylogenetic and ontogenetic skills. Although I have the impression that such a distinction may indeed be useful (Van Wieringen, 1986), it should not be conceived as an absolute one, but as a matter of degree. Particularly in a cultural skill like dancing, which served to illustrate such a skill, already existing autonomous characteristics or coordinative structures often have to be "overruled" in order to conform to "the rules of the game". The difficulty of such skills may be proportional to the degree in which such "overruling" is required. In natural skills, the emphasis may be more on exploiting coordinative structures and adapting them to the task at hand, then in overcoming them and creating completely new ones. Therefore, natural tasks might be less independent on cognitive involvement, on prescriptions for action in the sense of symbolic knowledge structures than are cultural ones.

Future research should be directed at the interplay of such prescriptions and the dynamic self-organising characteristics of the human effectors resulting in skilled behaviour.

Even if it will take a long time before we will be in a position to either prove or disprove, in a principled way, if the body becoming a dancer will indeed depend to a larger extent on prescriptions than does the leg becoming a walker, a research programme with such questions in mind seems feasible. A first exploration of this theme has been formulated by W.J. Beek (in press) and P.J. Beek (this volume), and experiments along the lines put forward there will start in due time in our laboratory.

Acknowledgements

Thanks are due to P.J. Beek and R.J. Bootsma for helpful comments on an earlier version of this paper.

References

Beaubaton, D., & Pailhous, J. (1987). Is the motor program in the body or in the mind? A cruel dilemma' (Comment on Zanone & Hauert). European Bulletin of Cognitive Psychology, 7, 130–135.

Beek, W.J. (in press). Synergetics and self-organisation: A response. In H.T.A. Whiting (Ed.), A natural-physical approach to movement control. Amsterdam: Free University Press.

Carello, C., Turvey, M.T., Kugler, P.N., & Shaw, R.E. (1984). Inadequacies of the computer metaphor. In M. Gazzaniga (Ed.), Handbook of Cognitive Neuroscience. New York: Plenum.

Harvey, N. (1985). Review of "Human motor actions: Bernstein reassessed". Edited by H.T.A. Whiting. (Oxford: North-Holland, 1984). Ergonomics, 28–11, 1589–1594.

Hoyt, D.F., & Taylor, C.R. (1981). Gait and the energetics of locomotion in horses. Nature, 292, 239–240.

Iran-Nejad, A., & Ortony, A. (1984). A biofunctional model of distributed mental content, mental structures, awareness, and attention. The Journal of Mind and Behavior, 5, 171–210.

Kelso, J.A.S. (1981). On the oscillatory basis of movement. Paper presented at the Psychonomic Society, Philadelphia, November 1981. Bulletin of the Psychonomic Society, 18, 63.

Kelso, J.A.S. (1984). Phase transition and critical behavior in human bimanual coordination. American Journal of Physiology: Regulatory, Integrative and Comparative Physiology, 15, R1000–R1004.

Kelso, J.A.S., Holt, K.G., Rubin, P., & Kugler, P.N. (1981). Patterns of human interlimb coordination emerge from the properties of non-linear, limit cycle oscillatory processes: theory and data. Journal of Motor Behavior, 13, 226–261.

Kelso, J.A.S., & Scholz, J.P. (1986). Cooperative phenomena in biological motion. In H. Haken (Ed.), Synergetic systems in physics, chemistry and biology. Berlin: Springer Verlag.

Kugler, P.J., Kelso, J.A.S., & Turvey, M.T. (1980). On the concept of coordinative structures as dissipative structures: I. Theoretical lines of convergence. In G.E. Stelmach & J. Requin (Eds.), Tutorials in motor behavior. New York: North-Holland.

Saltzman, E., & Kelso, J.A.S. (1987). Skilled actions: A task-dynamic approach. Psychological Review, 94, 84–106.

Schwerin von Krosigk, B. (1986). Der nackte Schauspieler: Der Entwicklung der Schauspieltheorie Jerzy Grotowskis. Berlin: Publica Verlag.

Thelen, E. (1987). We think; therefore, we move (comment on Zanone & Hauert). European Journal of Cognitive Psychology, 7, 195–198.

Turvey, M.T. (1986). Intentionality: A problem of multiple reference frames, specificational information, and extraordinary boundary conditions on natural law. (Comment on Sayre). The Behavioral and Brain Sciences, 9, 153-155.

Van Wieringen, P.C.W. (1986). Motor coordination: Constraints and cognition, A reaction to K.M. Newell. In M.G. Wade & H.T.A. Whiting (Eds.), Motor development in children: Aspects of coordination and control. Dordrecht: Martinus Nijhoff.

Von Holst, E. (1973/1937). The behavioral physiology of animals and man: The collected papers of Erich von Holst. Coral Gables: University of Miami Press.

Part III

LEARNING AND PERFORMING SKILLED MOVEMENTS

Cognition and Action in Skilled Behaviour
A.M. Colley and J.R. Beech (Editors)

"CATCH" QUESTIONS AND INCOMPLETE ANSWERS

H.T.A. Whiting, G.J.P. Savelsbergh and C.M. Faber
The Free University, Amsterdam

A series of experiments addressed to the task of one-handed catching are discussed in their historical perspective. The inadequacy of some of the solutions proposed to theoretical questions raised by experimentors are signalled. The information so gained is used to devise an experiment which would clarify some of these issues. Results of the experiment confirm the merit of using ability groups defined on some within-task criterion. In this way some clarification could be provided of the question, "Is it necessary to be able to see the hand as well as the ball" - "poor catchers" being shown to make more spatial errors when the hand was not visible. No sex differences were found in catching performance. The inclusion of UV light conditions in the experiment gave rise to interesting new hypotheses, which are discussed. In particular, it is postulated that successively degrading environmental information has differential performance effects on more or less experienced catchers.

In the late 1960s, early 1970s Whiting, with a succession of co-workers, was engaged in elucidating the question as to <u>whether it was necessary to keep the eye on the ball for successful catching</u>. More specifically, the research programme was addressed to the effect of restricting opportunities for picking up ball flight information on catching performance. What started out as a comparatively simple question turned out to be rather more complicated and to have many more practical theoretical implications than had been originally anticipated.

In retrospect this is, perhaps, not too surprising since already in 1974, Alderson, Sully, and Sully, in Whiting's laboratory, albeit utilising one standard ball velocity of 10 m/sec, had demonstrated that catching a ball involved both spatial and temporal predictions:

1. gross spatial orientation (getting the hand into the approximate spatial position for catching) - occurring some 200 ms before the ball reached the hand, followed by,

2. fine orientation (optimal spatial adjustment to meet oncoming ball), occurring 150-200 ms before contact with the palm, followed by,

3. grasp and hold, occurring 32-50 ms before contact.

The most significant aspect of Alderson et al.'s analysis was, however, in demonstrating the very narrow time window (+/- 30 ms) available, at that velocity, in which to make an effective grasp. Closing the fingers +/- 15 ms too early will result in the ball hitting the tips or back of the fingers and falling away. Closing the fingers +/- 15 ms too late will result in the ball hitting the hand and rebounding before the grasp action can be carried out.

In one of their earlier experiments, involving the catching of a ball in free flight under restricted temporal viewing conditions, Whiting, Gill, and Stephenson (1970) demonstrated increasingly better catching performance with increasing ball exposure time. Nevertheless, some subjects were able to produce very good performances when allowed to view the ball for only +/- 100 ms early in its flight path. The implications of this finding were not, however, completely clear since the reduced viewing periods of the ball were not manipulated with respect to their occurrence at different stages in the trajectory of the ball.

Why this might be an important question was signalled by Sharp very shortly after he had joined the research group. Sharp raised the interesting question as to whether there might be, in the experimental paradigm being used, a confounding effect of the amount of time for which the ball can be viewed and the amount of time for which it is in darkness - experimental manipulation of the one automatically bringing about a change in the other. This point is easier to follow by means of Figure 1, which presents a schematised view of the paradigm utilised in experiments to be subsequently discussed.

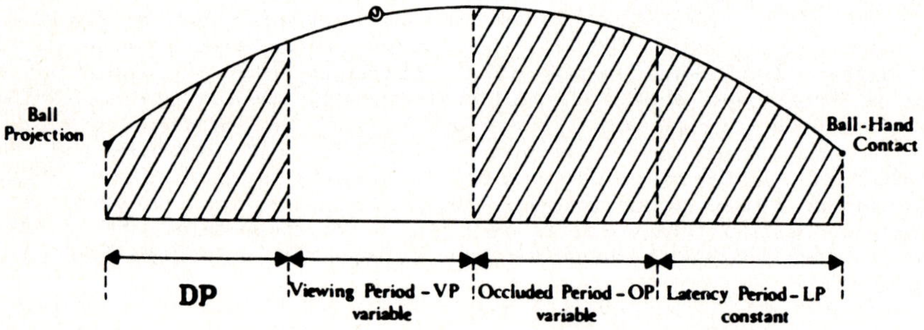

Figure 1

In a series of experiments (Sharp & Whiting, 1974, 1975; Whiting & Sharp, 1974) Sharp was able to confirm this confounding effect and to demonstrate that, within certain temporal boundaries (total times ranging from 20 ms to 400 ms only were manipulated), it was the total time available (a combination of viewing period - VP and occluded period - OP) which was important rather than VP or OP *per se*. Thus, increased performance, within these boundaries, could be brought about by increasing the VP or increasing the OP, while maintaining the total time constant. An interpretation of this finding offered at that time was in information-processing terms - providing an optimal amount of time for picking up ball-flight information followed by an optimal amount of time for processing that information.

This systematic relationship between catching performance and total time, however, was shown to break down for OP's greater than 80 ms. It would seem that the additional processing time gained by incrementing OP beyond 80 ms is outweighed by other factors, detrimental to performance. The simplest explanation is that these factors are concerned with motion prediction error. It is well known that motion prediction errors increase with prediction extent (Foot (1969, 1972), for example, showed that errors in predicting the point of coincidence of two moving targets increase linearly with the length of the prediction period, and Poulton (1963) showed that tracking error increases as the "required delay" between input and reproduction increases); while increasing OP may provide additional processing time, it also increases the time over which predictions must be extrapolated which, as it becomes longer, outweighs the advantage gained by the concomitant increase in processing time.

Two other interesting issues arose from this series of experiments. In the first place, it was apparent that, within the time boundaries utilised, performance was sub-optimal - on average, a maximum of 50% of the balls being caught - even though all subjects were capable of catching 100% of the balls in a condition which allowed the ball to be viewed throughout its total flight path (Sharp & Whiting, 1974). Secondly, performance showed a quantum leap when the total time available (OP + VP) exceeded 200 ms. The latter finding, it was suggested, was related to the two visual systems - the image-retina and the eye-head system - available for picking up ball flight information. The speed of objects passing across the field of view, the eye being stationary (image-retina system), is underestimated in comparison to conditions which allow smooth pursuit eye movements (Dichgans & Brandt, 1972). The eye-head movement detection system, which can be brought into play when the time available is in the region of 200 ms , provides more accurate information than the image-retina system. Sharp and Whiting (1975) produced some evidence in favour of this hypothesis by demonstrating superior catching performance of some subjects when ocular tracking was used. They do, however, draw attention to the limited scope of this, difficult to carry out, experiment and the need for replications.

The low performance of subjects in the experiment of Sharp and Whiting (1974) can be explained, it was suggested, by the particular combinations of OP and VP used in the experiment. When a whole range of possibilities, in this respect, was made available (Sharp & Whiting, 1975) it was possible to demonstrate near 100% catching performance for certain combinations of VP and OP.

These results give rise to a question which has yet to be experimentally addressed, namely, the most optimal position in the flight-path of the ball to provide information about ball flight. A likely candidate in this respect being the point of singularity defined by the turning point. Beek (1987) has produced some evidence in this respect in his study of jugglers.

These experimental findings of Whiting et al. lay relatively dormant in the literature until about 1982 when Smyth and Marriott sought to extend the paradigm by adding the additional question as to whether it was necessary to view the hand as well as the ball for successful catching. Their thesis was that, since articular proprioception is normally considered to provide accurate information about limb position, particularly in ball skills in which the eyes are thought to be occupied with tracking the ball, prevention of sight of the catching hand should, in principle, have no detrimental effect on catching performance.

Smyth (1986) points out that one of the limitations of the early studies of Whiting et al. was their failure to take into account the quality of the catch. Information, in this respect, would be provided by an analysis of the spatial and temporal errors made under the various restricted viewing conditions. The interesting question posed later by Smyth (1986), "is it a catch or a fumble", could not, with the evidence available, be adequately answered.

This is an important point and was appreciated by Whiting and his co-workers as early as 1970 and received limited experimental analysis by Sharp (1975):

> It must also be pointed out that in this experiment the task was to catch the ball. The quality of the catch was immaterial. In other situations in which, for example, the task involves doing something with the ball after it has been caught, the quality of the catch might well affect the efficiency with which the subsequent part of the task is carried out. Watching the ball for longer periods of time prior to its entering the hand might well influence the quality of the catch.
> (Whiting, Gill, & Stephenson, 1970)

Smyth and Marriott (1982) pursued this kind of analysis more systematically. They excluded vision of the hand by means of a matt black perspex screen fixed to the subject's head (with elastic) extending forward 25 cm on the right side of the subject's face and obscuring approximately 70° of the visual field. This, effectively, also prevented sight of the ball for the last +/- 150 ms of its flight. Care was taken to check for the intervention of a screen per se by having a condition in which a transparent screen of similar dimensions could be substituted. Subjects used were naive to this laboratory catching task and comprised both males and females. Smyth and Marriott were able to show that performance with the opaque screen was worse than with the transparent screen or a further condition in which no screen was utilised. The detrimental effect of a screen per se was evidenced by the significant difference between the number of balls caught under the transparent screen and the no-screen conditions. Analysis of the errors showed that more position than timing errors were made with the opaque screen, the reverse being true for the transparent screen and normal catching. The authors conclude that sight of the hand is necessary for efficient catching; errors made being mainly in the positioning of the hand rather than in timing of the grasp, i.e. subjects have inaccurate knowledge of the location of the hand.

More recently, Fischman and Schneider (1985) have returned to the question of the relationship between vision and proprioception in simple one-handed catching, adding the additional parameter of skill level. They utilised as subjects so-called experts - baseball and softball players (Experiment 1) - and novices (Experiment 2) in a similar paradigm to that of Smyth and Marriott, and utilised a similar velocity and distance (from ball projection machine to subject) but the screen they used was a black matt suspended board. They claim that their findings provide only limited support for Smyth and Marriott's (1982) contention that sight of the hand is necessary for successful one-handed catching. While Fischman and Schneider were able to show, in their first experiment, that catching performance without a screen (M = 19.00, $S.D.$ = 1.2; maximum possible 20 catches) was better than with a screen (M = 16.31, $S.D.$ = 2.2) there are a number of reasons why their findings do not necessarily support the contention of Smyth and Marriott concerning the necessity of being able to view the hand (Whiting, 1986).

In the first place, Fischman and Schneider failed to run a control condition involving a transparent screen, in spite of the fact that Smyth and Marriott had shown this to have a detrimental effect upon performance. Reference to Table 1 would suggest that the differences they find with and without the presence of an opaque screen might simply be explained in terms of the detrimental effect of a screen *per se* rather than having something to do with being unable to view the hand.

Table 1

Comparisons of catches and errors under the transparent and opaque screen conditions.

	Opaque	Transparent
% Catches:		
Fischman & Schneider	81.5	
Smyth & Marriott		75.2
% Position errors:		
Fischman & Schneider	5.6	
Smyth & Marriott		10.0
% Grasp errors:		
Fischman & Schneider	12.9	
Smyth & Marriott		14.8

The experimental populations in the two studies were very different. Any comparisons made, therefore, should only be based on the results of the *second* experiment of Fischman and Schneider and the experiment of Smyth and Marriott. In this respect, it is interesting that these authors, in contrast to Smyth and Marriott, report more grasp than position errors utilising the opaque screen. Since their classification scheme was the same as that of Smyth and Marriott, this raises the important point (signalled by Smyth, 1986) as to how far the two studies are comparable. This issue will not, however, be further addressed here.

The statement about the necessity of being able to see the hand is, in any case, too general since, presumably, subjects could not see their catching hand at all in either the study of Fischman and Schneider or that of Smyth and Marriott. Thus, the question arises, "at what stage in the total cycle, if at all, is it necessary to be able to see the hand?".

In the two studies in question, subjects were able to see the ball but not the hand until a period between 150 and 200 ms (the so-called latency period) before ball-hand contact. During the latter period they could not see either ball or hand. Fischman and Schneider's proposition that losing sight of the ball during the latency period affects the positioning phase of novice catchers, but not of experienced ones, even if true, needs to be qualified since in the study by Alderson, Sully, and Sully (1974), that they quote, the gross positioning (at least) of the hand takes place some 200 ms prior to ball-hand contact. If anything, therefore, it is the fine orientation, taking place 150-200 ms before contact, that is affected. No distinction is made by either Smyth and Marriott, or Fischman and Schneider, between these two spatial parameters.

Further qualifications would be necessitated by the findings of the study by Sharp and Whiting (1975) discussed above - a study not referenced by either Smyth and Marriott or Fischman and Schneider. Subjects (unselected, university students [N = 70] i.e. equivalent to those populations used in the Smyth and Marriott study and in the second experiment of the Fischman and Schneider study) were not able to see their catching hand under any of the conditions (since the room was in darkness) for at least the last 200 ms of ball flight. Nevertheless, under the block of conditions in which subjects could view the ball for periods of 480 ms, 440 ms, or 400 ms (Figure 2) their catching successes were 91.3%, 85.8% and 85.8% respectively ($\underline{M}$ = 87.6%)- equivalent to those obtained by Smyth and Marriott under normal catching conditions and, under the 480 ms condition, very close to the performance of Fischman and Schneider's experts.

It should be noted from the results of these last three conditions, that increasing the time in darkness before ball-hand contact by an additional period (OP) of 80 ms (i.e. so that the hand could not be seen for at least 280 ms before contact) only resulted in reduction in catching success from 91.3% to 85.8%. Clearly, not being able to see the hand, or the ball for that matter, during the last 280 ms of ball flight makes very little difference to the quantity of balls caught. Unfortunately, error analyses (positional or timing) were not carried out so that statements about the quality of the catch cannot be made.

A further critique to be levelled at the Fischman and Schneider study is that they confound their (so-called) cultural differences

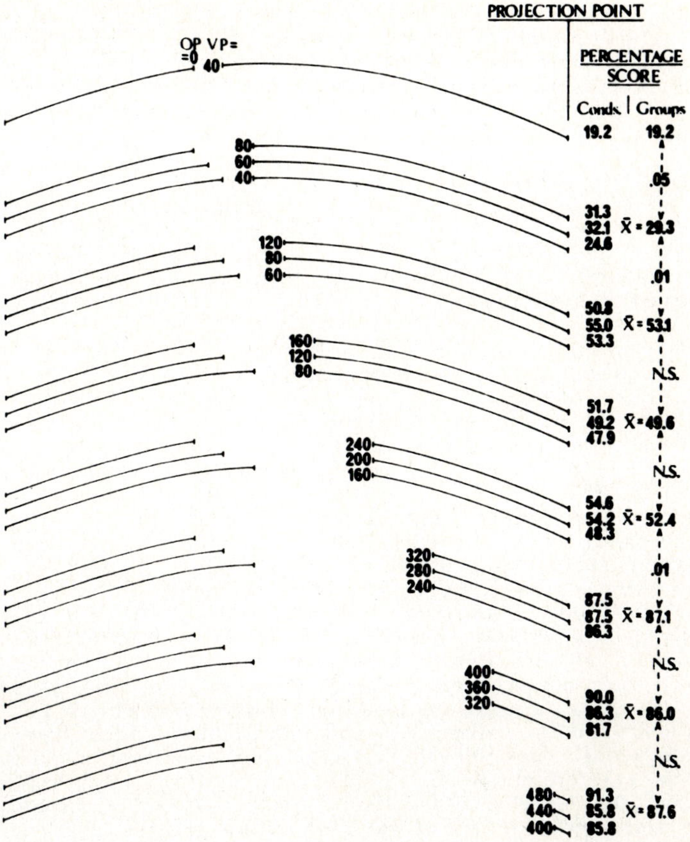

Figure 2

with in-task differences in catching ability. While in a study of Whiting, Alderson, and Sanderson (1973), that they cite, no significant differences in one-hand catching under restricted viewing conditions could be shown between cricketers (expert catchers) and non-cricketers. When the cricketers and non-cricketers were reclassified on the basis of a task-specific measure (one-handed catching within the laboratory task setting), into three ability groups, significant differences in catching performance between ability groups was apparent.

A final criticism levelled at both the Smyth and Marriott and Fischman and Schneider studies is that both used samples comprising male and female subjects. No comparisons of performance are presented and no suggestions made about possible interactions with ability and/or individual difference variables. Are there sex differences in catching ability and, if so, how are they manifested?

The above picture is further confused by a recent report of von Hofsten (1987) which maintains - contrary to Smyth and Marriott and Fischman and Schneider - that viewing the catching hand during the act does not seem to improve performance. In an experiment carried out with Pick, he claims, no differences were found between subjects catching a luminant ball with and without wearing a luminant glove on the catching hand. Unfortunately, von Hofsten provides no details of his experiments so that it is difficult, given the problems signalled in all the previous studies, to speculate upon the possible shortcomings in the experimental procedure, selection of subjects, etc.. Catching luminous balls in an otherwise dark room introduces other confounding factors such as figure-ground relationships and environmental structure.

Summary

In summary, a number of important catch questions have been raised and it is clear that the answers provided by existing studies are incomplete. If attention is restricted to those situations in which a ball in free flight as a consequence of an external agency is required to be caught, the central issue has to do with optimal temporal and spatial information about ball flight and spatial information about hand position. With respect to the first issue it is clear that some people are able to produce optimal catching performance when allowed only minimal (+/- 100 ms) exposure to ball flight information. There is, however, a lack of clarity about the quality of the catch under such conditions. A confounding factor in this respect, particularly if a computational standpoint is adopted, is the amount of time for which the ball is not exposed following an initial exposure period and, during which, computations on directional, positional, velocity and acceleration information might be carried out. If a "tau" standpoint (Lee & Young, 1986) is taken, the issue resolves itself into the effect of sampling "tau" earlier and earlier in the flight path of the ball.

Strictly speaking, the dark period (OP) is unimportant, although it would seem clear that having to "carry" tau information over a longer time period, i.e. increasing the perceptual-motor delay, independent of the question as to the accuracy of that information (for a decelerating object), would be a mitigating factor. Adopting either a "tau" or a computational standpoint leaves the issue of the most optimal moment at which to pick up information relatively open.

Being able to see or not see the hand appears to be a separate issue relating to spatial rather than temporal accuracy. It introduces similar issues with respect to optimal times when the hand should be in view and raises the general question of the mediating effects of expertise (c.q. within-task experience). Sex differences, given the existing studies, are unresolved and may reduce to expertise differences.

The effect of the different methodologies incorporated in the different studies - restricted opportunities for viewing, use of screening devices, catching a luminous ball in an otherwise dark room - give rise to their own confounding problems.

There are clearly a number of difficulties to resolve before more complete answers can be provided to the fundamental question raised many years ago by Whiting as to whether it is necessary to "keep the eye on the ball". As a first move in this direction the present authors have elected to carry out a series of experiments in which the methodology outlined by von Hofsten (fluorescent balls) is used to produce data which can be compared with that derived by using the screen procedure of Smyth and Marriott, and Fischman and Schneider. Within this paradigm sex differences and/or the mediating effects of within-task expertise can be explored. Only then can meaningful statements be made about the need to look at the hand and the nature of the errors which arise when this is prevented. The first of these experiments is reported below.

Experiment

Since the within-task ability variable seems to be crucial to sample selection and could, in itself, account for all of the differences found in the studies already cited, attention was focused on this aspect. Persistently Good and persistently Poor catchers were used to constitute the two comparative subject groups.

In an initial selection procedure, a sample of N=89 (57 male: 32 female) Ss were tested for their ability in one-handed catching. Balls were projected by machine with a velocity of V = 9.74 m/s from a distance of 6.4 m. (ball flight time = +/- 672 ms). No significant sex difference in the number of balls caught were apparent (t=1.07). On the basis of the constraints imposed by the distribution of Ss over the various numbers of successful catches from 11 to 30 out of 30, two groups were selected (Good catchers N=31: Poor catchers N=21). The Good catchers group had to achieve a score of 29 or 30 successful catches out of 30 while the Poor catchers group could range from 11 to 25 (i.e. less than 25 out of 30).

To ensure that Ss in groups were persistently Good or Poor catchers, they were tested again under full light conditions after a period of +/- 3 weeks (which reduced the groups of both good and poor catchers to N=15 (8 male: 7 female). They were tested yet again on the occasion of the experiment proper some eight weeks later. It was not found necessary to change the groups further except that one male subject in the group of poor catchers failed to complete the experiment thus reducing N to 14. The means and S.D.'s of number of catches for the two groups is given in Table 2.

There were no significant differences between the sexes within the final two groups, thus confirming the initially found absence of sex differences. In the Good catchers group only 5 of the 15 Ss caught less than 29 or 30 out of 30 (27, 21, 26, 28, 28) on one, only, of the three test sessions in full light. In the Poor catchers group only 3 of 14 Ss (one male S failed to complete the experiment) caught more than 25 out of 30 (26, 28, 27) on only one of the three test sessions in full light.

Apparatus

The accuracy of the tennis ball projection machine was such that

Table 2

Means and S.D.'s of catches (out of 30) for Good and Poor catchers. (Time interval: Test 1 - Test 2, ± 3 weeks: Test 2 - Test 3, ± 8 weeks)

	Good (N=15)		Poor (N=14)		t
	M	S.D.	M	S.D.	
Test 1	29.80	0.414	17.92	4.066	t = 10.87*
Test 2	28.66	2.469	18.75	5.365	t = 4.96*
Test 3	29.40	0.632	21.00	5.392	t = 5.79*
M =	29.29		19.22		

all balls fell within a circle of 30 cm diameter (centre 1.70 m above the floor) immediately behind the catching hand of the S. This was checked, and confirmed, after every two or three Ss. A tiny glowing red light on the machine indicated the projection point position of the ball. The experiment took place in an otherwise totally dark room.

Two video cameras were positioned in such a way that the catchers could be recorded from both side and frontal views. Ss wore a white surgical glove on the catching hand under all except the UVB condition when they wore a long sleeved black shirt and glove.

Conditions

Five conditions were used - three full light and two UV light.

Condition 1 - TEST - full light, ball and hand visible.

Condition 2 - TS - full light, ball and hand visible. A flexible plastic screen (50cm x 120cm) adjusted to the height of the S extending forward by 25 cm to the side of the S's face was interposed. The arm of the S was passed through a hole in the screen which was fixed with a pin to the S's clothing in the region of the shoulder.

Condition 3 - BS - full light, ball only visible (except for last +/- 150 ms). A flexible black plastic screen was substituted for the transparent screen.

Condition 4 - UVBH - Ultra violet light, ball and hand visible.

Condition 5 - UVB - Ultra violet light, ball only visible.

Procedure

All Ss received the five conditions in random order with the constraint that the two UV conditions (randomised) always followed one another. For each light condition ten training trials were given prior to the test and for the UV conditions 30 training trials, following a ten minute dark adaptation period. During the latter period a ball was on display illuminated by the UV source. Between each condition was a rest period of +/- 3 minutes. Following the dark adaptation period it was checked that the Ss could see their hand by manipulating an artificial hand, in the region of where their catching hand would be, and questioning them about what they could see. Ss were unable to note any distinguishing features.

Dependent variables

1. Number of balls caught out of 30.
2. Position errors - a failure to make contact with the ball in the region of the head of the metacarpals.
3. Grasp errors - ball makes contact with the metacarpal region but grasp is too early or too late.

Analysis of position and grasp errors was based on:

i) For conditions Test:TS:BS - video recordings.

ii) For conditions UVBH:UVB - responses of Ss, who were told that if the ball came on to the metacarpals but they failed to catch it they were to report this as good. To test the validity of this method a small group of Ss (3 of each group) went through the same procedure in the light condition. Their responses were compared with the actual video analyses. Ss in these conditions practised this kind of response during all practice trials.

Results

Means and S.D.'s of number of catches (out of 30) under the five conditions for good and poor catchers are presented in Table 3 and for position errors and grasp errors in Tables 4 and 5 respectively.

Table 3

Means and S.D.'s of catches (out of 30) under the five conditions for Good and Poor catchers (Test:TS:BS:UVBH:UVB)

	Good (N=13)		Poor (N=14)	
	M	S.D.	M	S.D.
Test	29.29	.961	19.22	4.146
TS	28.26	1.870	17.35	7.890
BS	27.86	3.159	18.35	5.943
UVBH	24.80	5.185	9.71	7.269
UVB	22.60	5.475	7.21	6.104

Skill (2: Good and Poor) x subjects (N=29) x conditions (5) ANOVAS for the three dependent variables - number of catches, position errors and grasp errors - were carried out. In all three ANOVAS significant ($p < .01$) main effects for skill and conditions and a significant interaction ($p < .01$) skill x conditions were found. Post hoc tests (Newman-Keuls) were carried out and the most interesting significant comparisons are reported and discussed separately for the three dependent variables.

Table 4

Means and S.D.'s of number of position errors for Good and Poor catchers under all five conditions.
(Test:TS:BS:UVBH:UVB)

	Good (N=15)		Poor (N=14)	
	M	S.D.	M	S.D.
Test	.06	.25	4.42	3.10
TS	.80	.94	6.21	4.62
BS	1.20	1.56	8.28	4.14
UVBH	3.00	3.50	12.57	5.47
UVB	4.13	3.99	15.50	4.76

Table 5

Means and S.D.'s of number of grasp errors for Good and Poor catchers under all five conditions
(Test:TS:BS:UVBH:UVB)

	Good (N=15)		Poor (N=14)	
	M	S.D.	M	S.D.
Test	.53	.64	4.64	3.20
TS	.93	1.28	6.14	4.57
BS	.86	1.35	3.35	2.59
UVBH	2.20	2.07	8.21	4.75
UVB	3.26	1.98	6.28	3.73

1. Number of catches

For the category Good catchers, no significant differences were found between the number of catches made under the full light condition (TEST) and those made under either of the screen conditions (TS, BS). Neither was there a significant difference between the number of catches made under the two screen conditions (TS, BS). A similar finding was also apparent for the category Poor catchers. It would seem that preventing the viewing of the hand by using a black (flexible) screen does not affect the number of catches made by subjects classified either as Good or Poor catchers. This is contrary to the findings of both Smyth and Marriott (1982) and Fischman and Schneider (1985). It is not clear whether these differences are attributable to the type of screen used or the more precise sub-categorisation of subjects.

The inclusion of the UV light conditions (UVHB, UVB) was justified by the finding of significant differences between the number of catches made under the full light (TEST) condition and those made under the UVB condition for both groups of subjects and under the UVHB condition for subjects categorised as Poor catchers ($p < .01$).

2. Position errors

For the category Good catchers the results obtained and the comparison between the effects of the various conditions reflect precisely those reported for number of catches. The only difference was that now the two conditions full light (TEST) and UVHB were also significantly different ($p < .05$). In a similar way, the performances of the Poor catchers reflected their performance on number of catches with the exception that prevention of the viewing of the hand via a black screen (BS) resulted in significantly more position errors as compared to those obtained under the full light (TEST) condition, i.e. preventing sight of the hand resulted in significantly more position errors. The presence of a screen per se (TS), contrary to the findings of Smyth and Marriott (1982), had no detrimental effect.

3. Grasp errors

For the category Good catchers the only significant difference ($p<0.05$) found was that between the full light (TEST) condition and the UVB condition. This was, in itself, surprising since if it is assumed that grasp errors have to do with a failure to accurately make use of the "time to contact" variable as specified by tau (Lee & Young, 1986) - the inverse of the rate of retinal expansion brought about by the approaching ball - it is difficult to understand why this should be more difficult under the UV condition than under the full light condition. This finding merits further experimental investigation. The same argument might be used with respect to the performance of the Poor catchers who also showed significantly more ($p < .01$) grasp errors under the UVHB condition than under the full light (TEST). There were, however, unlike the performance of the Good catchers, no significant differences between the full light (TEST) and the UVB condition. It is possible that the extra information available in the UVHB condition constitutes a distraction for this category of catchers. Some support for this suggestion is provided by the finding of significantly ($p < .05$) more grasp errors for these subjects in the presence of the transparent screen (TS) as compared to the presence of the black screen (BS) - the latter probably forcing them to pay more attention to "time to contact" information. This is another interesting issue worth pursuing.

General Discussion

While the findings reported here provide limited support for those of Smyth and Marriott (1982) and Fischman and Schneider (1985), they also show that classifying subjects on the basis of a within-task criterion of performance does lead to different findings. Thus, preventing sight of the hand by the use of a (flexible) screen does result in more position errors for relatively Poor catchers but a transparent screen per se has no significant effect. Preventing sight of the hand by the use of a (flexible) black screen has no effect on the grasp errors of either good or bad catchers. A word of caution must, however, be expressed here. Since the number of position errors increases significantly when viewing the hand is prevented (BS), it is not clear to what extent these would also result in grasp errors so that this finding may, in fact, be artefactual.

For reasons already discussed, the inclusion of the UV conditions give rise to interesting new hypotheses. An additional interesting general issue also presents itself. From Tables 3 and 4 can be seen that (except for the conditions TS and BS for Poor catchers in Table 3 - differences which are not significant) there is a trend towards deterioration in performance through the conditions (as presented) from TEST to UVB. Since this order might also be construed to represent a successive degradation of environmental information, the interesting idea presents itself that the detrimental findings apparent under some conditions are the result of the paucity of environmental information that has differential effects on more or less experienced catchers. This issue is currently being explored. The fact that this trend is not apparent for grasp errors can be accounted for in the manner suggested under 3. above.

References

Alderson, G.J.K., Sully, D.L., & Sully, H.G. (1974). An operational analysis of a one-handed catching task using high speed photography. Journal of Motor Behavior, 6, 217-226.

Beek, P.J. (1987). Exploring the dynamics of juggling. In A.M. Colley & J.R. Beech (Eds.), Cognition and action in skilled behaviour. Amsterdam: North-Holland.

Dichgans, J., & Brandt, T. (1972). Visual-vestibular interaction and motion perception. Bibliographia Opthalmologica, 82, 327-338.

Fischman, M.G., & Schneider, T. (1985). Skill level, vision and proprioception in simple one-handed catching. Journal of Motor Behavior, 17, 219-229.

Foot, H.C. (1969). Visual prediction of the point of coincidence of two moving targets. Ergonomics, 12, 723-733.

Foot, H.C. (1972). Intermittent viewing in a study of visual prediction. Perceptual and Motor Skills, 34, 223-226.

Hofsten, C. von (1987). Catching. In H. Heuer & A.P. Sanders (Eds.), Perception and action. Berlin: Springer-Verlag.

Lee, D.N., & Young, D.S. (1986). Gearing action to the environment. In Experimental Brain Research Series 15. Berlin: Springer-Verlag.

Poulton, E.C. (1963). Sequential short-term memory: Some tracking experiments. Ergonomics, 6, 518-522.

Sharp, R.H. (1975). Skill in fast ball games: some input considerations. Unpublished Ph.D. thesis, Department of Physical Education, University of Leeds.

Sharp, R.H., & Whiting, H.T.A. (1974). Exposure and occluded duration effects in a ball-catching skill. Journal of Motor Behavior, 3, 139-147.

Sharp, R.H., & Whiting, H.T.A. (1975). Information-processing and eye-movement behavior in a ball-catching skill. Journal of Human Movement Studies, 1, 124-131.

Smyth, M.M. (1986). A note: is it a catch or a fumble? Journal of Motor Behavior, 18, 492-496.

Smyth, M.M., & Marriott, A.M. (1982). Vision and proprioception in simple catching. Journal of Motor Behavior, 14, 143-152.

Whiting, H.T.A., Gill, B., & Stephenson, J. (1970). Critical time intervals for taking in flight information in a ball-catching task. Ergonomics, 13, 265-272.

Whiting, H.T.A., & Sharp, R.H. (1974). Visual occlusion factors in a discrete ball catching task. Journal of Motor Behavior, 6, 11-16.

Whiting, H.T.A., Alderson, G.J.K., & Sanderson, F.H. (1973). Critical time intervals for viewing and individual differences in performance on a ball-catching task. International Journal of Sports Psychology, 4, 155-166.

Whiting, H.T.A. (1986). Isn't there a catch in it somewhere? Journal of Motor Behavior, 18, 486-491.

Cognition and Action in Skilled Behaviour
A.M. Colley and J.R. Beech (Editors)

THE ACQUISITION OF SKILLED HANDWRITING : DISCONTINUOUS TRENDS IN KINEMATIC VARIABLES

Ruud G.J. Meulenbroek and Gerard P. van Galen
University of Nijmegen

The inference of movement control strategies from recorded writing signals is illustrated by presenting the recordings and corresponding absolute velocity profiles of the first attempts in writing an unfamiliar grapheme by an adult subject. A number of kinematic variables derived from these recordings are discussed and used as dependent variables in an experiment. Primary school children from grade two to six wrote the letters of a cursive alphabet in a paced writing task. Movement time, absolute velocity, curvature and writing dysfluency measurements of produced grapheme segments were measured. The changes in these kinematic variables during primary school revealed a discontinuity in writing development. The results show that during the acquisition process a temporary decline in performance measures can be observed as a result of feedback-controlled movement strategies. During the learning of the handwriting skill a feedback-controlled movement strategy is gradually replaced by an open-loop movement strategy.

Inferring control strategies from recorded writing movements

In the early stage of learning a skill, feedback is assumed to shape the relevant schema (Schmidt, 1975; 1976) or representations of the movement patterns involved, while in a later stage feedback processes have a monitoring function and do not interrupt the execution of planned movements. The detection of movement corrections and interruptions is often used as a technique to investigate how skilled movements are learned, controlled and coordinated. Clear examples of the inference of control strategies from recorded movements are the studies of Hay (1979, 1984) and von Hofsten (1979, 1980). By analysing the displacement functions of aimed reaching movements Hay and von Hofsten have demonstrated that 5-year-old children use an open-loop ballistic movement strategy, 7-year-old children use a closed-loop feedback controlled movement strategy and 9- and 11-year-old children manage to integrate these two control strategies.

In comparison with discrete aiming or pointing tasks, cursive handwriting is a more complex skill which can be characterised by a continuous flow of precise, distally performed, curved movements. Nevertheless, handwriting is often considered as a series of composite aiming movements (e.g. Meulenbroek & van Galen, 1986; Wann, 1986). When writing movements are performed skilfully, each aiming movement corresponds with an upstroke or a downstroke of a grapheme. Strokes can be straight or curved trajectories. An illustration of this type of analysis of handwriting is depicted in Figure 1.

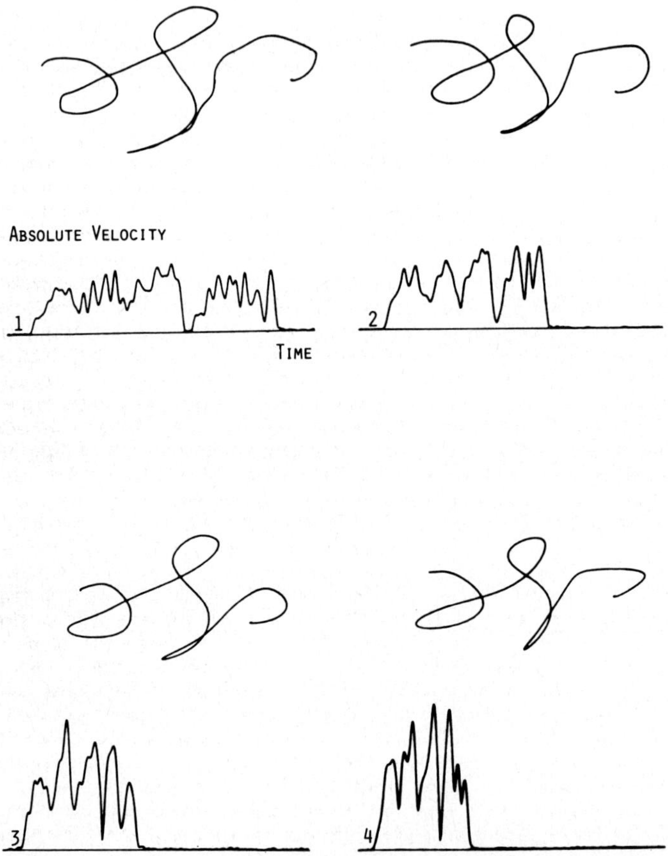

Figure 1. The first four attempts at writing an unfamiliar grapheme by an adult subject. Writing movements were recorded with a sample frequency of 105.2 Hz and filtered with a low-pass filter of 12 Hz. Below each recorded writing sample the corresponding absolute (tangential) velocity function is depicted.

An adult subject was asked to study an unfamiliar grapheme carefully for a few minutes. Then he was asked to write the grapheme a number of times without being able to see the original model. His writing movements, performed with a normal ballpen on standard writing paper, were recorded by means of a Calcomp digitizer and a PDP-11/45 computer, with a sample frequency of 105.2 Hz. The recorded signals were filtered with a low-pass filter of 12 Hz and displayed for inspection. Figure 1 depicts the first four attempts of the subject writing the unfamiliar grapheme. Below each attempt the absolute (tangential) velocity of the pen-point movements as a function of time is depicted. Typical changes can be observed in these velocity profiles: 1) the time needed to perform the unfamiliar grapheme decreases with the number of attempts (the velocity profile becomes narrower), 2) the highest velocity within each attempt increases, and 3) the number of velocity-peaks starts to correspond with the number of up- and downstrokes which are needed to perform the grapheme. The grapheme recordings show furthermore 1) a decrease in writing size, and 2) sudden curvature changes within up- and downgoing parts of the grapheme which are present in the first two, but absent in the last two, attempts. From these aspects of the recorded writing movements and their corresponding tangential velocity profiles we deduce that the first attempt was probably controlled by a closed-loop movement strategy resulting in slowly performed, large-sized, frequently interrupted movements and that the fourth attempt was controlled by an open-loop movement strategy resulting in rapidly performed, somewhat smaller and uninterrupted ballistic movements. However, this deduction must be made with care because there is no information in these recordings which reflects the sources and time characteristics of involved kinaesthetic and/or visual feedback processes.

The writing movements of young children show a large number of interruptions within up- and downstrokes of produced graphemes. Figure 2 contrasts graphemes (and corresponding velocity profiles) performed by a 7-year-old child (on the left-hand side) with those performed by an adult (on the right-hand side). The child produced the writing patterns with a large number of motoric impulses whereas the adult produced in both patterns five motoric impulses to realize the five strokes of each pattern.

The acquisition of cursive writing movements

In a study of repetitive writing behaviour of first, second and third grade primary-school children (Meulenbroek & van Galen, 1986) we studied the microstructure of the stroke production process from a developmental viewpoint. We found that the acquisition of the writing skill probably occurs in discontinuous stages in a similar way to that described for aimed reaching tasks by Hay (1979, 1984). In our study the youngest children performed relatively fast movements with few interruptions. The writing performance of second-grade children was slower and showed frequent interruptions. Grade three children achieved a moderate writing speed and their frequency of movement interruptions decreased. In the following experiment we tried to verify these observations in a letter writing task performed by primary-school children.

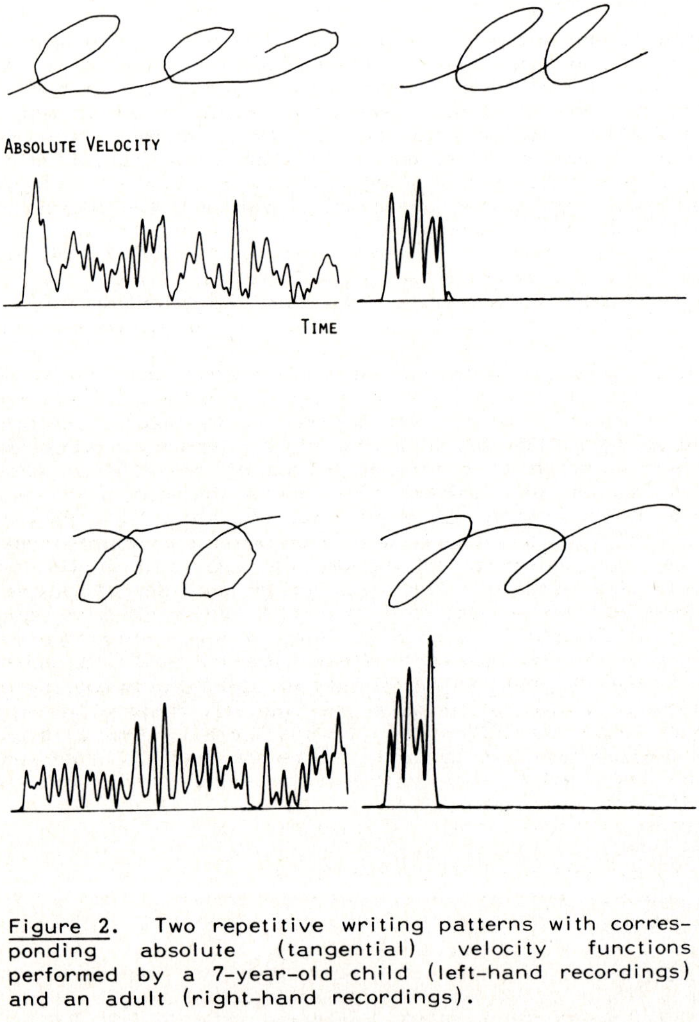

Figure 2. Two repetitive writing patterns with corresponding absolute (tangential) velocity functions performed by a 7-year-old child (left-hand recordings) and an adult (right-hand recordings).

Method

Subjects

Seventy-five normal children from an ordinary urban primary school in Nijmegen served as subjects in this experiment. They were selected from grades two to six, each selected group consisting of fifteen children. The mean age and range of ages for the five groups given in years and months were respectively: 8;0 (7;4 - 9;0), 8;10 (8;5 - 9;6), 10;0 (9;5 - 10;6), 11;1 (10;7 - 11;9) and 12;0 (11;5 - 12;9).

Procedure and apparatus

All subjects performed the experiment in an airconditioned, moderately lit, sound-proofed van. Each subject was seated on a school chair in front of a school desk, both adjusted to the body size of the subject. Visual stimuli were projected on to the writing surface by means of a slide-projector and a special mirror. The projection contained no double reflections. On each slide the contours of two adjacent, horizontally placed bright squares and one bright letter was depicted. The mirror above the school desk was placed in such a manner that the projected body of the smallest letters was 5 mm. The letter was always presented in the centre of the left-hand square. The subject had to write the correct cursive grapheme in the centre of the right-hand square. Left-handed subjects were allowed to write the grapheme to the left of the stimulus-field.

The subject was instructed to write the correct cursive grapheme as soon and as fast as possible whenever a new letter was presented in the left-hand square. An Apple-2 microcomputer controlled the slide projection and the recording of the writing movements. The latter were sampled at a rate of 100 Hz by means of an Apple-2 XY tablet and a slightly thicker than normal ballpen which were both attached to the microcomputer. The XY tablet and the projected stimuli were rotated 10 degrees anti-clockwise for right-handers and 10 degrees clockwise for left-handers to ensure an optimal writing posture of the subject. The experimenter was seated on the right-hand side of the subject and observed the writing movements by means of a TV monitor placed in front of him. This monitor could not be seen by the subject. After the subject had completed a grapheme the experimenter stopped the sampling period, which had a maximum duration of six seconds, and a high tone was presented as an indication for the subject to shift the non-ruled writing paper (A4 format) upwards to such a degree that the just written letter came to be situated above the two squares. An inter-trial rest period of about 20 seconds was used to store the latency and the sampled writing movements on a diskette.

Each subject performed two series of 26 trials in which each letter of the alphabet occurred once. In each series a different order of letters was used.

Data analysis

Data analyses were performed by means of a VAX-11/750 computer. Each recorded grapheme was divided into up- and downstrokes by means of an interactive computer analysis system. A distinction was made between the entry and exit strokes of a grapheme and the strokes which made up the body of the letter itself. Because it was reasoned that in normal handwriting the movement kinematics of entry and exit strokes are influenced by preceding and following letters, these strokes were excluded from the analyses.

Of each grapheme segment (64 per alphabet) the following measures were calculated : duration, distance, mean and maximum velocity, minimum and maximum curvature and the number of absolute velocity inversions per unit length. An example of the analysis of one

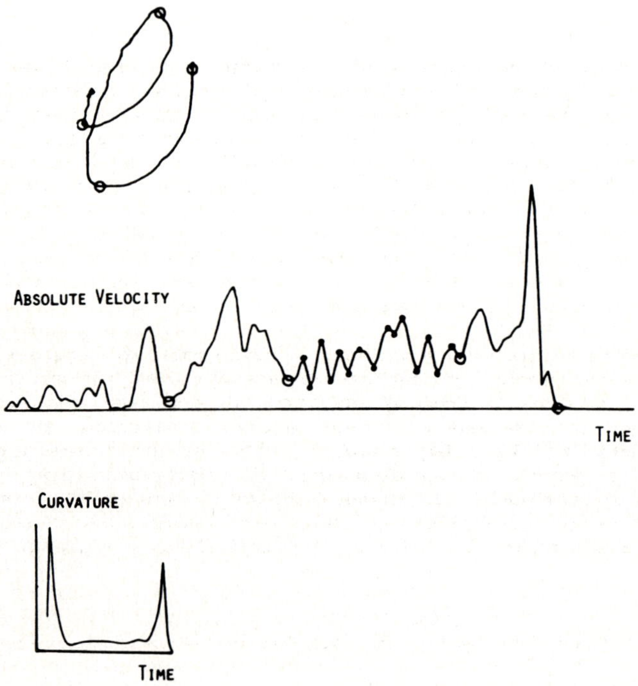

Figure 3. Example of the data analysis of one record. The grapheme 'e' (cut in three segments; open circles) and the corresponding absolute velocity function of the writing movements (middle graph). Movement time, distance, velocity and writing dysfluency (i.e. number of velocity inversions [filled circles] per unit length) were calculated on the basis of the absolute velocity pattern. Curvature measurements of the central segment of the grapheme 'e' were determined from the curvature function (lower graph) which was derived by dividing the angular and absolute velocity functions.

record is depicted in Figure 3. The curvature function of each grapheme segment was derived by dividing the angular and absolute velocity functions. This procedure is fully described by Maarse,

Teulings, and Bouwhuisen (1985). The number of absolute velocity inversions per unit length (with exclusion of the velocity dips at the borders of the cut segments) was regarded to reflect the dysfluency with which grapheme segments were produced. It was reasoned that when during the production of a grapheme segment more than one inversion occurs in the absolute velocity pattern, motoric impulses interrupt the ballistic manner in which a handwriting stroke is normally produced (Meulenbroek & van Galen, 1986).

Results

Figure 4 depicts the changes of the different kinematic variables as a function of grades. The leftmost graph depicts the mean movement time of the analysed grapheme segments. A decreasing trend can be observed which levels off at grade five. Trend analysis revealed a significant linear trend ($\underline{F}(1,70)=65.28$; $\underline{p} < .001$) as well as a significant cubic trend ($\underline{F}(4,70)=4.65$; $\underline{p} < .05$). The second graph shows significant linear and cubic trends in the mean writing velocity data (respectively: $\underline{F}(4,70)=15.21$; $\underline{p}<.01$ and $\underline{F}(4,70)=4.32$; $\underline{p}<.05$). Writing velocity decreases from grade two to three. From grade three, writing velocity increases up to grade six. Similar results were found in the maximum velocity data.

The dysfluency data are depicted in third graph of Figure 4. Grade three children wrote the cursive letters with the highest number of velocity inversions. From grade three to grade six, a decrease of dysfluency is observed. Trend analysis revealed a significant linear trend ($\underline{F}(4,70)=9.04$; $\underline{p} <.001$). The maximum curvature of the grapheme segments is depicted in the fourth graph of Figure 4. Again a discontinuous developmental trend can be observed. The linear trend ($\underline{F}(4,70)=11.91$; $\underline{p}<.001$) and cubic trend ($\underline{F}(4,70)=7.20$; $\underline{p}<.01$) were significant. While the maximum curvature of grapheme

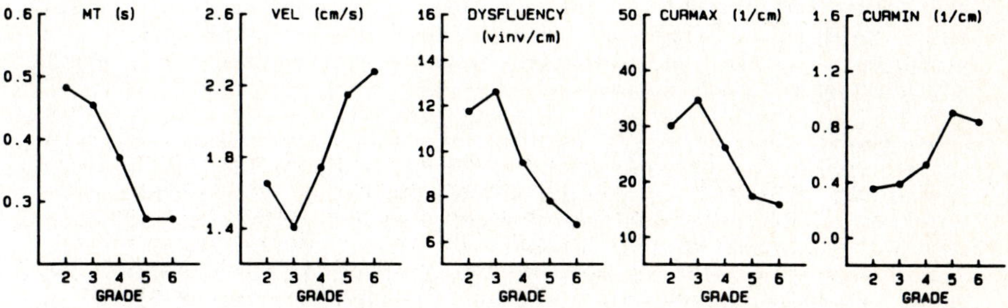

Figure 4. Changes in the analysed kinematic variables of grapheme segments as a function of grades.
MT = movement time (s);
VEL = Mean Writing Velocity (cm/s);
DYSFLUENCY = Number of Velocity Inversions per cm;
CURMAX = Maximum Curvature (1/cm);
CURMIN = Minimum Curvature (1/cm).

segments decreases from grade three to grade six the minimum curvature data show a reversed developmental trend (rightmost graph of Figure 4). The minimum curvature increases linearly from grade two to grade five ($F(4,70)=30.60$; $p<.001$).

Discussion

In this experiment primary-school children wrote single cursive graphemes as fast as possible after visual presentations of single letters. The acquisition of handwriting skill was investigated by analysing a number of kinematic variables of the cursive grapheme segments thus produced. Evidence was found for a discontinuity in development of the writing skill during primary school. Our observations correspond with earlier findings of Hay (1979, 1984) and von Hofsten (1979, 1980) concerning the development of other motor skills and those of Meulenbroek and van Galen (1986) concerning repetitive writing behaviour. A decline in performance was observed from grade two to grade three. Writing velocity decreased, movements became more dysfluent, and large curvature changes during the stroke production process occurred more often. The changes in these kinematic variables are probably due to the use of visual and kinesthetic feedback processes which interrupt the normally smooth production of grapheme segments. However, it may be possible that the grade three children tried to produce the shapes of the graphemes more accurately than the children in the other grades. No attempt was made in this experiment to determine the shape accuracy of the graphemes.

Another explanation of the discontinuity in writing development has been put forward by Wann (1986). Wann stated that at this point in the acquisition of the writing skill, writing pressure could be responsible for the dysfluency of stroke production. When writing pressure is high the increase in the number of inversions in the absolute velocity profile does not necessarily reflect the involvement of feedback processes. Therefore, in future studies, shape accuracy and pen-point pressure should be taken into consideration, together with kinematic variables which reflect the underlying control strategies, to make the inference of control strategies from recorded writing signals more valid.

From grade three to grade six writing performance became gradually faster, more fluent and more efficient with respect to grapheme curvatures. As far as the curvature measurements are concerned it appeared that older children wrote cursive graphemes with less straight grapheme segments and less dramatic curvature changes. The straight writing movements were replaced by slightly more curved movements, probably corresponding with the natural curvature of stationary movements of the hand and fingers (Maarse, Schomaker, & Thomassen, 1986).

The point at which performance temporarily declines during the development of motor skills seems to differ depending on the skill in question. With reaching (Hay, 1979) and with drawing simple repetitive writing patterns (Meulenbroek & van Galen, 1986) the decline was observed in 7-year-olds. With cursive handwriting, we have demonstrated a decline in performance in grade three children with a mean age of ten years. It seems that as the skill which has to be mastered becomes more complex, the discontinuity in the acquisition process is observed at a later age.

References

Hay, L. (1979). Spatial-temporal analysis of movements in children: Motor programs versus feedback in the development of reaching. Journal of Motor Behavior, 11, 189-200.

Hay, L. (1984). A discontinuity in the development of motor control in children. In W. Prinz & A.F. Sanders (Eds.), Cognition and motor processes. Berlin: Springer-Verlag.

Maarse, F.J., Shomaker, L.R.B., & Thomassen, A.J.W.M. (1986). The influence of changes in the effector coordinate system on handwriting movements. In H.S.R. Kao, G.P. van Galen, & R. Hoosain (Eds.), Graphonomics: Contemporary research in handwriting. Amsterdam: North-Holland.

Maarse, F.J., Teulings, H.L., & Bouwhuisen, C.F. (1985). Signaalverwerking toegepast in schrijfonderzoek. In F.J. Maarse, W.E.J. van den Bosch, P. Wittenburg, & E.A. Zuiderveen (Eds.), Computers in de psychologie. Lisse: Swets & Zeitlinger.

Meulenbroek, R.G.J., & van Galen, G.P. (1986). Movement analysis of repetitive writing behaviour of first, second and third grade primary school children. In H.S.R. Kao, G.P. van Galen, & R. Hoosain (Eds.), Graphonomics: Contemporary research in handwriting. Amsterdam: North Holland.

Schmidt, R.A. (1975). A schema theory of discrete motor skill learning. Psychological Review, 82, 225-260.

Schmidt, R.A. (1976). The schema as a solution to some persistent problems in motor learning theory. In G.E. Stelmach & J. Requin (Eds.), Tutorials in motor behavior. Amsterdam: North-Holland.

von Hofsten, C. (1979). Development of visually directed reaching: the approach phase. Journal of Human Movement Studies, 5, 160-178.

von Hofsten, C. (1980). Predictive reaching for moving objects by human infants. Journal of Experimental Child Psychology, 30, 369-382.

Wann, J.P. (1986). Handwriting disturbances: Developmental trends. In H.T.A. Whiting, & M.G. Wade (Eds.), Themes in motor development. Dordrecht: Martinus Nijhoff.

Cognition and Action in Skilled Behaviour
A.M. Colley and J.R. Beech (Editors)

TEMPORAL AND SPATIAL ANTICIPATION IN TWELVE-YEAR-OLD BOYS AND GIRLS

Martinus Buekers, Jan Pauwels and Paul Meugens
Catholic University of Leuven

In the past decade anticipation behaviour has been investigated in detail. These experiments have mostly examined one of two components of anticipation behavior — temporal anticipation, where subjects have to make a motor response coincident with some external event, — or spatial anticipation, where subjects are asked to predict as fast as possible the direction or the landing point of a moving object. The separation of these two factors might suggest that anticipation skill has two independent components. However, the existing literature does not provide clear evidence concerning this independence. An experiment was therefore performed in which twelve-year-old subjects (17 girls and 17 boys) were submitted to two different tests, a temporal anticipation task and a spatial anticipation task. In the temporal anticipation task the subjects had to give a motor response (finger-lift) at the moment when a moving stimulus arrived at a stable target. Error scores (total error and variable error) were calculated to the nearest ms. In the spatial anticipation task the subjects had to predict the trajectory of a flying ball, as fast as possible, by indicating one out of four possible landing areas. Accuracy and time scores (ms) were recorded. The results showed no significant differences between boys and girls for spatial anticipation. However, for temporal anticipation the variable error scores showed a significant sex difference. The correlation between total error and response times was very low (rho = .10) indicating that there is no relationship between spatial and temporal anticipation performance. Consequently the statement that anticipation can be divided into two separable components appears to be defensible.

Anticipation is clearly important in the performance of sports. This is not only the case for open skills (e.g. volleyball), in which the players continually have to make temporal and spatial judgements. To a large extent, closed skills (e.g. gymnastics) also rely on the ability of the performer to predict the future organisation of any movement. Poulton (1957) was the first to distinguish between effector, receptor and perceptual anticipation. Subsequently other definitions have been used, resulting in a variety of terms like transit reaction, timing, anticipatory timing, coincidence timing, anticipation, coincidence–anticipation, etc. Since these definitions are largely a function of the experimental task, they can be considered as operational definitions.

In spite of the practical value of these operational definitions, the division of anticipation into different well-defined components is to be preferred, because it offers a useful conceptual framework for fundamental research. Konzag and Konzag (1980) have made a distinction between "external" and "internal anticipation. In a broad sense, external anticipation can be defined as the prediction of external events, while internal anticipation describes the prediction of the performer's own movements. Both sorts of anticipation contain three different components (Figure 1): event anticipation (what will happen?), spatial anticipation or spacing (where will it happen?) and temporal anticipation or timing (when will it happen?).

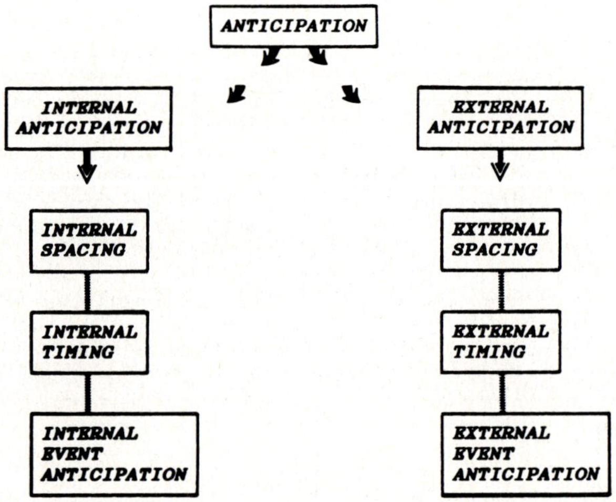

Figure 1. Different components of anticipation behaviour.

The different components of anticipation can be defined as follows:

— Internal event anticipation is the prediction of which action has to be undertaken in order to match the environmental demands.
— External event anticipation is the prediction of which action will occur in the environment, on the basis of external cues.

— Internal timing is the temporal prediction concerning the proper movement.
— External timing is the temporal prediction concerning the external events.

— Internal spacing is the spatial prediction concerning the actor's own body.
— External spacing is the spatial prediction concerning external cues.

Using this framework, external anticipation can be defined as the prediction of which action will occur, and the temporal and spatial predictions concerning this action. Similarly, internal anticipation can be defined as the prediction of which action has to be undertaken, and the temporal and spatial predictions concerning this "proper" movement.

Since these different aspects of anticipation are closely linked in everyday skills and sports, many experiments have been conducted using tasks in which more than one component is present. The studies of Whiting and co-workers (Whiting, Gill, & Stephenson, 1970; Whiting, Alderson, & Sanderson, 1973; Whiting & Sharp, 1974) are representative of this approach. More recently Smyth and Marriott (1982) and Fischman and Schneider (1985) investigated spatial and temporal accuracy in one-hand catching. However, since these studies are not primarily interested in the relationship between spatial and temporal anticipation, experimental evidence concerning this relationship is rather limited.

In contrast to this, a lot of attention has been directed to sex differences in the external timing component of anticipation performance. However, the conclusions drawn from these studies are not straightforward, for some authors (Haywood, 1980; Stadulis, 1971) have failed to find a significant sex difference, whereas other studies (Bruce, 1966; Dunham, 1977) have shown significantly better performances for the male subjects. Wrisberg and Mead (1983) have argued that in young children, sex differences only appear when the coordination of large muscle groups is required. Therefore sex differences seem to be the result of motor rather than perceptual differences. The finding that sex differences are highly task-specific was confirmed in a number of experiments (Bard, Fleury, Carriere, & Bellec, 1981; Hoffman, Imwold, & Koller, 1983; Jensen, Picado, & Morenz, 1981).

In the present study an attempt was made to answer two questions. First, is there a relationship between the performance on an external timing and an external spacing task? Since these two aspects of anticipation behaviour seem to be firmly linked in everyday skills, a positive correlation was expected. The second question is related to gender effects. Although no differences would be expected in a simple external timing task, the findings of Fleury (1974) and Maccoby and Jacklin (1974) indicate that boys perform better than girls in spatial prediction tasks.

Method

Subjects

The subjects were 12-year-old boys (n=17) and girls (n=17), from a primary school in Heverlee. Permission for participation was obtained from the parents and school authorities before the start of the experiment.

Task 1 : External timing

Apparatus and task

The components of the apparatus were a runway and a response-circuit. The runway (Figure 2) consisted of 640 LED's (red bar graph displays MV57164) attached end to end. The connected parts, which had a total length of 130 cm, were fixed in an aluminium rail, which was fastened in a wooden panel. A control-device (micro-computer 6502 uP, 1Mhz clock) was programmed to light up the successive lamps within the desired duration. In this experiment, the stimulus light moved from the left to the right and the speed of the stimulus was 65cm/s.

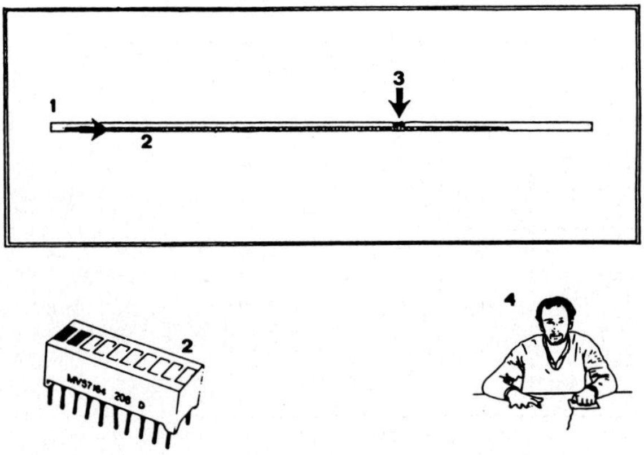

Figure 2. Schematic view of the test situation for the external timing task.

1) Runway 2) LED's

3) Target 4) Response-circuit

The response-circuit consisted of a movable plate and a stable sensor, placed on a table. The table was standing in front of the runway at a distance of 4 m. The subject placed the index of the preferred hand on the sensor and the other hand on the plate.

Subjects were asked to make a movement (finger-lift) at the exact moment when the moving light arrived at a stationary target. When the subject's finger was lifted from the sensor the circuit was interrupted, resulting in an error score (deviation from the target in ms).

Procedure

The subject was seated in front of the display, at a distance of 4 m, and asked to place the index of the preferred hand on the sensor and the other hand on the plate. After further instruction on the task, three familiarization trials were given, followed by the 30 test trials. Temporal error (deviation from the target in ms) was recorded for each trial. For each subject, total error (TE = the total amount of deviation of the responses about the target) and variable error (VE = the standard deviation of the responses about the subject's mean response) were calculated for the 30 trials.

Task 2 : External spacing

Apparatus and task
A "Jetball" ball-launcher was used to project, in a controlled way, volleyballs to one of four possible landing-areas (Figure 3). An electronic timer was activated at the moment when the ball was launched, and stopped at the moment when the subject called the number of the landing-area. Accuracy scores and response times (to the nearest ms) were recorded.

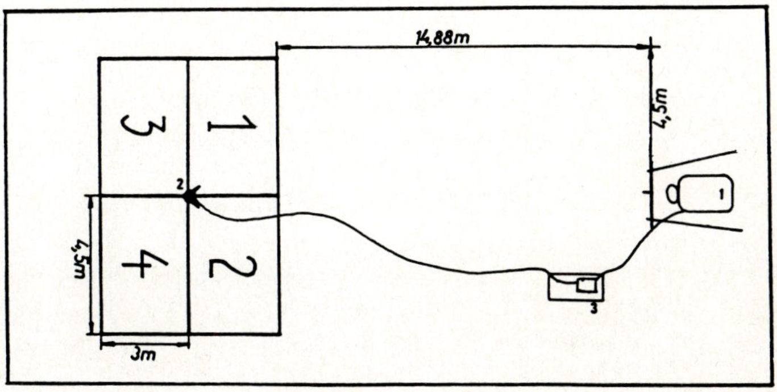

Figure 3. Schematic view of the test situation for the spacing task.
1) ball-launcher
2) subject (facing the ball-launcher) with microphone
3) timer.

The subject had to predict as fast as possible the landing-area of a ball, launched towards him or her from a distance of 18 m. In order to do so, the subject shouted (in a microphone) a number corresponding to one out of four possible landing-areas (Figure 2).

Procedure
The subject was placed at the intersection of the four landing-areas with a hand-held microphone. After familiarisation with the task, in which the subjects had to learn the numbers corresponding to the landing-areas, 20 trials were given in a random order (5 trials for each landing-area).

Each subject performed the timing task and the spacing task on the same day. Both tasks were balanced for order across subjects.

Results

External timing

For each subject, mean total area (TE) and mean variable error (VE) were calculated for the 30 trials. For total error, group means were 59.82 ms (boys) and 65.47 ms (girls). Variable error group means were 48.29 ms for the boys and 52.88 ms for the girls.

T-tests showed a significant difference for variable error, $t(32) = 1.69$, $p < .05$ but not for total error, $t(32) = 1.08$, $p < .05$.

External spacing

Table 1 shows the means and standard deviations for response times and accuracy scores. The differences between boys and girls were not significant for the response times, $t(32) = 0.50$, $p < .05$ nor for the accuracy scores, $t(32) = 0.15$, $p < .05$.

Table 1

Means and standard deviations for response times (to the nearest ms) and accuracy scores (number of right predictions).

	Gender	Mean	S.D.
Response times (ms)	Boys	1190	210
	Girls	1240	334
Accuracy scores	Boys	16.18/20	2.15
	Girls	16.08/20	2.04

Further 2(sex) X 4(landing-areas) analyses of variance, with repeated measures on the last factor, revealed a significant main effect of landing-areas for the time scores, $F\ (3,96) = 16.07$, $p < .01$, and a significant main effect of landing-areas for the accuracy scores, $F\ (3,96) = 13.22$, $p < .01$.

Tukey *a posteriori* comparisons indicated that the areas situated in front of the subject were predicted faster ($p < .01$) than those situated at the back of the subject (Figure 4). For the accuracy scores the area situated at the left back of the subject was predicted less accurately ($p < .01$) than the other areas (Figure 5). No other means were significantly different.

Spatial-temporal relationship

Spearman's rank order correlation coefficient was calculated, comparing total error scores for the timing task with time scores for the spacing task. The low correlation (rho = 0.10) supports the notion that the two experimental variables are independent.

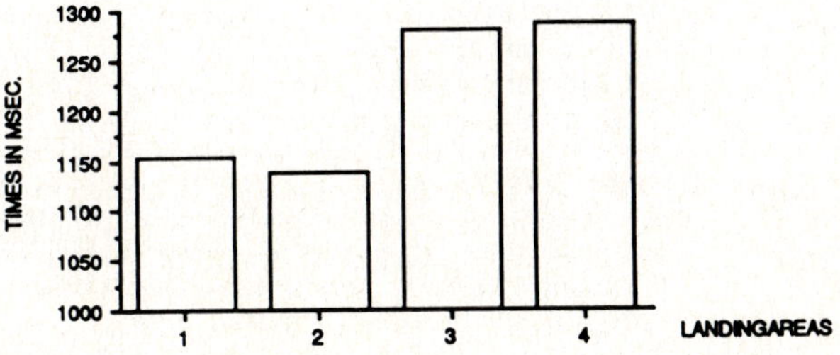

Figure 4. Mean response times for the landing-areas 1 and 2 (in front of the subject) and 3 and 4 (at the back of the subject).

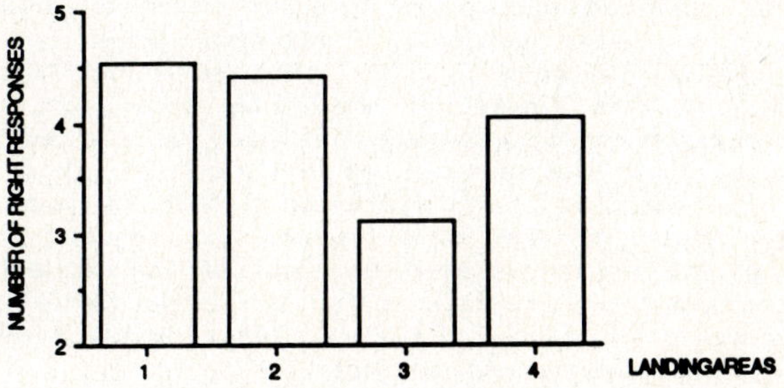

Figure 5. Mean number of right responses for the different landing-areas.

Discussion

In contrast to the hypothesis that no gender effect would show up in a simple external timing task, significant differences were found for variable error, suggesting the existence of a gender effect in anticipation performance even though the task was merely a perceptual one. Hence these results are in line with the findings of Wrisberg, Paul, and Ragsdale (1979), who showed a significantly higher response consistency (smaller VE) in males than in females. Previous work of Buekers, Pauwels, and Sunaert (1986) has indicated that the gender effects are present across different age groups ranging from 6 to 10 years old. Taking these results into account together with the Bruce (1966) and Dunham (1977) studies, it seems that even in a simple external timing task non-age-specific sex differences are present. However, for accuracy scores the present findings are in contrast with the Wrisberg, Paul, and Ragsdale (1979) findings. Although the boys attained a higher performance level than the girls, this difference failed to be significant. This might indicate that the sex differences are caused by a lack of consistency of performance in the female subjects.

The statement that boys perform better than girls in spatial prediction tasks was not confirmed in this experiment. Both groups were able to predict the right landing-area of the launched balls in about 80% of the trials. Findings from a previous study (Buekers & Pauwels, 1981) showed that 18-year-old subjects predicted the landing-area correctly in 83% of trials. The fact that the performance level of 12-year-old children is comparable with the results of 18-year-old subjects is noteworthy. However, time scores indicate that almost 60% of the ball flight had to be seen before the prediction was made. Compared with the older subjects, who needed only 47% of the ball flight, this decision time is rather high. Clearly, the younger subjects need a longer prediction time in order to attain the same accuracy level as older subjects. Although young performers can make valid spatial judgements they need sufficient time to do so. A consequence of this limitation would be that, for example, the initiation of a movement to a served ball may be started rather late, resulting in a (too) late arrival at the position where a hit or a catch has to be executed. A distinction has to be made with regard to the flight path of the ball, since the results indicate that predictions for the areas situated in front of the subject were faster and more accurate than predictions for the areas behind the subject. Earlier experiments (Buekers & Pauwels, 1981) revealed the same effect for older and more experienced subjects.

The second point of interest in this experiment was the question as to whether anticipation behaviour can be divided into two independent skills. The results suggest that external timing and external spacing may indeed be independent. The fact that sex differences only appeared in the timing task and not in the spacing task might be seen as one indication of this, but the strongest support comes from the very low correlation (rho = .10) between the two time scores for the total experimental group. Perhaps then, time and space are not processed in the same way. However, in game situations both components of anticipation behaviour are crucial. For example, in order to catch a ball, a player must not only be on time, he has to be on time <u>and</u> in the right place. One could argue that in more experienced groups (competition players) the correlation between the two components in question would be higher. Results from an experiment by Devos (1985) indicate that the opposite is the case.

Findings from a number of studies strongly suggest that anticipation behaviour can be divided into different components. Our results suggest that, among these, external spacing and external timing must be considered as separate skills.

References

Bard, C., Fleury, M., Carriere, L., & Bellec, J. (1981). Components of the coincidence-anticipation behavior of children aged from 6 to 11 years. Perceptual and Motor Skills, 52, 547-556.

Bruce, R.D. (1966). The effects of variation in ball trajectory upon the catching performance of elementary school children. (microform) Eugene, Oregon: Microform Publications.

Buekers, M. & Pauwels, J. (1981). Anticipatie in volleybal: snelheid en nauwkeurigheid van de predictie van een balbaan. Hermes, 15, 187-198.

Buekers, M., Pauwels, J., & Sunaert, A. (1986). Geslachts en leeftijdsverschillen inzake en invloed van feedback op de ontwikkeling van de anticipatievaardigheid bij kinderen. Hermes, 18, 277-286.

Devos, L. (1985). Anticipatie: de invloed van volleybal-vaardigheid op timing en spacing. Unpublished Masters Thesis, Leuven: K.U. Leuven.

Dunham, P. (1977). Age, sex, speed and practice in coincidence—anticipation performance of children. Perceptual and Motor Skills, 45, 187-193.

Fischman, M.G. & Schneider, T. (1985). Skill level, vision, and proprioception in simple one-hand catching. Journal of Motor Behavior, 17, 219-229.

Fleury, M. (1974). Perception et mouvement II: perception de l'espace. Mouvement, 9, 149-167.

Haywood, K.M. (1980). Coincidence—anticipation accuracy across the life span. Experimental Aging Research, 6, 451-462.

Hoffman, S.J., Imwold, C.H., & Koller, J.A. (1983). Accuracy and prediction in throwing: a taxonomic analysis of children's performance. Research Quarterly for Exercise and Sport, 54, 33-40.

Jensen, B.E., Picado, M.E., & Morenz, C. (1981). Effects of precision of knowledge of results on performance of a gross motor coincidence—anticipation task. Journal of Motor Behavior, 13, 9-17.

Konzag, I. & Konzag, G. (1980). Anforderungen an die kognitieven Functionen in der psychischen Regulation sportlicher Spielhandlungen. Theorie und Praxis der Korperkultur, 29, 20-31.

Maccoby, E.E. & Jacklin, C.N. (1974). The psychology of sex differences. Stanford, Ca: Stanford University Press.

Poulton, E.C. (1957). On prediction in skilled movements. Psychological Bulletin, 54, 467-478.

Smyth, M.M. & Marriott, A.M. (1982). Vision and proprioception in simple catching. Journal of Motor Behavior, 14, 143-152.

Stadulis, R.E. (1971). Coincidence anticipation behavior of children (microform) Eugene, Oregon: Microform Publications.

Whiting, H.T.A., Alderson, G.J.K., & Sanderson, F.H. (1973). Critical time intervals for viewing and individual differences in performance of a ball-catching task. International Journal of Sports Psychology, 4, 155-164.

Whiting, H.T.A., Gill, E.B., & Stephenson, J.M. (1970). Critical time intervals for taking in flight information in a ball-catching task. Ergonomics, 13, 265-272.

Whiting, H.T.A. & Sharp, R.H. (1974). Visual occlusion factors in a discrete ball-catching task. Journal of Motor Behavior, 6, 11-16.

Wrisberg, C.A. & Mead, B.J. (1983). Developing coincident timing skill in children: a comparison of training methods. Research Quarterly for Exercise and Sport, 54, 67-74.

Wrisberg, C.A., Paul, J.H., & Ragsdale, M.R. (1979). Subject gender, knowledge of results, and receptor anticipation. Research Quarterly, 50, 699-708.

Cognition and Action in Skilled Behaviour
A.M. Colley and J.R. Beech (Editors)

CLUMSINESS OR PERCEPTUO-MOTOR DYSFUNCTION?

Judith I. Laszlo, Phillip J. Bairstow, Jon Bartrip
Institute of Child Health, University of London

Ursula T. Rolfe
St. Louis University Medical Center

The task orientated approach in management of clumsiness was focussed on symptom alleviation. The process orientated approach, here described, aims at causal diagnosis and focal therapy. Forty children, attending mainstream Junior schools were chosen by teachers for participation in the study. The selected children were considered by the teachers to have motor difficulties which interfered with their progress at school, i.e. they were clumsy. Kinaesthetic perception, and spatial and temporal programming processes were assessed. Children in the experimental groups were trained in all or some of the processes in which they were found to be deficient. Training time ranged from 1.5 to 3 hours per child, spread over a two-week period. The Control Group received training along the lines of traditional remedial teaching. The results showed that: first, adequate kinaesthetic perceptual ability is necessary in motor behaviour; second, improvement in deficient processes resulted in significant improvement in general motor performance and acquisition of complex skills; third, the emotive label of clumsiness can be eliminated by the diagnostically valid term of perceptual-motor dysfunction; and fourth, traditional training in the Control Group did not result in improved motor performance.

This chapter describes the use of a new process-orientated method of diagnosis and treatment for clumsy children. Clumsiness is most often identified by teachers and parents when the child reaches seven or eight years of age. On average up to 10% of children attending mainstream Junior schools are labelled clumsy (Gubbay, 1975); 80% of clumsy children are boys. Typically, clumsiness is manifested by difficulties in the acquisition of complex motor skills such as efficient use of knife and fork, dressing, hand-writing and playing sport. In severe cases the child repeatedly bumps into furniture, drops and overturns objects, walks and runs in an ungainly fashion. Some clumsy children exhibit introverted behaviour patterns. In order to avoid accidents and injury, withdrawal to a corner offers the safest solution.

The many difficulties the clumsy child encounters in the home and school can adversely affect his or her emotional and social development. Parents, however patient, respond with irritation to repeated slow, awkward and inelegant actions, often expressing their impatience through verbal criticism or even physical punishment. Many parents are unaware of the developmental disorders underlying clumsiness and assume that the child is merely careless and lazy. At school bad performance of paper-pencil skills are criticised by the teachers, inept sport performance by classmates. The child is accused of untidiness and lack of application. The teacher's disapproval and peer ridicule erodes self-confidence and self-esteem. Indeed, these secondary consequences of clumsiness may persist into adult life. While adults (but not children) can restrict their choice of occupational and leisure activities to those they are able to perform without difficulties, the low self-esteem might hinder their mature emotional and social functioning.

The serious consequences of clumsiness are well recognised by paediatricians, psychologists and many educationalists and hence various diagnostic tests and remedial teaching methods have been developed in an effort to help the clumsy child. Methods often employed focus on the tasks the children have difficulty performing. The diagnostic tests, formal (e.g. Gubbay, 1975; Stott, Moyes & Henderson, 1972) or informal, consist of motor items. The diagnosis may confirm the difficulties which lead to the referral by the teacher or parent, but this task-orientated approach does not investigate the cause of the child's difficulties. Treatment focuses on remedial teaching of the tasks the child is unable to perform, together with "general motor exercises" such as trampoline practice.

In contrast to the task-orientated approach, the process-orientated approach, to be described, is based on theoretical foundations. It is aimed at diagnosing the cause of the difficulties underlying overt symptoms.

The closed-loop model, proposed by Laszlo and Bairstow (1985a) was used to identify the perceptual and motor processes which underlie the acquisition and performance of all perceptuo-motor skills. It is argued that defective development of such processes could result in poor performance of a number of skilled acts. Here only a brief description of the closed-loop model will be given, citing only some key references which provide evidence for the relative independence of the relevant processes.

The closed-loop system is characterised by the cooperative action of perceptual and motor processes. The performance of perceptuo-motor tasks depends, in the first instance, on input from the environment and from the position of body parts in space. Two functionally distinguishable, though interconnected, central units can be defined: the Central Processing Unit is responsible for processing and storage of information while the Motor Programming Unit is responsible for the activation of the muscles. In the Central Processing Unit a motor plan of action is formulated. In formulating this plan the input is taken into account along with memory traces stored from previous attempts at the task or related tasks, motivation and the goal to be reached. The plan is transmitted to the Motor Programming Unit where it is translated into specific motor unit activation patterns, resulting in the output, i.e. the movement itself.

The output is monitored through the sensory feedback loop which connects output to the Central Processing Unit, and enables error detection and error correction. Acquisition of a skill depends on practice of the skill. With each repetition the memory traces of previous attempts are retrieved, and the information generated by the present attempt, including error information, is processed and stored. Thus the task-relevant memory traces are enriched, leading to improvement in the motor plan and consequently the motor programme becomes refined and more appropriate.

Only some of the processes described can be assessed in isolation. These fall into two classes: sensory-perceptual and motor. The sensory channels include kinaesthesis, vision, hearing and touch. Kinaesthesis signals the relative position of body parts, the extent, direction, speed and force of movements. It is of fundamental importance in the acquisition and performance of all motor tasks, it is the major component of memory for motor tasks (Bairstow & Laszlo, 1978a, 1978b) and has a major role in error detection and hence correction (Laszlo & Bairstow, 1985a). The contribution of the other sensory channels depends on the demands of the task, e.g. vision is important in handwriting, hearing in violin playing.

The motor factors include control of the direction and extent of movement — spatial programming (Georgopoulos, Schwartz, & Kettner, 1986; Passingham, 1985) and the speed at which the movement is performed — temporal programming (Sittig, Denier van der Gon, & Gielen, 1985). The last process to be considered for assessment is motor planning. Planning is aimed at formulating the mode of action. It integrates multi-sensory information, and knowledge about the goal (Cole & Abbs, 1986).

The process-orientated approach was applied first to kinaesthetic function. The Kinaesthetic Sensitivity Test (KST) (Laszlo & Bairstow, 1985b) was constructed to investigate two aspects of kinaesthetic information processing: kinaesthetic acuity and kinaesthetic perception and memory. Developmental trends were established for both test items (Bairstow & Laszlo, 1981; Laszlo & Bairstow, 1980). Further, it was shown (Laszlo & Bairstow, 1983) that children who performed the kinaesthetic test items at or below the 25th percentile for their age could be trained to improve their kinaesthetic ability. Following training, evidence of improvement in paper-pencil skills was found.

The success of the kinaesthetic training study encouraged the development of the process-orientated Perceptual-Motor Abilities Test (PMAT). With the aid of this test the developmental trends in perceptual and motor processes were charted (Laszlo & Bairstow, 1985a). The purpose of the present study was twofold. Firstly, in order to ascertain the usefulness of the test as a diagnostic instrument, the PMAT was to be given to clumsy children. It was hoped that dysfunction in specific perceptual and motor processes could be diagnosed and the child's ability profile established. Secondly, the effectiveness of the training programmes were to be investigated. Specific training programmes were devised for individual processes with the view of increasing the functional level of the process. It was argued that improvement of a defective process would lead to acquisition and better performance of those tasks which are dependent on the improved process. Thus, if successful, the process-orientated approach would, through improvement in a limited number of processes, facilitate acquisition and skilful performance on many tasks. In contrast, with the task-orientated approach, every task the child finds difficult to perform must be practised separately and it can be argued that continued deficiency in any one process could persist and hinder improvement in motor skills dependent on it.

Method

Subjects

Forty children attending six mainstream Junior schools participated in the study. The selection of the children was carried out by the headteachers or class teachers. At the first meeting with the headteachers the purpose of the study was described in general terms and their cooperation was sought in selecting children whose motor development was considered to lag behind their intellectual development. Three headteachers involved class teachers in the selection process, while the remaining three headteachers made the choices themselves. Class teachers selected about 10% of the total number of children in the school, headteachers recommended far fewer children. Altogether, 47 children were referred. Of the 38 chosen by the class teachers four were not included in the study while three children out of nine referred by headteachers were unsuitable.

The final sample comprised 31 boys and 9 girls. Four were left-handed. The mean age was 9 years 3 months with a range of 7 years 5 months—11 years 3 months at the time of the first testing session.

Experimental Design and Procedure

The summary of the experimental protocol is given in Table 1. Prior to testing, the class teachers filled in a questionnaire for each child selected from their class. The questionnaire is attached in Appendix 1 (Section a). Questions relevant to Academic Attainment, Motor and Social Behaviour were answered on a five point rating scale. The questionnaires were collected from the teachers before the first testing session, but were not evaluated till all testing had been completed.

The first testing session was carried out at the Department of Developmental Paediatrics (The Wolfson Centre). Each child was accompanied by parent/s. A paediatric medical and developmental history was obtained using a parent questionnaire, and each child was given a physical and neurological examination by a paediatrician. None of the children were found to suffer from identifable neurological disorders. Three children were reported to have had seizures at some time, but were not under medication at the time of the study. The examination included vision and hearing. Four children were

Table 1

Summary of Research Design

Groups	Stage 1 Test 1	Stage 2 Training In	Stage 3 Re-test	Stage 4
1	Teacher's Questionnaire TOMI PMAT Neurological Examination	Kinaesthetic Acuity and/or Kinaesthetic Perception and Memory and/or Spatial programming and/or Temporal programming	TOMI PMAT	Teacher's Follow-up Questionnaire
2	Teacher's Questionnaire TOMI PMAT Neurological Examination	Kinaesthetic Acuity and/or Kinaesthetic Perception and Memory	TOMI PMAT	Teacher's Follow-up Questionnaire
3	Teacher's Questionnaire TOMI PMAT Neurological Examination	Spatial programming and/or Temporal programming	TOMI PMAT	Teacher's Follow-up Questionnaire
4	Teacher's Questionnaire TOMI PMAT Neurological Examination	Tracing, Drawing, Spatial Puzzles, Miming and Fine and Gross Motor Tasks	TOMI PMAT	Teacher's Follow-up Questionnaire

referred to the optician because they needed spectacles. Each child performed the PMAT and the Test of Motor Impairment (TOMI); (Stott, Moyes & Henderson, 1984). The TOMI, a task-orientated test, was included in the study to obtain an assessment of the child's motor status through a test which is unrelated to the PMAT. The TOMI was selected from the available range of tests because it is easy to administer and can be scored objectively.

On completion of this testing session the PMAT raw scores were transformed to Z scores for each test item and an ability profile was drawn up for each child. On the basis of the PMAT scores a decision of whether the child should participate in the study was reached. The criterion of inclusion was that on at least three of the test items, the child's error score was above one standard deviation from the mean score for his age. The children with the highest four rank scores were allocated randomly into four groups; the next highest rank scores were allocated similarly. This procedure was repeated until all subjects were placed into four groups. Restriction to randomness was imposed by placing only those children who showed high error scores on kinaesthetic acuity and/or kinaesthetic perception and memory into Groups 2 and 3. As 30 children (75%) were kinaesthetically deficient the rank order grouping could be maintained.

The groups differed from each other on the type of training provided (see Table 1). In Group 1 children were trained in all areas in which they were found deficient; in Group 2 only kinaesthetic training was given, though the children had performed poorly in spatial and/or temporal programming as well; in Group 3 only spatial and/ or temporal programming were trained, kinaesthetic training was withheld; Group 4 training did not relate to diagnosed deficiencies but included practice in fine and gross motor skills.

After training the children were retested on the PMAT and TOMI at the Wolfson Centre.

Teachers were asked to complete a similar questionnaire to the one they filled in at the beginning of the study approximately 8-12 weeks after the children were retested. In addition to the five point rating scale, on various aspects of school attainment, motor and social behaviour, they were asked to rate the general improvement of the children in these three areas on a three point scale (Appendix 1, Section b).

Test and Training Procedure

1. PMAT

This test has been described in detail by Laszlo and Bairstow (1985a). Here only a short description of the test items are listed, grouped according to the process or processes each item was designed to measure, and the scoring method used for each item is specified.

a. Planning and spatio-temporal programming:

i. The Ward game. The child is required to roll 20 small billiard balls along a modified billiard table aiming at the middle flap of a seven flap target assembly which moves from side to side at the far end of the table. The graded scores are recorded during performance. The mean aiming error score is calculated.

b. Spatio-temporal programming:

i. The Video game is not included in this report. Tracking and target interception tasks given in the present study were performed on a more sophisticated computer system than was used in 1985. Detailed analysis of the difficulties the children encountered in these tasks is being assessed at present.

ii. Ball catching - whole body interception task. Four balls, graded in size, are released from the top of a chute. The chute setting varies from 15°-35° in five even steps. The child waits behind a line 3 m from the chute until the ball is released, then runs forward to catch the ball before it hits the ground. The number of missed balls out of the total is recorded.

c. Planning and spatial programming:

i. Ball handling - manual dexterity. Eighteen balls of sizes varying from cricket balls to small marbles are to be put from one small bucket into another, one at a time, with one hand as fast as possible. Time taken for completion of the task is recorded.

ii. Drawing. Line drawings of a square, placed in oblique orientation, and a horseshoe, have to be copied. Instructions stress the need for exact replication of the models both in size and shape. The score is calculated by placing the model over the drawing and calculating the mm^2 area of non-overlap.

d. Spatial programming:

i. Tracing. The same figures as in the drawing task are given, outlined first by parallel lines 3 mm apart, then by single lines. Tracing between the lines and over the single line is performed. When tracing between the parallel lines an error is recorded if the drawn line crosses either of the parallel lines. In single line tracing an error is recorded if the child's line deviates by 1 mm from the drawn line. If the deviation is wider than 1 mm, the length of the deviation is also measured and each 5 mm length is given one error score.

ii. Dotting - paper-pencil aiming task. Eleven black 1 mm dots were printed at increasing distances from each other. The child is required to touch each dot with a red felt tip pen, completing the task as fast as possible. An error is recorded when the red dot is discernable outside the printed dot.

e. Sensory processing:

i. Static kinaesthesis-posture. The child lies on his back. A toy "Pink Panther", the limbs of which are bent into the posture the child is to imitate, is held above the child. While looking at the pink panther (without looking at his own limbs) the child is asked to place his arms and legs 'exactly like pink panther has his'. The number of the child's joints not in the required position are counted and recorded.

ii. and iii. Kinaesthetic acuity and kinaesthetic perception and memory are the two test items included in the Kinaesthetic Sensitivity Test (Laszlo & Bairstow, 1985a, 1985b). This test is commercially available, hence only a brief description of these test items will be included. Kinaesthetic acuity is measured by moving the hands of the child up two ramps under a masking box. The ramps are set at different angles. The child has to indicate which arm was moved higher. The number of incorrect judgements out of a total 32 trials is recorded.

Kinaesthetic perception and memory. Six closed, "nonsense" patterns are presented to the child by passively guiding his hand, holding a stylus, under a masking box. The patterns are reorientated by the tester, the masking box is removed and the child attempts to replace the pattern into its original position. The degree of error between original and final orientation is recorded, and the mean error over the six patterns calculated.

iv. Visual and kinaesthetic velocity discrimination. The scores obtained for these items did not discriminate between the normative and present samples. Thus the results of this task were not included in the analysis.

f. Balance:

i. Heel to toe and one-legged stands are performed with and without visual input. In each of the eight positions the child is required to stand for 10 s. Error is calculated by subtracting the total score from 80.

2. TOMI

This is in wide use, thus it is not necessary to describe it here. The single score, which is derived from summing the objective scores of all test items, indicates the severity of the child's motor impairment.

The total testing time per child for PMAT, TOMI and the video game averaged 1 hour 45 mins. In the first stage (Table 1) neurological examination and the self-concept questionnaire (the latter will be described in another publication) added, approximately, a further hour to the testing time. Children said that they enjoyed the PMAT and video game. Except in one case the entire testing programme could be completed in one session.

3. Training

Training was carried out in the schools over a 2—2$\frac{1}{2}$ week period. The children were seen every day, except when they were absent from school. The mean number of training sessions per child was nine. This mean varied between groups: in Group 1 the mean number of sessions per child was 10.2; in Group 2, 7.7; in Group 3, 9.3; and in Group 4, 8.6. The low average number of sessions in Group 2 was due to the fact that some children completed their kinaesthetic training in 3–4 sessions. The average training time spent in each group was: 3 hr 15 min in Group 1; 1 hr 36 min in Group 2; 2 hr 37 min in Group 3; and 2 hr 12 min in Group 4.

All training tasks were graded in difficulty. At the beginning of training the tasks attempted by the child were made as easy as possible. Gradually the task difficulty was increased. Thus exposure to failure was minimal and during the course of training the child could monitor his progress.

a. Spatial programming:

i. Ball aiming task. A football, a smaller ball and a tennis ball were thrown into three boxes - large, medium and small. First the large box was used with the child standing at 1 m distance from the box. The distance was gradually increased to 3 m. The procedure was repeated with the medium and then the small boxes. Only when the easier task was being performed reliably and confidently was the next level of difficulty introduced.

ii. Pencil-paper aiming task. A set of eight puzzle pictures were produced by an artist. The figures to be found were defined by numbered circles or dots. Grading of task difficulty was achieved by using 3 mm target circles in all eight drawings, then repeating the set with 1 mm target dots. Across the series of drawings variance in line length between targets and the frequency of oblique lines increased gradually. The child was asked to connect the numbered circles or dots with straight lines, while making sure to "hit" each target.

iii. Dressing an 18" Snoopy. Seven complete outfits were provided. Fasteners on the outfits varied from large to small buttons, poppers of decreasing sizes, and hooks and bars.

b. Temporal programming:

i. A toy train, with variable speed controlled engine, was pulling one, two or three open carriages. Children were trained to remove and replace small dolls from the moving carriages. First one doll was manipulated, and the train was going slowly. Gradually the speed was increased to maximum. At slow speed again, a second doll and carriage was introduced, and the speed increased. At the final level of difficulty six dolls were used. In order to decrease the spatial demands children moved the dolls when the train was just in front of them.

ii. Drum beat. The child attempted to keep time with a metronome while beating a toy drum. First the preferred, then the non-preferred hand was used, followed by both hands together and finally alternating the hands. The speed of the metronome beat was gradually increased.

iii. Hang-ball. The ball was placed in a net, which was suspended from a hook in the ceiling. The child hit the ball with a large plastic racket to start the ball swinging, and then tried to hit it every time the ball swung back. The speed of the hang-ball movement depended on the force with which the child hit the ball at each swing. The number of successful hits before a miss were counted.

c. Kinaesthetic training (Laszlo & Bairstow, 1983, 1985a):

i. Kinaesthetic acuity. The runway apparatus and masking box were used in training. In the first session the runways were set at 20° difference from each other, with the masking box covering the runways. The child's hands, holding the two pegs, were guided up and down the runways as many times as was necessary for the child to decide which hand went up higher. Even with this large separation between runways, the dyskinaesthetic child found this task very difficult. Typically, by the end of the 10-minute session, the child could discriminate the 20° difference confidently. On the next day 18° runway separations were given, and when this difference was perceived, angle separation was reduced by 2° steps. Training was terminated when 8° separation was discriminated reliably, i.e. four correct answers out of five.

ii. Kinaesthetic perception and memory. The same apparatus as was used for testing was used in training except for the patterns. The children were trained on four simple patterns, graded in difficulty. In the first session the pattern was a straight line, which was shown to the child, then placed on the turntable under the masking box. The child's hand, holding the stylus, was moved back and forth along the line five times. The orientation of the line was changed, after having removed the child's hand from the pattern, the masking box was removed. The child attempted to reorient the line to its perceived position. The child worked with the straight line until it was repositioned correctly (to within 15° error) four times out of six. This procedure was repeated with the remaining three training patterns.

d. Control group tasks:

i. Paper-pencil tasks. Copying of eight line drawings. Each figure was copied repeatedly, verbal knowledge of results were given. Copying of regular continuous patterns were practised also.

ii. Spatial puzzles. Shape identification and a number of maze puzzles demanded line drawings.

iii. Fine manipulative skills. The "Labyrinth" game and electronic basket-ball game were practised. Both games were scored automatically while in use.

iv. Gross motor skills included walking along an obstacle course with eyes open or blindfolded; imitating postures; acting out simple situations.

4. Retest:

Children were brought to the Wolfson Centre by the parent(s). The PMAT, TOMI and video- game were administered as in the first testing session. In order to minimize possible boredom effect the children were promised a small prize for sustained effort and good performance.

Results

One-factor ANOVA with repeated measures was performed on the subjects' index scores for the first PMAT. The groups did not differ significantly from each other ($\underline{F}(3,27)=0.04$, ns).

The Test-Retest results on the PMAT over the four groups were subjected to a 4 (Groups) x 2 (Test-Retests) x 11 (Tasks) ANOVA, with repeated measures on two factors using Z scores. Table 2a gives the summary of the ANOVA results.

Four individual ANOVAs, one for each group (2 (Test-Retest) x 11 (Tasks)) with repeated measures on both factors were performed. The results of these analyses are in Table 2b.

Figure 1 is the graphical representation of the effects of the training regimes.

The results depicted in Figure 1 are confirmed by the statistical analyses. It was shown that at the beginning of the study the level of perceptuo-motor dysfunction (PMD) was not dissimilar across groups. The group means ranged from 1.43 to 1.63 standard deviations from the normative mean.

The differential effect of training regimes was reflected in the significant Groups x Test-Retest interaction (Table 2a) and by the significant Test-Retest main effects in the individual ANOVAs for Groups 1 and 2, in contrast to the non-significant main effects obtained for Groups 3 and 4 (Table 2b). The significant Tasks x Test-Retest interaction showed that the performance level of test items were affected differentially by the training regimes.

Two Wilcoxon matched-pairs signed-ranks tests were carried out comparing the TOMI scores of Test and Retest. The results of Groups 1 and 2, and 3 and 4 were combined for these analyses. Only for Groups 1 and 2 were a significant improvement in the TOMI scores found (Table 2c).

The relationship between PMAT and TOMI scores was examined by calculating Spearman's Rank Order Correlation Coefficients separately

Table 2

Summary of the Results of the Statistical Analyses

a) PMAT results over all groups: 4 (groups) x 2 (Test-Retest) x 11 (Tasks) ANOVA, repeated measures on last two factors.

FACTOR	df	F	p
Groups	3,36	0.29	NS
Test-Retest	1,36	27.69	<0.01
Tasks	10,360	55.21	<0.01
Groups x Test-Retest	3,36	6.35	<0.01
Groups x Tasks	30,360	1.64	<0.02
Test-Retest x Tasks	10,360	2.93	<0.01
Groups x Test-Retest x Tasks	30,360	1.23	NS

b) PMAT results for individual groups: 2 (Test-Retest) x 11 (Tasks) ANOVA, repeated measures on both factors.

FACTOR		GROUP 1		GROUP 2		GROUP 3		GROUP 4	
	df	F	p	F	p	F	p	F	p
Test-Retest	1,9	31.94	<0.01	21.38	<0.01	0	NS	1.45	NS
Tasks	10.90	16.15	<0.01	39.28	<0.01	2.79	<0.01	20.48	<0.01
Test-Retest x Tasks	10.90	2.45	<0.05	7.52	<0.01	1.56	NS	2.86	<0.01

c) TOMI: Wilcoxon's matched pairs signed-ranks test on Test-Retest for Groups 1 & 2 and Groups 3 & 4.

GROUPS	N	T	p
1 & 2	18	31.5	< 0.01
3 & 4	19	75.5	NS

for the first Test and for Retest. The correlation coefficients were: rho = 0.655, $p < 0.001$, (N=40), for the first Test, and rho = 0.660, $p < 0.001$, (N=40), for the Retest. Thus both tests were shown to define the children's relative placement regarding their performance, in a similar way.

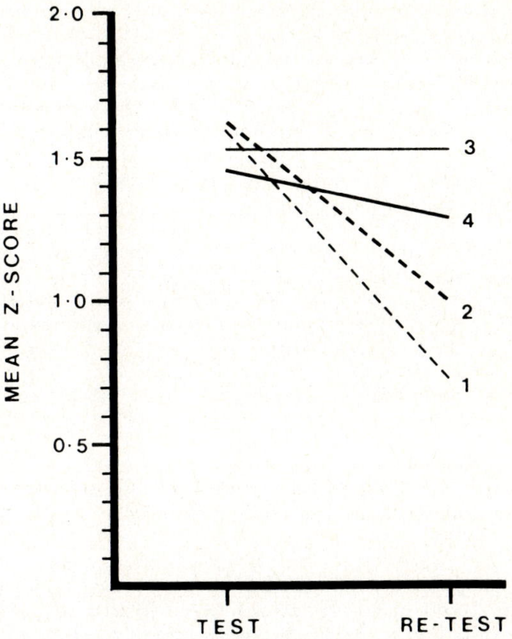

Figure 1. The effects of the training regimes on Groups 1—4.

The teachers' ratings collated from the questionnaires which were given prior to the first testing session showed that all the children referred were judged to perform motor skills below average level. However, the teachers found the five point rating scales difficult to complete. Thus a three-point general improvement scale, representing a summary of the original format, was added to the follow-up questionnaire (see Appendix 1b). Teachers were asked to use ratings of: Improved, No change, or Got worse, for Academic Attainment, Motor Behaviour and Social Behaviour. Only two children were rated "got worse" and both of these ratings were for Social Behaviour. These two ratings were included in the "No change" cell. Three 2 x 2 chi square tests (Improved/No change x Groups 1 and 2/Groups 3 and 4) were performed, one for each questionnaire category. For Motor Behaviour $\chi^2=7.96$, $df=1, p< 0.01$ indicating differential improvement. That is, according to the teachers, children from Groups 1 and 2 improved, while the others did not. On the other hand, neither Academic Attainment nor Social Behaviour yielded significant χ^2s (χ^2 = 0.0001; and 0.139 respectively).

Discussion

The results strongly support the original hypothesis: process-orientated diagnosis and therapy does alleviate PMD.

There was preliminary evidence that deficient kinaesthetic function can be improved quickly and effectively (Laszlo & Bairstow, 1983). Kinaesthetic training was shown to be effective in this study also. Improvement in kinaesthetic sensitivity was not confined to the limbs which were used in training (both arms in kinaesthetic acuity, preferred arm in kinaesthetic perception and memory). The fact that ball catch and posture, whole body tasks, improved in Group 2, ($F(1,9)=9.83, p<0.05$) comparing test-retest, shows that kinaesthetic processing improved generally.

Prior to the present study training in programming had not been attempted. The fact that all six children, from Group 1, who received training in spatial and/or temporal programming only, did improve, indicates the effectiveness of this technique. Although Figure 3 shows a slight advantage for Group 1 over Group 2 on retest, implying that in addition to kinaesthetic training, spatio-temporal training enhances progress, the difference was not significant statistically.

The significant improvement in motor behaviour shown by the teachers' follow-up questionnaire strongly suggests that process-orientated training generalizes to everyday skills which are different from the training tasks.

One is now in a position to compare the process with the task-orientated method, looking at practical considerations. In the former the child is trained over a 2—2½ week period, for a total of 2–3 hours; in the latter, remedial treatment might extend over years. Within a short time the child can observe improvement in his own performance of simple tasks, such as those included in the TOMI. For more complex tasks, e.g. handwriting, skill development depends on practice, in order to learn, from basic elements, the total skill. The process-orientated method cannot provide the child with a blue-print for performance but with the necessary abilities to acquire complex skills; hence the delay in seeking the teachers' opinion on the child's progress in the follow-up questionnaire.

The two diagnostic methods generate different diagnostic labels. Task-orientated tests yield global indices of motor proficiency or motor impairment, i.e. the child is diagnosed as normal or clumsy. Yet to label a child "clumsy" is neither informative nor helpful; it is a superficial, derogatory term which might upset the child emotionally. Parents and teachers often assume that clumsiness is the child's fault - there is nothing wrong with the child but lack of application. The process-orientated diagnosis need not resort to a general label. The diagnosis pin-points the underlying cause of the problem. It is not the child who is clumsy - rather the child suffers from a diagnosable perceptual or motor dysfunction. The term "perceptual-motor dysfunction" has many advantages over "clumsiness": it clarifies the actual cause of the problem, it has no emotional overtones and it implies a clinical cause rather than degrading the child.

The results of this investigation have theoretical implications. The fact that children in Group 2 improved but those in Group 3 did not, shows that kinaesthetic perceptual ability is a necessary prerequisite for acquisition and performance of motor skills.

Neurophysiological evidence (Cole & Abbs, 1986; Georgopoulos et al., 1986; Passingham, 1985; Sittig et al., 1985) has been reported recently which showed that spatial and temporal programming parameters are, to a certain extent, independently controlled. Support for these findings was obtained in the present study. In some of the children only one programming process was found to be deficient, in others the level of dysfunction differed markedly between spatial and temporal programming. Some of our findings were contrary to expectations. When the study was planned, it was predicted that PMD children would exhibit similar PMAT profiles, i.e. PMD presents a predictable combination of dysfunction, varying only in degree. All clumsy children show similar motor patterns (they are all clumsy) but the underlying cause of their difficulties is far from uniform. The most frequently observed dysfunction, that of dyskinaesthesia, affected 73% of the PMD children.

It is often said that left-handers are clumsy. Yet the frequency of left-handedness (10%) was no higher in our sample than in the population. It seems that left-handedness cannot be considered a causative factor of PMD.

We found no evidence supporting the popular notion that clumsiness is related to intelligence. Children in our sample represented the full range of intellectual ability found in mainstream schools. One 11-year-old boy was transferred to a school for children with moderate learning difficulties. From one school the three brightest boys (teachers' opinion) from the top class were referred to us. All three were suffering from PMD. While it is unquestionable that PMD is a hindrance to the bright child, it is especially valuable to offer help to the intellectually less able. Improvement in perceptuo-motor function in these children will broaden their response repertoire and will enable them to gain satisfaction from physical activities.

The training sessions were enjoyed by the children. The training programmes, in which the demands on the children were increased gradually, provided a unique situation for them. They were not exposed to failure, they performed successfully, and were able to monitor their own progress. The task in which sudden improvement was most clearly perceived was kinaesthetic acuity. They expressed their delight by exclamations such as: "I can feel it!" "This is easy." One of the boys, who was unable to perform the task during the first testing session, tried to solve the problem by attempting to peep into the masking box. During his third training session he said with a smile: "I don't have to try cheating any more. I can feel it." The kinaesthetic perception and memory task was acquired more gradually than kinaesthetic acuity, and required longer training time. The Control Group children did enjoy the training, and although they were deprived of observing improvement in their performance, the inclusion of games into the programme helped to keep motivation at a high level.

In a number of cases the change in social and emotional behaviour was quite dramatic. Two examples will be described. One 10-year-old girl who, prior to training, seldom talked, had no friends and refused to participate in games, became a "chatterbox" according to the teacher. She even surprised us by playing some practical jokes.

She found a friend and started playing games. One boy, aged 11 years, was selected into the school football team one month after he completed kinaesthetic acuity training. His success on the football field was not reflected in improved social behaviour. Indeed, he was one of the two children who were rated in the teachers' follow-up questionnaire as "Got worse". Perhaps with improved motor performance and self-confidence, the competence in expressing his aggression became more efficient!

The teacher's role in the management of PMD children cannot be over-emphasised. They proved to be able to recognise children who have motor difficulties reliably (see section on Subjects). Their assessment on children's motor function was not biased by the child's intellectual ability. Parents on the other hand were poor judges of motor competence. Most of the parents interviewed at The Wolfson Centre during the first testing session were surprised at the teacher's assessment. Though many described their child as "messy", "slow" and "uncoordinated" they were certain that this was "normal". It might be argued that parents could cope better with the day-by-day problems of the child suffering from PMD, if they knew that the child has a diagnosed condition, rather than just being careless or lazy. They might feel less irritated, and could provide more support.

The teacher's role in the management of PMD children is not confined to referral for treatment. After training has been completed, praise for even small improvements in complex skills, such as handwriting, is essential. Without support and encouragement from both teachers and parents the child might lose motivation. Unrealistic expectations of an immediate "cure" can also be damaging. This was demonstrated in the case of a 9-year-old boy, who improved markedly on the PMAT and TOMI on retest (this was the only child not referred by his teachers, but by his mother). According to his mother, soon after training, his handwriting became tidy and legible. However, his teacher continued to call him "clumsy" whenever he failed to meet her expectations. The boy became withdrawn and his handwriting deteriorated.

Only with cooperation between therapist, teachers and parents can optimal improvement be achieved. It is the therapist's responsibility to: a) explain to the teachers and parents that the child is suffering from a diagnosable and treatable disorder; and b) that support for the child will be needed in the months following intervention.

Acknowledgements

The research was supported by a grant from the Medical Research Council and a grant from Action Research for the Crippled Child. Our thanks go to the children and staff of Whting Hill, Coppetts Wood, Clitterhouse, Montem, St. Marks, and St. George the Martyr Junior Schools; to Professor K.S. Holt; and to Eric Brown for producing interesting and stimulating drawings used in training.

References

Bairstow, P.J., & Laszlo, J.L. (1978a). Perception of movement patterns. Recognition from visual arrays of distorted patterns. Quarterly Journal of Experimental Psychology, 30, 311-317.

Bairstow, P.J., & Laszlo, J.I. (1978b). Perception of movement patterns. Recall of movement. Perceptual and Motor Skills, 47, 287-305.

Bairstow, P.J., & Laszlo, J.I. (1981). Kinaesthetic sensitivity to passive movements in children and adults, and its relationship to motor development and motor control. Developmental Medicine and Child Neurology, 23, 606-616.

Cole, K.J., & Abbs, J.H. (1986). Coordination of three-joint digit movements for rapid finger-thumb grasp. Journal of Neurophysiology, 55, 1407-1423.

Georgopoulos, A.P., Schwartz, A.B., & Kettner, R.E. (1986). Neuronal population coding of movement direction. Science, 233, 1416-1419.

Gubbay, S.S. (1975). The clumsy child. A study of Developmental Apraxia and Agnostic Ataxia. London: Saunders.

Laszlo, J.I., & Bairstow, P.J. (1980). The measurement of kinaesthetic sensitivity in children and adults. Developmental Medicine and Child Neurology, 22, 454-464.

Laszlo, J.I., & Bairstow, P.J. (1983). Kinaesthesis: Its measurement, training and relationship to motor control. Quarterly Journal of Experimental Psychology, 35, 411-421.

Laszlo, J.I., & Bairstow, P.J. (1985a). Perceptual motor behaviour: Developmental assessment and therapy. London: Holt, Rinehart and Winston.

Laszlo, J.I., & Bairstow, P.J. (1985b). Kinaesthetic Sensitivity Test. Perth, Australia: Senkit Pty Ltd. London: Holt, Rinehart and Winston.

Passingham, R.E. (1985). Premotor cortex: Sensory cues and movement. Behavioural Brain Research, 18, 175-185.

Sittig, A.C., Denier van der Gon, & Gielen, C.C.A.M. (1985). Separate control of arm position and velocity demonstrated by vibration of muscle tendon in man. Experimental Brain Research, 60, 445-453.

Stott, D.H., Moyes, F.A., & Henderson, S.E. (1972). Test of Motor Impairment. Guelph, Ontario: Brook Educational Publishing.

Stott, D.H., Moyes, F.A., & Henderson, S.E. (1984). Test of Motor Impairment. Guelph, Ontario: Brook Educational Publishing.

Appendix 1

Questionnaire

Section A

Name of teacher :

Name of child :

School attainment :

	Very poor 1	2	Average 3	4	Very good 5
Oral expression					
Reading					
Number work					
Reasoning					
Attention span					

Motor behaviour :

Drawing—painting					
Handwriting					
Manual activities					
Dressing					
Ball skills					

Social behaviour :

Friendly, outgoing					
Popular with peers					
Cooperative, helpful					
Active in playground					

Section B

Overall has the child improved over the last 2 months in :

	Improved	No change	Got worse
School attainment			
Motor behaviour			
Social behaviour			

General comments (if any) :

Cognition and Action in Skilled Behaviour
A.M. Colley and J.R. Beech (Editors)

DISCUSSION: IDENTIFYING CRUCIAL ELEMENTS IN SKILLS

Kenneth Flowers
University of Hull

Taken together, these chapters demonstrate the wide range of component processes involved in perceptuo-motor skills, and the wide-spread integrated activity which must take place in performing even seemingly simple controlled actions. Two concern perceptual anticipation and two motor expression, but in all cases the interface between input and output processes is so close that it is difficult to separate them. Both the Whiting, Savelsbergh and Faber, and the Laszlo et al. studies suggest that the development of good levels of skill may depend on some crucial components of perceptual learning, a lack of which may prevent effective motor performance, i.e. that some components may be identified which are crucial for the development of skilled as distinct from unskilled movement. Laszlo et al. suggest the intriguing possibility that such components can be not only identified by appropriate techniques, but treated if deficient.

Whiting et al. in their elegant and meticulous investigation of the visual information required to catch a ball suggest that skilled subjects need an opportunity to calculate the flight of the ball for some minimum period up to 200 ms before contact with the hand. The fact that this period need not involve sight of the ball throughout is instructive; it suggests that subjects need a certain amount of time to extrapolate the flight trajectory, but that it can be done from quite little information. This may be because the flightpath involved in this experiment appears to have been relatively consistent and its extrapolation therefore easily learnt (at least by good catchers); once this is done the trajectory can be anticipated accurately even without further information in real time - provided the ball stays on the calculated path. If so, one might query the rationale of the experiment, in that, if one is dealing with well-practiced subjects and a trajectory that is predictable, it may not matter too much exactly when the information is given, and the whole question of when and where the latest sight of the ball can occur for accurate catching becomes less and less important. As Gregory (1970) has pointed out, the great advantage of switching to a predictive mode of behaviour based on an internal model of external events is that it frees the subject from the constraints of real-time information processing delays and incomplete or interrupted data inputs.

It is also interesting that the Whiting model includes a 200 ms minimum blind period before the point of impact which does not seem to impair catching efficiency - presumably because all the calculations have to be done before then. This replicates Bartlett's "point of no return" in movement, the basic minimum reaction time necessary to initiate or adjust a movement from immediate sensory information. Here, if the trajectory were to change during the last 200 ms the subject would presumably be unable to adjust for it; as Bartlett pointed out, this is the objective of the bowler at cricket or baseball. Such a change would catch the catcher (or batsman) out whichever mode of response (reacting directly to the stimulus in real-time or attempting to anticipate it) the subject adopts.

This raises the intriguing question as to whether the difference between good and poor catchers in the experiment here reflects a difference in the ability to calculate the flight path from the data available, or rather slowness in information processing; that is, do poor catchers need more time to process the data or more information in order to be able to extrapolate the path accurately, or possibly more practice to improve their predictions? If the first, perhaps their minimum reaction time would be more than 200 ms; if the second, perhaps the OP command of the task would need to be longer. If they are simply bad at the calculations, could they improve with appropriate training as Laszlo et al.'s children did?

Laszlo et al., in their important study, show that kinaesthesis may be just as crucial as vision in accurate motor performance. Is there a separate internal model of one's body based on kinaesthetic sensation similar to that for external events, or is it a matter of correlating proprioception to vision so that external events monitored by vision can be accurately mapped on to proprioceptive sensation? And are visual-spatial awareness and body sense separate perceptual domains with regard to action? It would be interesting to know how accurate these impaired children were on tasks of judging spatial relations not involving their own movements. The results here have a bearing on the question of what is learned in developing skill and in what order, and whether there is a hierarchy or simply a set of parallel component processes.

Like Whiting et al., Buekers, Pauwels and Meugens argue that spatial and temporal aspects of anticipation are calculated separately but it is not clear from their data whether there is a priority for the spatial aspect or not. Bairstow (in Part 1 of this book) also claims that subjects calculate spatial position and movement parameters of a moving target separately, and there is some evidence from neurology that different parts of the brain may be involved in the two calculations. Posterior areas of the cortex appear to be involved in spatial awareness while frontal areas subserve the calculation of timing and coincidence of events. Also, Stein (1987) has suggested that the cerebellum may be concerned with generating velocity of movements rather than their spatial position, that is, with a predictive feedforward function. Both Whiting et al.'s results here and Smyth and Marriott's (1982) results imply that spatial and temporal estimation are separate, since a screen which interferes with spatial perception produces, if anything, more spatial than timing errors (rather than both, as would occur if spatial anticipation was a pre-requisite for timing accuracy), but this is not incontrovertible. The data of Buekers et al. does not provide much information on this point, as their temporal task did not test spatial ability very much. It would be interesting to see how subjects perform with a curving or more complicated trajectory where space and time parameters are both more than minimally demanding.

Meulenbroek and Van Galen have produced one result which is potentially very provocative for our ideas of skill, namely that young children seem to begin writing actions in a ballistic mode and then change to a feedback-controlled strategy as their skill develops. If they had shown simply that skill improves as children get older and more practiced, and that this involves switching from a feedback mode to a ballistic one, their results would be of less interest. But the initial ballistic strategy of their youngest children raises some intriguing questions. Normally one assumes that the development of skill involves proceeding from an initial real-time-monitored strategy of performance to a pre-programmed ballistic strategy with practice: thus ballistic movements are built up as the result of learning. But if young children begin with ballistic attempts at the actions required, it suggests that they have some kind of crude inbuilt programs for action which they then refine during learning. Assuming that this result is not, as the authors note, possibly an artefact, it raises the question as to whether skills are "built up" or "refined out" from crude early attempts. Are these young writing movements similar to early walking reflexes which can be observed in young babies and then disappear, to re-emerge as part of an integrated walking pattern later on in development?

Meulenbroek and Van Galen raise the question of whether ballistic and feedback control are separate ways of performing or simply functional modes of operation of the motor system. Neurologically there is quite a lot of evidence now that the nervous system comprises a federation of control mechanisms providing parallel and alternative means of initiating and controlling movements. The pyramidal pathways seem to have evolved "on top of" earlier pathways for the control of limb movements, for example, so that the movements of hand manipulation may be made independently of those of the arm and the trunk, and differently from hand movements made as part of general upper limb action. Similarly, control of breathing during speech and singing appears to be taken over by pyramidal pathways, while breathing at other times is left to more automatic mechanisms subserved by older phylogenetic systems. Could it be, therefore, that different ways of performing movements reflect different underlying subsystems of the nervous system, and that if skill is broken down into components these will be found to correspond to divisions in the brain?

References

Gregory, R.L. (1970). On how little information controls so much behaviour. Ergonomics, 13, 25-35.

Smyth, M.M., & Marriott, A.M. (1982). Vision and proprioception in simple catching. Journal of Motor Behavior, 14, 143-152.

Stein, J. (1987). Paper presented to Fifth Annual Meeting of the Brain Research Association, Edinburgh.

Part IV

COGNITIVE PROCESSES IN SKILLED PERFORMANCE

Cognition and Action in Skilled Behaviour
A.M. Colley and J.R. Beech (Editors)

INTERNAL CONSISTENCY OF THE CONCEPT OF AUTOMATICITY

Jim G. Phillips and Barry G. Hughes
University of Wisconsin

While attention theorists have examined the internal consistency of the concept of automaticity by asking how attentional demands covary with intentional control, the relationship between attention demands and awareness is not clear. The current experiments used the internal consistency of two-process models of attention as a null hypothesis, and considered the functional relationship between controlled and automatic processes. Three experiments manipulated subjects' awareness and knowledge, and related these manipulations to aspects of performance traditionally considered to be controlled or automatic. It was found that variations in awareness and knowledge were not related to processes that have traditionally been considered controlled. Manipulations of subjects' awareness or knowledge consistently affected how they executed their movements, suggesting executive processes such as awareness, are coordinated with automatic processes such as movement execution. It was recommended that theoretical models of automaticity consider how automatic processes are coordinated with controlled processes.

Automaticity is a central concept in explanations of skill acquisition. However, like a number of other constructs in psychology, accounts of automaticity are beset by the problems of explanatory circularity and the lack of internal consistency. Three experiments will be briefly discussed in terms of the internal consistency of the concept of automaticity. These experiments also have some bearing upon the relationship between verbalisable knowledge and performance.

Although the concept of automaticity has been invoked to explain skill, this concept has often been criticised for its circularity (Allport, 1980; Neisser, 1980; Stelmach & Hughes, 1983). This criticism is not unique to theories of skill and automaticity. Whenever cognitive psychologists explain skilled performance in terms of mental operations, there is the possibility that these mental operations are inferred from the very same performance to be explained. For example, an increase in reaction time (RT) may be explained in terms of additional processing operations, but any additional processing operations are inferred from increases in RT; in this case there is no independent definition of processing operations. To circumvent this problem, theorists have examined the internal consistency of their explanations. For example, structural theories of attention have tried to localise processing delays at one particular stage of information processing (Broadbent, 1982), while generalised capacity models of attention have related processing delays to additional phenomena associated with information processing (Posner, 1978), such as intentional control and awareness.

This paper will focus upon the concept of automaticity, as it is invoked to explain the reductions in cognitive effort and conscious involvement with skilled performance. Generalised capacity, or two-process models of attention (Posner & Snyder, 1975; Schneider & Shiffrin, 1977) have accounted for an independence of attention demands from performance in terms of two mutually exclusive modes of information processing; one that is controlled and one that is automatic. Controlled processing is associated with three conjoint properties: high capacity demands, intentional control, and awareness. Automatic processing, on the other hand, is associated with low capacity demands, is obligatory, and does not involve awareness.

Two-process models of attention have been criticised for their deceiving simplicity, as they neatly explain all information processing, and limitations to performance, by way of this simple dichotomy. However, Broadbent (1982), Cheng (1985), Neumann (1984), and Ryan (1983) have all challenged the definitions used by two-process models of attention, arguing that unless these properties consistently distinguish between controlled and automatic processing, any distinction is merely a redescription of the observation that some tasks require more attention than others.

The concept of automaticity has also been empirically shown to lack consistency. For example, experiments examining the relationship between attention demands and intentional control have found that processes that are considered obligatory (i.e. under stimulus control), such as the Stroop effect, can also be influenced selectively by attention (Francolini & Egeth, 1980; Kahneman & Chajczyk, 1983; Lowe & Mitterer, 1982). Obligatory processes have been found to require attention (Paap & Ogden, 1981), and attention demanding processes have been shown to have obligatory properties.

The lack of a consistent relationship between attention demands, awareness, and intentional control also challenges a classical view of consciousness (James, 1890), which assumes (e.g. Dennett, 1978; Lundh, 1979; Posner, 1978) that attention, awareness, and intentional control are synonymous, or assumes less strongly, that these aspects of consciousness covary along a single dimension. Similarly, models of attention involving a central processor assume that attention demands and intentional control are synonymous (c.f. Allport, 1980; Welford, 1980). However, the observed lack of internal consistency suggests that there is a dimension of attentional demands that can be independent of a dimension of intentional control, or awareness. Attention, awareness, and intentional control may reflect independent functions or orthogonal dimensions (Logan, 1985; Mandler, 1975) that may be dissociated (Hilgard, 1977; McLeod, 1977; Wickens, 1980).

A dichotomous classification between controlled and automatic processing is thus not adequate. Faced with this problem, the researcher has two possible choices: either dispense with the notion of automaticity, or to focus more effort on coming to grips with the multidimensional nature of cognitive-motor performance. The mechanisms relating attention, intentional control, and awareness should be examined.

Paradigms considering the relationship between performance and awareness can provide additional methods of operationalising these issues. Information processing approaches have assessed the relationship between verbalisable knowledge and performance (e.g. Annett, 1986; Bransford et al., 1982; Broadbent, FitzGerald, & Broadbent, 1986). One advantage of these methods is that both variables are readily assessed and manipulated. However, although information processing paradigms allow more accurate assessment of factors influencing performance (Smith & Miller, 1978; White, 1980), they rely upon retrospective judgements (Ericsson & Simon, 1980; White, 1982), and so their treatment of awareness is post hoc. The current experiments employed more a priori manipulations of awareness (e.g. Carver & Scheier, 1981; Dixon, 1987), focussing upon awareness of specific task details (Eisler, 1982). Individual differences in awareness were assessed and awareness was experimentally manipulated.

Given that attentional demands, intentional control, and awareness may not be consistently related, three experiments examined processes that have traditionally been considered controlled and automatic on the basis of their attention demands; namely, the preparation and execution of fast movements respectively. For example, Schmidt (1972) suggested the faster the movement, the less likely it is to involve attention for ongoing control. In addition, experimenters have assumed that a two-choice fast aiming movement is programmed in advance (Klapp, 1975; Klapp, Wyatt, & Lingo, 1974), and that the reaction time provides an indication of the amount of processing required to prepare a movement. In other words, in faster movements preparatory processes require capacity, are controlled, and thus should be more affected by manipulations of awareness. This test of the consistency of the relationship between awareness, and controlled and automatic motor processes, would provide converging evidence for other studies examining automaticity in fast movements.

Three experiments considered the consistency with which manipulations of awareness or knowledge affect controlled and automatic processes. An orthogonal model would suggest that manipulations of awareness would not affect controlled processes, because awareness, attention, and intentional control, are independent functions. On the other hand, two-process models of attention suggest that controlled processes should be consistently more susceptible to manipulations of awareness, since awareness, attention, and intentional control, are considered related functions. Thus, for two-process models of attention to be consistent, manipulations of awareness should have greater effects upon processes involving attention or intentional control.

Experiment 1

It has been traditionally assumed that two-choice movement tasks require attention for the preparation of the movement (Klapp et al., 1974), and that faster movements do not involve attention for ongoing control (Schmidt, 1972). Thus, for a fast two-choice movement task, the reaction time (RT) is assumed to reflect controlled processes, and the movement time (MT) is assumed to reflect automatic processes. Since two-process models of attention consider that awareness and attention are related functions, a manipulation of awareness should affect processes involving attention, and therefore a manipulation of awareness should have its strongest effects upon preparatory processes.

In this experiment the effects of manipulations of awareness upon a fast aiming movement were examined. Awareness was manipulated by instructing subjects to monitor either a controlled process (by rating the duration of RT), or an automatic process (by rating duration of MT). This explicit manipulation of awareness was called the direction of set. Individual differences in awareness were also examined by separating subjects into accurate and inaccurate raters of performance. This implicit manipulation of awareness was called the accuracy of set. It was hypothesised that if awareness and attention demands are related, then manipulations of awareness should have a greater effect upon reaction times.

Method

The experiment involved a 2x8 (rating task x practice) design. To manipulate awareness, subjects either rated RT, or rated the duration of a fast movement.

Sixteen students (mean age 21.9) served as subjects. In this auditory two-choice reaction time task, subjects moved a graphics pen horizontally 15cm to the left or right to hit a 2.5cm diameter target situated upon a Tectronix graphics tablet. Subjects started each trial by placing the graphics pen in a start position. After a random delay, a 4800 Hz tone was presented in either ear, signifying the direction to which subjects should move the pen. Subjects were encouraged to hit the targets, and to move faster than 250 ms. After each trial, subjects either rated the duration of their reaction time or the duration of their movement time upon a seven-point scale (1 being very fast, 7 being very slow). Subjects always rated the same aspect of performance within a block of trials. There were two blocks of 26 practice trials, followed by 16 blocks of experimental trials, with the two rating tasks interleaved by block throughout. Stimulus presentation, recording of reaction time, movement time, and positioning accuracy were controlled by a PDP 11/34 computer.

Results and Discussion

The accuracy of set was examined as a between-subjects factor. Subjects' correlations between rated performance and actual performance were averaged and rank-ordered. Subjects were then assigned to groups on the basis of a median split. This produced a 2x8x2 (accuracy of set x practice x direction of set) design.

The effectiveness of subjects selection and of the rating task may be seen in the correlations between reaction time, movement time, and subjects' ratings (of RT or MT). Table 1 shows that accurate raters had higher correlations between RT and ratings of performance, $F(7,7)=13.442$, $p < .05$. Correlations between MT and ratings of performance were higher when subjects were rating movement time, than when they were not rating movement time, $F(1,14)=4.932$, $p<.05$.

Manipulations of awareness did not affect reaction times. Accuracy of set did not affect RT, $F(1,14)=2.345$, $p>.05$. Direction of set did not affect RT either, $F(1,14)<1$. There were no interactions of practice with other factors, showing that practice had independent effects on performance. The direction of set by accuracy of set interaction approached significance, $F(1,14)=3.186$, $p<.10$. Accurate raters tended to be slower when rating their reaction times, while there was little difference for inaccurate raters.

Movement times were more affected by manipulations of awareness. While the effect of accuracy of set was not significant, $F(1,14)=1.613$, $p>.05$, there was a significant effect of direction of set, $F(1,14)=8.336$, $p<.05$. Subjects tended to move faster when rating the duration of their movements (mean = 222.9 ms), than when rating the duration of their reaction times (mean = 235.1 ms).

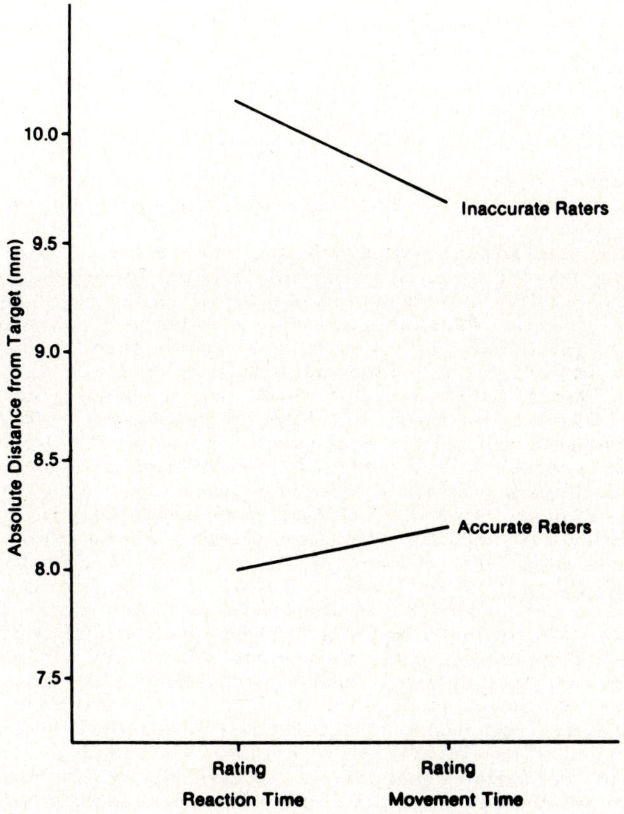

Figure 1. The effects of accuracy of rating, and rating task, upon movement accuracy.

The finding that movements were more affected by manipulations of awareness was supported by analysis of absolute positioning error. There were no effects of accuracy of set, $F(1,14)=1.079$, $p>.05$, or direction of set, $F(1,14)<1$. However, there was an interaction between accuracy of set and direction of set, $F(1,14)=4.869$, $p<.05$. As may be seen in Figure 1, accurate raters had smaller absolute errors when rating reaction times, while inaccurate raters had larger absolute errors when rating reaction times.

Manipulations of awareness had greater effects upon the execution of fast movements, rather than upon preparatory processes. These results are not consistent with two-process models of attention, which suggest that controlled processes should be more likely to be affected by manipulations of awareness.

Table 1

Average correlation between rating and performance.

	ACCURATE RATERS		INACCURATE RATERS	
Rating Task	Rating RT	Rating MT	Rating RT	Rating MT
Performance				
RT	0.455	0.369	0.182	0.200
MT	0.475	0.552	0.379	0.430

Experiment 2

In order to provide converging evidence for Experiment 1, Experiments 2 and 3 manipulated subjects' knowledge of experimental tasks. Two-process models assume that controlled processing is associated with awareness and more detailed knowledge of a task (e.g. frequency judgements, Fisk & Schneider, 1984). If awareness is associated with controlled processing, then an increased awareness of task relevant knowledge will reduce the extent of automatic processing. The more a subject knows about details influencing movement task difficulty, the less automatic that movement should be. To create some task relevant information, the difficulty of a task was varied. The degree of awareness was then examined by varying subjects' knowledge of this task relevant information.

In a precueing task such as that employed by Rosenbaum and Kornblum (1982), the reliability of precues was varied to alter the difficulty of response preparation. Subjects' awareness of the manipulation of precue reliability could then be assessed and manipulated. For two-process models to be consistent, awareness of manipulations of precue reliability should have greater effects upon reaction times.

Method

To manipulate awareness, the procedure consisted of four phases: an initial phase to familiarise subjects with the equipment, a practice phase, experimental phase 1 (during which subjects were not told of the manipulation of precue reliability), and experimental phase 2 (when subjects were told of the manipulation of precue reliability).

Sixteen subjects (mean age 27 years) were presented with 24 trials in a choice reaction task to familiarise themselves with the apparatus. In an auditory two-choice reaction time task, subjects moved a graphics pen forward horizontally from a start button, through 15cm to the left or right, to hit a 2.5cm diameter target situated upon a Tectronix graphics tablet. In each of the practice and experimental phases, subjects performed two blocks of trials of a precue task, in which the same movement was required. Two blocks of 24 practice trials were followed by two blocks of 48 experimental trials. A precue signal (1000 Hz) provided information about the ear to which the imperative signal (2000 Hz) would be presented. The imperative signal occurred 1, 1.5, or 2 seconds after the precue, and signified the target to which subjects moved. In some blocks of trials the precue predicted the imperative accurately 58.3% of trials, while in other blocks of trials the precue was accurate 75% of trials. Subjects were asked to use the precue to prepare their movement, but were warned that the precue was not always correct. Subjects were encouraged to have both fast RT and MT. Stimulus presentation, recording of reaction time, movement time, and positioning accuracy were again controlled by a PDP 11/34 computer.

After two blocks of experimental trials subjects were told of the manipulation of precue reliability, and asked to rate how reliable the precues were in each condition upon an 11-point scale from 0% to 100%. In the second experimental phase, subjects were given two blocks of 48 trials in which they were told whether the precue would be accurate on 58.3% or 75% of trials.

Results and Discussion

To create a between-subjects factor, the rated proportion of precues for the 58.3% condition was subtracted from that of the 75% condition. Subjects were then ranked and split at the median into two groups: those who judged which task had more correct precues (aware), and those who did not (unaware). The design was then a 2x2x2x2 (quality of awareness x direction of awareness x cue reliability x cue validity) with quality of awareness as a between-subjects factor.

The extent of advance preparation may be seen when subjects have to cancel a previously prepared response, and prepare another response. Differences in RT and MT, between correctly precued and incorrectly precued responses, may thus be used as indices of the degree of advance preparation.

The manipulation of task difficulty was successful. Cue reliability and cue validity had significant interactive effects upon reaction time $F(1,14)=8.742$, $p<.02$. There was a change in the degree of preparation only when the precue was reliable. However, there was no effect of quality of awareness, $F(1,14)<1$, and neither was there an effect of direction of awareness, $F(1,14)=3.009$, $p>.05$. An expected interaction between quality of awareness and precue reliability and precue validity only approached significance, $F(1,14)=3.375$, $p<.09$. Subjects who were aware of changes of task difficulty only tended to be influenced by task difficulty.

As expected (Rosenbaum, 1980), varying the difficulty of preparation had no effects per se upon movement times. The effects of precue reliability, $F(1,14)=2.758$, $p>.05$, and precue validity, $F(1,14)=2.441$, $p>.05$, were not significant. However, manipulation of awareness did affect movement times, in conjunction with variations in the difficulty of preparation. As may be seen in Figure 2, subjects who were aware of manipulations of task difficulty were slower when precues were more reliable, $F(1,14)=6.702$, $p<.03$. In addition, there was an interaction between direction of awareness, precue reliability, and precue validity, $F(1,14)=6.431$, $p<.03$. When subjects were aware of variations in task difficulty, incorrect precues slowed movements.

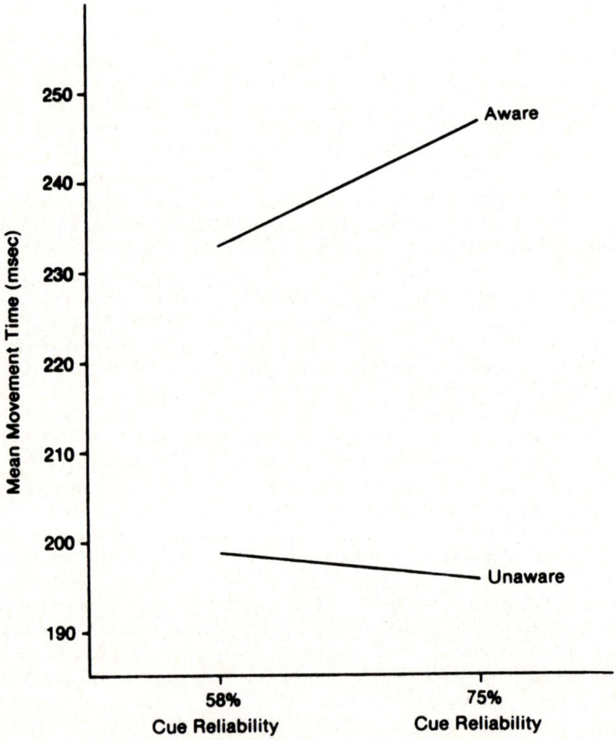

Figure 2. The interactive effect of quality of awareness, and cue reliability, upon movement time.

Again, the results are not consistent with two-process models of attention, since controlled processes were less affected by manipulations of awareness. Variations in difficulty of the precue task affected reaction times; however, knowledge of these variations affected response execution. When subjects knew precues were reliable, subjects responded to an incorrect precue with slower movements.

Experiment 3

Whereas Experiment 2 examined the effects of awareness of difficulty of response preparation, Experiment 3 examined the effects of awareness of difficulty of response execution. The effects of awareness upon the ability to modify an automatic process (that is, the execution of a rapid movement) was examined. A manipulation of task difficulty was required. As fast movements are more readily modified early in their execution (Gottsdanker, 1973; Williams, 1971), this experiment manipulated the proportion of time that an early modification of a movement would be required. If awareness is associated with controlled processing, then awareness of manipulations of the difficulty with which movements could be modified should have greater effects upon reaction times.

Method

As in Experiment 2, there were four phases to the experiment: a baseline phase (used to calculate modification signal position), a practice phase, experimental phase 1 (untold of the manipulation of modification signal positions), and experimental phase 2 (told of the manipulation of modification signal positions). As before, the experiment was controlled by a PDP 11/34 computer.

Sixteen subjects (mean age 19.7 years) shifted a graphics pen from a start button through a set of 9 infra-red photocells spaced at 3cm intervals. On hearing an initiation signal (1000 Hz), subjects moved to one of two 2.5cm diameter targets situated upon a Tectronix graphics tablet, 35.5cm or 47.5cm from the start button. Subjects were given a block of 20 trials to the near target, and a block of 20 trials to the far target. The median RT when subjects moved to the near target was used to calculate the first modification signal position.

There were two blocks of 27 practice trials, followed by two blocks of 54 experimental trials in which subjects were required to move to the near target. On 4/9ths of trials, a modification signal (2000 Hz) would require subjects move to the far target. There were three alternative positions at which a modification signal could occur within a block of trials. The first and last positions were fixed: Position 1 was at an ISI corresponding to half the median RT as derived from the baseline task, position 3 occurred 10 ms after subjects moved through the fourth photocell. Between blocks of trials the difficulty with which a movement could be modified was manipulated, the second modification signal position varied in its proximity to the beginning of the movement: Position 2a occurred 15 ms after subjects released the start button, Position 2b occurred 10 ms after subjects moved through the second photocell.

After the first two blocks of experimental trials, subjects were told of the manipulation of modification signal positions, and asked to rate upon a 12-point scale, for each condition, where during the movement did the modification signals occur; 0 representing the start of the movement, 9 representing the near target, and 11 being the far target. In the second experimental phase, subjects were given two blocks of 54 trials in which they were told where within each block of trials the modification signals could occur.

Results and Discussion

To create a between-subjects factor, the distances on the rating scale between modification signal positions 1, 2 and 3 were calculated for each condition. The eight subjects with the greatest rated changes in the variable modification signal position (in the correct direction) were assigned to the Aware group. The design was then a 2x2x2x2 (quality of awareness x direction of awareness x task difficulty x modification signal position). To simplify analyses, only the fixed modification signals were examined. Reaction time and two measures of intermediate movement time were analysed. The first intermediate movement time (MT1) was measured from the time subjects lifted the graphics pen from the start button, to the time they moved through the third photocell (a distance of 17.5cm). The second intermediate movement time (MT2) was measured from when the graphics pen moved through the ninth photocell to when it hit the near target (a distance of 3cm), or to when it hit the far target (a distance of 15cm).

Reaction time was not affected by task difficulty, $F(1,14) < 1$, but varied with modification signal position, $F(1,14)=9.217$, $p < .01$. Subjects responded faster when the modification was required during the movement latency (mean = 285.5 ms), than during execution (mean = 308.4 ms) suggesting subjects might delay their movement until a modification signal occurred. There was no effect of quality of awareness, $F(1,14) < 1$, or direction of awareness, $F(1,14) < 1$. Knowledge of task difficulty did not influence preparation.

As subjects had to move further when they modified a movement in this task, a successful modification may be seen as a speeding up of movement (Megaw, 1974). The first intermediate movement time varied with modification signal position, $F(1,14)=7.612$, $p < .02$. Subjects modified their movements and moved faster when modifications were required at position 1 (mean = 107.5 ms), than when modifications were required at position 3 (mean = 112.7 ms). There was no effect of task difficulty on MT1, $F(1,14)=1.248$, $p > .05$. Direction of awareness did influence MT1, $F(1,14)=7.696$, $p < .02$. Subjects moved slower when told of task difficulty (mean = 113.5 ms), than when not told (mean = 106.8 ms). Directing awareness towards task difficulty altered the speed of the initial phase of the movement.

The faster the second intermediate movement time, the more successful was the modification of the movement. As predicted, the second intermediate movement time varied with modification signal position, $F(1,14)=650.319$, $p < .01$. Subjects had faster movements when modifications were required at position 1 (mean = 270.3 ms), than at position 3 (mean = 475.5 ms). There was an interaction between task difficulty and modification signal position in their effects on

MT2, $F(1,14)=10.487$, $p<.01$. Subjects moved faster when modifications were required at position 3, if more modifications occurred at the end of the movement. Quality of awareness interacted with task difficulty in their effects on MT2, $F(1,14)=8.64$, $p<.02$. As may be seen in Figure 3, aware subjects were faster towards the end of the movement, when more modifications were required towards the end of the movement. Manipulations of awareness had greater effects upon the execution of movement, rather than upon preparatory processes.

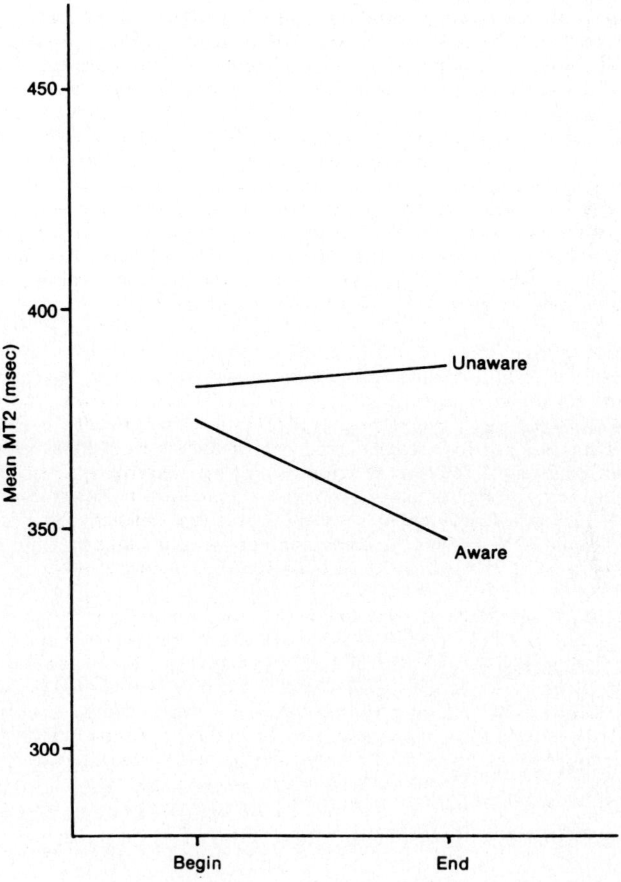

Figure 3. Interactive effects of quality of awareness, and task difficulty, upon MT2.

General Discussion and Conclusions

It was found that variations in awareness and knowledge did not have their strongest effects upon processes that have traditionally been considered to be controlled. This did not support a two-process model, and tends to suggest that attention, intentional control, and awareness, reflect independent orthogonal executive processes (Logan, 1985; Mandler, 1975). However, variations in awareness and knowledge showed some consistent effects on processes traditionally considered to be automatic, and so a strictly orthogonal model was not supported either. Variations in subjects' awareness or knowledge affected the execution of movements. This suggests that executive processes such as awareness are coordinated with automatic processes such as movement execution. These results are also consistent with the view that mental processes are not subject to introspective access, whereas their results are (Miller, 1962).

While these data are not compatible with two-process models of attention, it does not suggest that there is no relationship between these properties. These results have implications for mechanisms explaining the development of automaticity. Theories of automaticity must eventually explain the dissociation between performance and conscious involvement, as well as how behaviours that do not involve awareness, or that are obligatory, are coordinated with conscious behaviours.

There are a number of mechanisms proposed to explain automaticity. Some accounts discuss means of reducing the amount of processing required for a task (e.g. Annett, 1985; Cheng, 1985; Schneider & Shiffrin, 1977), while others view the site of processing as more important (Kahneman & Treisman, 1984; Underwood, 1982). However, these mechanisms all emphasise the role of attention, and assume that explanations of attention will also explain intentional control and awareness. The lack of a strong consistent relationship between attention, intentional control, and awareness, shows this assumption is unwarranted.

It is suggested that characteristics such as attentional demands and awareness do not lie at one end of a single dimension, but that they are linked functionally. Future research in automaticity should consider coordination within goal-directed behaviours (e.g. Marsden, Rothwell, & Day, 1983; Underwood, 1985). The determination of the mechanisms by which automatic behaviours are coordinated with controlled, goal-directed behaviours remains a most outstanding problem in this area.

Acknowledgements

Data was collected by the first author while at the Psychology Department at Flinders University, South Australia. The authors would like to thank Dr. Denis Glencross of the Psychology Department of Flinders University for his comments on a previous draft of this paper.

References

Allport, D.A. (1980). Attention and performance. In G.L. Claxton (Ed.), Cognitive psychology: New directions. London: Routledge.

Annett, J. (1985). Motor learning: A review. In H. Heuer, U. Kleinbeck, & K. -H. Schmidt (Eds.), Motor behavior: Programming, control and acquisition. Berlin: Springer-Verlag.

Annett, J. (1986). On knowing how to do things. In H. Heuer & C. Fromm (Eds.), Experimental Brain Research Series 15. Berlin: Springer-Verlag.

Bransford, J.D., Stein, B.S., Vye, N.J., Franks, J.J., Auble, P.M., Mezynski, K.J., & Perfetto, G.A. (1982). Differences in approaches to learning: An overview. Journal of Experimental Psychology: General, 111, 390-398.

Broadbent, D.E. (1982). Task combination and selective intake of information. Acta Psychologica, 50, 253-390.

Broadbent, D.E., FitzGerald, P., & Broadbent, M.H.P. (1986). Implicit and explicit knowledge in the control of complex systems. British Journal of Psychology, 77, 33-50.

Carver, C.S., & Scheier, M.F. (1981). Attention and self-regulation: A control-theory approach to human behavior. New York: Springer-Verlag.

Cheng, P.W. (1985). Restructuring versus automaticity: Alternative accounts of skill acquisition. Psychological Review, 92, 414-423.

Dennett, D.C. (1978). Toward a cognitive theory of consciousness. Minnesota Studies in the Philosophy of Science, 9, 201-228.

Dixon, P. (1987). The structure of mental plans for following directions. Journal of Experimental Psychology: Learning, Memory, and Cognition, 13, 18-26.

Eisler, H. (1982). On the nature of subjective scales. Scandinavian Journal of Psychology, 23, 161-171.

Ericsson, K.A., & Simon, H.A. (1980). Verbal reports as data. Psychological Review, 87, 215-251.

Fisk, A.D., & Schneider, W. (1984). Memory as a function of attention, level of processing, and automatization. Journal of Experimental Psychology: Learning, Memory, and Cognition, 10, 181-197.

Francolini, C.M., & Egeth, H.A. (1980). On the non-automaticity of "automatic" activation: Evidence of selective seeing. Perception and Psychophysics, 27, 331-342.

Gottsdanker, R. (1973). Psychological refractoriness and the organisation of step-tracking responses. Perception and Psychophysics, 14, 60-70.

Hilgard, E.R. (1977). Divided consciousness: Multiple controls in human thought and action. New York: Wiley.

James, W. (1890). The principles of psychology. London: Macmillan.

Kahneman, D., & Chajczyk, D. (1983). Tests of the automaticity of reading: Dilution of Stroop effects by colour-irrelevant stimuli. Journal of Experimental Psychology: Human Perception and Performance, 9, 497-509.

Kahneman, D., & Treisman, A. (1984). Changing views of attention and automaticity. In R. Parasuraman & D.R. Davies (Eds.), Varieties of attention. Orlando: Academic Press.

Klapp, S.T. (1975). Feedback versus motor programming in the control of aimed movements. Journal of Experimental Psych-

ology: Human Perception and Performance, 104, 147-153.
Klapp, S.T., Wyatt, E.P., & Lingo, W.M. (1974). Response programming in simple and choice reactions. Journal of Motor Behavior, 6, 263-371.
Logan, G.D. (1985). Executive control of thought and action. Acta Psychologica, 60, 193-210.
Lowe, D.G. & Mitterer, J.O. (1982). Selective and divided attention in a Stroop task. Canadian Journal of Psychology, 36, 684-700.
Lundh, L.G. (1979). Introspection, consciousness, and human information processing. Scandinavian Journal of Psychology, 20, 223-238.
Mandler, G. (1975). Consciousness: Respectable, useful, and probably necessary. In R.L. Solso (Ed.), Information processing and cognition: The Loyola symposium. Hillsdale, New Jersey: Erlbaum.
Marsden, C.D., Rothwell, J.C., & Day, B.L. (1983). Long-latency automatic responses to muscle stretch in man: Origin and function. In J.E. Desmedt (Ed.), Motor control mechanisms in health and disease. New York: Raven Press.
McLeod, P. (1977). A dual task response modality effect: Support for multiprocessor models of attention. Quarterly Journal of Experimental Psychology, 29, 651-677.
Megaw, E.D. (1974). Possible modification to a rapid on-going programmed manual response. Brain Research, 71, 425-441.
Miller, G.A. (1962). Psychology: The science of mental life. Harmondsworth: Penguin.
Neisser, U. (1980). The limits of cognition. In P.W. Jusczyk & R.M. Klein (Eds.), The nature of thought: Essays in honor of D.O. Hebb. Hillsdale, New Jersey: Erlbaum.
Neumann, O. (1984). Automatic processing: A review of recent findings and a plea for an old theory. In W. Prinz & A.F. Sanders (Eds.), Cognition and motor processes. Berlin: Springer-Verlag.
Paap, K.R., & Ogden, W.C. (1981). Letter encoding is an obligatory but capacity-demanding operation. Journal of Experimental Psychology: Human Perception and Performance, 7, 518-527.
Posner, M.I. (1978). Chronometric explorations of mind. Hillsdale, New Jersey: Erlbaum.
Posner, M.I. & Snyder, C.R.R. (1975). Attention and cognitive control. In R.L. Solso (Ed.), Information processing and cognition: The Loyola symposium. Hillsdale, New Jersey: Erlbaum.
Rosenbaum, D.A. (1980). Human movement initiation: Specification of arm, direction, and extent. Journal of Experimental Psychology: Human Perception and Performance, 7, 180-195.
Rosenbaum, D.A. & Kornblum, S. (1982). A priming method for investigating the selection of motor responses. Acta Psychologica, 51, 223-243.
Ryan, C. (1983). Reassessing the automaticity-control distinction: Item recognition as a paradigm case. Psychological Review, 90, 171-178.
Schmidt, R.A. (1972). The index of preprogramming (IP): A statistical method for evaluating the role of feedback in simple movements. Psychonomic Science, 27, 83-85.
Schneider, W. & Shiffrin, R.M. (1977). Controlled and automatic human information processing: 1. Detection, search, and

attention. Psychological Review, 84, 1-66.

Smith, E.R., & Miller, F.D. (1978). Limits on perception of cognitive processes: A reply to Nisbett and Wilson. Psychological Review, 85, 355-362.

Stelmach, G.E., & Hughes, B.G. (1983). Does motor skill automation require a theory of attention? In R.A. Magill (Ed.), Memory and control of action. Amsterdam: North-Holland.

Underwood, G. (1982). Attention and awareness in cognitive motor skills. In G. Underwood (Ed.), Aspects of consciousness, Vol.3. London: Academic Press.

Underwood, G. (1985). Eye movements during the comprehension of written language. In A.W. Ellis (Ed.), Progress in the psychology of language, Vol.2. London: Erlbaum.

Welford, A.T. (1980). The single-channel hypothesis. In A.T. Welford (Ed.), Reaction times. London: Academic Press.

White, P. (1980). Limitations of verbal reports of internal events: A refutation of Nisbett and Wilson and of Bem. Psychological Review, 87, 105-112.

White, P. (1982). Beliefs about conscious experience. In G. Underwood (Ed.), Aspects of consciousness, Vol.3. London: Academic Press.

Wickens, C.D. (1980). The structure of attention resources. In R.S. Nickerson (Ed.), Attention and performance VIII. Hillsdale, New Jersey: Erlbaum.

Williams, L.R.T. (1971). Refractoriness of an extended movement to directional change. Journal of Motor Behavior, 3, 289-300.

Cognition and Action in Skilled Behaviour
A.M. Colley and J.R. Beech (Editors)

DEFICIENT PROCESSING IN LEARNING AND PERFORMANCE

Elizabeth Limons and John B. Shea
The Pennsylvania State University

Two experiments investigated the assumption made by Shea and Zimny (1983) in their recently proposed theoretical framework for contextual interference that recognition and recall performance are at least partially separable and can be independently manipulated. In both experiments, recognition training prior to acquisition resulted in fewer tasks being recalled for the recognition training condition than for the non-task recognition and no-recognition training conditions. We offer an explanation in which recognition training enabled subjects to solely use identification processes to keep the tasks in working memory and allow subsequent motor performance. These identification processes, however, did not provide detailed enough knowledge of the tasks to support recall performance (i.e. deficient processing). These findings are interpreted within a parallel-distributed processing view of learning and performance.

Current motor skills research conducted within the action systems approach can be characterized by an emphasis on the learner-environment/task functional relationship. While there are various existing interpretations of direct action, in general this approach has emphasized sophisticated kinematic understanding at the expense of any account based on mental processes. In fact, action system theorists have rejected the notion of mental representation and all other mechanisms that have been traditionally identified with a constructionist approach to cognition. The criticism that psychology is burdened by an ever increasing number of mechanisms is not a new one and previous attempts at limiting these mechanisms have not been especially successful. Certainly, the inability of the action theorist to provide a satisfactory account for learning in the absence of representations (Sheridan, this volume) poses a major obstacle for this approach. In order to offer such an account, the action theorists will eventually be forced to incorporate some form of representation into their thinking. Until this is done, the account for skill learning which offers the greatest explanatory power, is offered through a constructionist interpretation.

Recent constructionist conceptualizations have moved away from traditional conceptions of representation and memory and have emphasized more dynamic accounts. One such alternative is that offered by distributed processing models (Baddeley, 1986; Pew, 1984). Such models may be hierarchical (Rosenbaum, Kenny, & Derr, 1983) and are inherently parallel in nature. These distributed models might provide the common ground for resolution of the motor-action controversy (see Meijer & Roth, 1988). In fact, coordinative structures can be viewed as special instances of this kind of control system (Pew, 1984).

In this paper, we will present two experiments in which the results are interpreted within a parallel-distributed framework. The experiments were designed with the intent that they would provide insight into the mechanisms underlying an effect known as contextual interference (Battig, 1979), in which sequencing of tasks across trials affects subjects' processing capabilities. Shea and Morgan (1979) were the first to report this effect where subjects received either random (high contextual interference) practice during task acquisition or blocked (low contextual interference) practice during acquisition. Random practice, while depressing performance during acquisition, facilitated performance during retention, and blocked practice, while facilitating performance during acquisition, depressed performance during retention. Since then, many researchers (Lee & Magill, 1983; Shea & Zimny, 1983) have replicated the results of this study and proposed differing perspectives concerning the locus of the contextual interference effect.

Two such researchers, Shea and Zimny (1983) have offered an account for contextual interference where blocked subjects perform mostly intraitem processing of a task; in other words, they elaborate only on information within the task itself. Random subjects, however, are not only able to elaborate within the task itself, but can make interitem comparisons between tasks. Elaboration at the interitem level or with existing well-known knowledge from outside the experimental situation (Shea & Zimny, 1987) is thought to aid recall memory by providing multiple routes for retrieval of the task. In this way if one set of connections becomes inaccessible, then others can be used. If specifics of a task are forgotten it might be possible for the learner to reconstruct them from the knowledge that is still available (Reder, Charney, & Morgan, 1986). Moreover, this process of reconstruction can lead to the establishment of new retrieval routes which can improve later retention.

A common finding in contextual interference experiments is that both blocked and random acquisition groups perform well on recognition tests but only the random group performs well on recall tests of retention (Shea & Zimny, 1983). Shea and Zimny postulated that recognition is primarily dependent upon intraitem elaborative types of processing, while recall performance necessitates inter- as well as intraitem elaborative types of processing. If this is true, then the processing required for tests of recall and recognition can to some extent be independently manipulated.

Although the experiments presented in this paper were designed with the intent of validating the differential processing hypothesis proposed by Shea and Zimny through the manipulation of recognition training during acquisition, we will focus our discussion on the somewhat unexpected findings of these experiments which we interpret in terms of deficient processing.

Experiment 1

Methods

Subjects

Seventy-two right-handed students at the Pennsylvania State University, University Park participated in the experiment.

Apparatus

Subjects were tested on an apparatus similar to that described by Shea and Morgan (1979). Briefly, it consisted of a plywood platform with six freely movable plywood barriers attached to the top surface. A button switch was located on the midline and front of the apparatus. Directly behind the start button were two holes and a rubber tennis ball rested in the first hole. A red warning light and three clear stimulus lights were mounted at the rear of the apparatus. Directly behind the lights an upright plywood barrier was constructed to shield the subject's view of the experimenter's activity. Diagrams of the task(s) to be performed were displayed on this barrier.

Tasks

Subjects performed three tasks. These tasks were performed with the right hand, and consisted of releasing the start button in response to the onset of a stimulus light and picking-up the tennis ball. While holding the ball, the subject then knocked down four barriers in one of the following orders, as shown in Figure 1: (a) left middle, right rear, left bottom, and right middle (Task 1); (b) left middle, right bottom, left rear, and right rear (Task 2); (c) right middle, left rear, right bottom, and right rear (Task 3). After knocking down the barriers the subject placed the ball in the second hole in the top surface of the apparatus. Each of the tasks was paired with a different stimulus light.

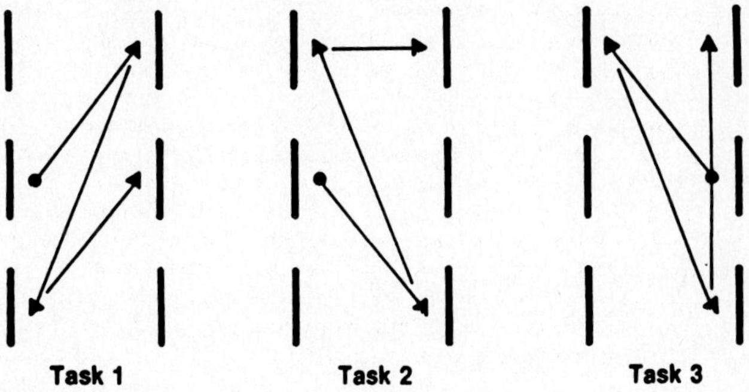

Figure 1. Tasks performed by subjects on the apparatus.

Design and Procedures

Figure 2 outlines the experimental protocol used for Experiment 1. Two levels of contextual interference (low contextual interference, or blocked versus high contextual interference, or random) were crossed with three levels of recognition training (no recognition training, NT: recognition training with patterns depicting the tasks performed in acquisition, T: and recognition training with patterns depicting tasks not performed during acquisition, TNT). This design resulted in six independent groups which were the blocked-NT, blocked-T, blocked-TNT, random-NT, random-T, and random-TNT groups. Subjects were randomly assigned to these groups.

<table>
<tr><th>Group</th><th>Pre-Training</th><th>Acquisition</th><th></th><th>Retention Tests</th></tr>
<tr><td>Blocked/
No Recognition Training
(B-NT)</td><td>None</td><td>54 trials blocked practice</td><td rowspan="6">TEN MINUTE FILLED INTERVAL</td><td>Cued Recall
Uncued Recall
Performance
Recognition</td></tr>
<tr><td>Random/
No Recognition Training
(R-NT)</td><td>None</td><td>54 trials random practice</td><td>Cued Recall
Uncued Recall
Performance
Recognition</td></tr>
<tr><td>Blocked/
Recognition Training with Task Patterns
(B-T)</td><td>Task patterns to 100% recognition</td><td>54 trials blocked practice
Recognition test following trials 18 & 36</td><td>Cued Recall
Uncued Recall
Performance
Recognition</td></tr>
<tr><td>Random/
Recognition Training with Task Patterns
(R-T)</td><td>Task patterns to 100% recognition</td><td>54 trials random practice
Recognition test following trials 18 & 36</td><td>Cued Recall
Uncued Recall
Performance
Recognition</td></tr>
<tr><td>Blocked/
Recognition Training with Non-task Patterns
(B-TNT)</td><td>Non-task patterns to 100% recognition</td><td>54 trials blocked practice
Recognition test following trials 18 & 36</td><td>Cued Recall
Uncued Recall
Performance
Recognition</td></tr>
<tr><td>Random/
Recognition Training with Non-task Patterns
(R-TNT)</td><td>Non-task patterns to 100% recognition</td><td>54 trials random practice
Recognition test following trials 18 & 36</td><td>Cued Recall
Uncued Recall
Performance
Recognition</td></tr>
</table>

Figure 2. Experimental Protocol for Experiment 1.

All groups received a total of 54 acquisition trials on the three tasks in three sets (acquisition phases) of 18 trials. Subjects in the blocked condition (blocked-NT, blocked-T, and blocked-TNT groups) always completed 18 trials on one task before another task was first introduced. The order in which the tasks were presented was counterbalanced across subjects. Subjects in the random condition (random-NT, random-T, and random-TNT groups) were given acquisition trials in an unsystematic sequence such that six trials on each of the three tasks were included in each phase of 18 trials. The sequencing of trials for each task within each phase of acquisition provided that no more than two trials on the same task would occur consecutively.

Subjects in the T condition (blocked- and random-T groups) were given recognition training before acquisition practice trials in which they were required to study three diagrams depicting the tasks they would practice for 5 s each. They were then given a recognition test in which they were asked to identify the three diagrams they had just studied from among six other nonstudied task diagrams. Subjects in the TNT condition (blocked- and random-TNT groups) were given recognition training in the same way as the T condition, with the exception that the three studied diagrams depicted tasks different from those practiced during acquisition. In addition, recognition tests for the task diagrams studied before acquisition practice were given between each phase of acquisition practice. Subjects were not allowed to study the task patterns before these tests, however. Subjects in the NT condition were not given recognition training or recognition tests between acquisition practice phases.

All subjects received identical tests for retention following a 10 min filled retention interval. Subjects were first given a cued recall test in which they performed one trial for each task in response to the stimulus light with which the task was paired during acquisition. The diagrams of the tasks were not present, and task presentation order was counterbalanced across subjects in each group for this test. Subjects were then given an uncued recall test in which they were given 10 s to perform each of the acquisition tasks in any order they chose. As in the cued recall test, the diagrams of the task were not present during this test. However, subjects were not required to pair the task with an appropriate stimulus light for this test. In this respect performance of this test required less knowledge specification of the tasks than the cued recall test. Following the uncued recall test, subjects were given a performance test which was identical to that of acquisition practice. Subjects performed the tasks in response to appropriate stimulus lights with the task diagrams present. Six trials (2 per task) were presented in a blocked sequence and six trials (2 per task) were presented in a random sequence for this test. In addition, the order of task presentation and the presentation order of the blocked-random test sequences were counterbalanced across subjects in each group. Finally, subjects were given a recognition test. This test consisted of identifying the three task diagrams practiced during acquisition from among six other distractor task diagrams.

Results

The total time (TT) in seconds between the onset of the stimulus light and the completion of the subject's response by placing the ball in the second hold of the apparatus was used as the measure of skill for acquisition trials and the retention performance test. In addition, the number of trials on which errors were made was recorded for each subject.

The TT scores for the 18 trials of each task were averaged into 6 blocks of 3 trials for analysis. In addition, the 12 TT scores for each task in the blocked and random testing sequences for the retention performance test were averaged for analysis. The number of errors made during acquisition and retention performance were also analysed. The percentage of correctly recalled/recognized tasks was analysed for the cued, uncued, and recognition tests. In all analysis the rejection region was $p < .05$.

Figure 3 shows mean TT measures for the contextual interference-recognition training groups computed in 3 trial blocks for each acquisition phase. The analysis conducted on TT measures showed that TT was significantly less for the blocked (M=1.80s) than for the random (M=2.73s) contextual interference condition. As can be seen in Figure 3, TT for the random condition decreased at a faster rate across trial blocks in each acquisition phase than it did for the blocked condition. TT decreased markedly for all groups over trial blocks for the first phase of acquisition, but decreased little over trial blocks for the second and third phases of acquisition. In addition, TT was significantly slower for the T (M=5.60s) than for the NT (M=2.28s) and TNT (M=2.87s) recognition training conditions on Trial Block 1 only for Phase 1. The differences between the NT and TNT conditions were not significant across trial blocks. For Phase 2, TT was significantly slower for the T (M=2.78s) and TNT conditions (M=2.87s) than for the NT (M=2.23s) condition on Trial Block 7 only. The differences between the T and TNT conditions on Trial Blocks 7-12 were not significant. In Phase 3 there were no significant differences in TT among the recognition training conditions on Trial Blocks 13-18.

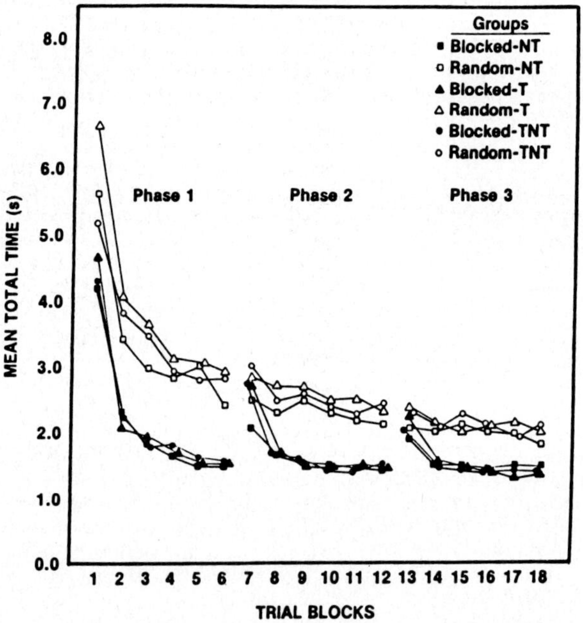

Figure 3. Acquisition mean total time measures for the six blocks of three trials for each acquisition phase in Experiment 1.

The analysis of mean percentage correct measures for the cued recall retention test showed significant main effects of contextual interference where the random condition correctly recalled more tasks (M=44%) than the blocked condition (M=21%). The main effect of recognition training was significant. Figure 4 shows the mean percentage correct measures for recognition training conditions for the cued and uncued recall retention tests collapsed over contextual interference. Both the NT (M=37%) and TNT (M=40%) groups correctly recalled more tasks than the T groups (M=20%), although the NT and TNT groups did not differ significantly from each other.

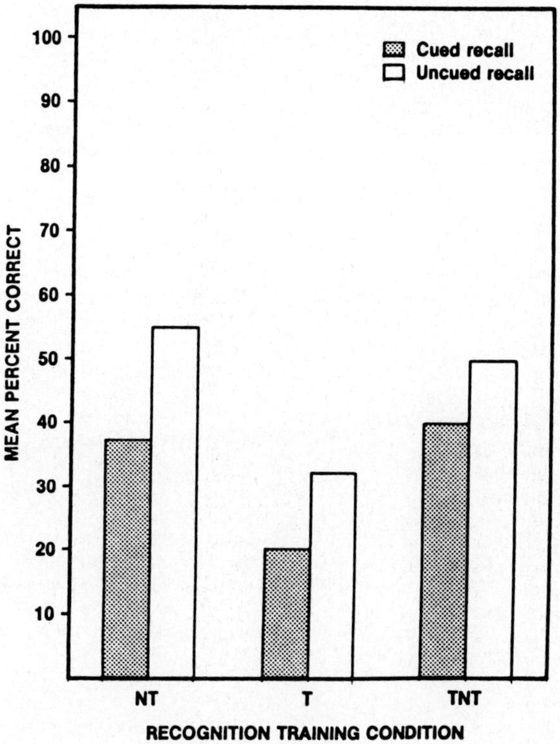

Figure 4. Mean percentage correct for recognition training conditions for cued and uncued recall tests in Experiment 1.

The analysis of mean percentage correct measures for the uncued recall retention test showed that the main effect of contextual interference was significant. Subjects in the random condition recalled more correct tasks (M=58%) than those in the blocked condition (M=34%). The effects of recognition training were also significant. Figure 4 shows that in both the NT (M=54%) and TNT (M=50%) conditions more tasks were correctly recalled than in the T condition

(M=34%). The NT and TNT conditions did not significantly differ from each other, however.

The analysis of TT measures for the performance retention test showed that subjects in the random acquisition condition (M=2.07s) performed significantly faster than those in the blocked acquisition condition (M=2.51s). In addition, subjects in the T condition (M=2.39s) performed more slowly than those in either the TNT (M=2.31s) and NT (M=2.16s) conditions. In contrast to the cued and uncued recall retention test findings, however, the effect of recognition training was not significant. In addition, the analysis of mean number of errors made for the performance retention test showed a main effect of contextual interference, where subjects in the random condition (M=.08) committed fewer errors than those in the blocked condition (M=.38).

Finally, all groups (M=97%) obtained close to 100% correct on the recognition retention test. This accounted for all comparisons in the analysis of these measures being nonsignificant.

Discussion

Findings from this experiment provide support for the separability of recognition and recall test performance through the use of recognition training procedures. Recognition performance was established at 100% prior to the acquisition trials for the T and TNT conditions and remained at this level throughout acquisition and at the final recognition retention test. This training did not alter the usual contextual interference finding of better recall for the random than for the blocked condition, however. Of notable importance was the finding that subjects in the T recognition training condition performed significantly worse on cued and uncued recall tests of retention than subjects in the NT and TNT conditions, whose performance was similar. These findings were consistent across both the random and blocked contextual interference conditions. In addition, analysis of acquisition TT data showed that subjects in the T condition performed more slowly than subjects in the NT and TNT conditions during the first three trials of each acquisition phase. Subjects in the NT and TNT conditions performed similarly on these trials.

These findings can be interpreted within Shea and Zimny's (1983) model of elaborative/distinctive processing, focussing on processing at the intra- and interitem level. Analysis of retention data in this study showed that for tests of uncued and cued recall, subjects in the T recognition condition demonstrated less knowledge concerning the three test patterns than did subjects in the NT and TNT conditions. However, since both random and blocked contextual interference conditions were affected consistently by recognition training, it would appear that some processing employed by both groups was affected by such training. In terms of intra- and inter-item processing, only intraitem comparisons are said to be utilized by both contextual interference conditions. That is, the blocked condition primarily uses intraitem processing, and the random condition utilizes both intra- and interitem processing. Thus, it is reasonable to assume that recognition training with the same test patterns practiced during acquisition has a detrimental affect on subjects' capacity to perform intraitem processing. Further support for this hypothesis comes from results of acquisition data analysis, which showed that during Acquisition Phase 1, the T recognition condition performed the first trial block (first three trials) more slowly than the NT and TNT conditions. It would seem then that during these three trials, intraitem processing for the T condition somehow differed from this processing in the NT and TNT conditions. Since just prior to the first three trials of Acquisition Phase 1, subjects received recognition training, it can be argued that this training required subjects to engage in deficient processing (Dellarosa & Bourne, 1985). In other words, these subjects did not reap as full benefits from intraitem comparisons as those subjects who either received no, or different, recognition training. Viewing patterns just prior to acquisition performance enabled subjects to mostly use identification operations in order to keep the task in working memory and allow subsequent motor performance. It was this initial perceptual matching process (Anderson, 1983), following recognition training on the same patterns that were performed during acquisition, that accounted for slower performance times on the first three trials of Acquisition Phases 1 and 2. Furthermore, even though these identification processes were not sufficient to produce the full intraitem processing functions which aided in retention performance, they were sufficient to allow performance of the tasks when diagrams were present, as well as superior recognition performance. For random contextual interference conditions, these identification processes did allow for subsequent interitem comparisons between tasks which produced the contextual interference effects found in this and previous experimental investigations. This interitem processing, however, was not as detailed when more knowledge of the tasks was available, as it was when no recognition training was provided.

It has recently been proposed that the more similar the processes used during acquisition are to those required in a later test, the more performance in this later test will be facilitated (Lee, 1987; Morris, Bransford, & Franks, 1977). This interpretation would suggest that cued and uncued recall for the TNT condition should have been similar to that for the T condition, because the TNT subjects received recognition training, albeit with tasks dissimilar from those practiced in acquisition. This training might have been predicted to lead subjects in the TNT condition to perform processing sufficient for recognition but not sufficient for cued and uncued recall performance. This was clearly not the case, since cued and uncued recall performance for this condition was similar to that of the NT condition. It therefore appears that it was not just recognition training <u>per se</u> that caused poor retention performance, but it was how the subject utilized the recognition training information. Most likely, subjects in the TNT condition did not engage in deficient processing as did subjects in the T condition, because the former could not perform perceptual matching during acquisition trials. Thus subjects in the TNT condition performed processing similar or identical to the subjects in the TNT condition, and remained unaffected by recognition training.

Experiment 2

We explained the effects of recognition training on retention in Experiment 1, by stating that the processing performed by the T condition across the 54 acquisition trials was insufficient for the full intra- and interitem processing necessary for recall purposes. In addition, we stated that the longer performance times for the T and TNT conditions than for the NT condition on the first block of acquisition trials, was due to a vertification process by which subjects determined whether or not the acquisition tasks were the same as those for which they had received recognition training. The outcome of this verification process determined the quantification of processing performed across the remainder of the acquisition trials. According to this explanation, recall for the groups in Experiment 1 was more dependent on the amount of processing performed throughout acquisition than on the verification process per se. It is possible, however, that the verification process might have been solely responsible for the obtained recall differences among conditions. That is, the verification process might have distracted subjects from performing the appropriate amounts of intra- and interitem processing necessary for recall purposes. The finding that performance was slower for the T than for the TNT and NT conditions for the first block of acquisition trials, in combination with the finding that the T condition recalled fewer tasks than the TNT and NT conditions, lends credence to this speculation.

Experiment 2 was conducted to determine if the processes responsible for the recall findings in Experiment 1 were present throughout the acquisition trials, or were localised in the first block of acquisition trials. It was reasoned that informing subjects just prior to the acquisition trials that they would be performing tasks which were the same as those for which they had just received recognition training, would eliminate the need for a verification process on the part of T condition subjects. The effectiveness of this instruction in eliminating the verification process would be evidenced by a reduced performance time on the first acquisition trial block. If recall performance was dependent on processing performed across all acquisition trials, the number of correctly recalled tasks would not differ between T condition subjects who received instructions concerning the identity of the acquisition and recognition tasks (TI condition), and subjects who did not receive these instructions (the T condition). If recall performance was solely dependent on processing performed on the first block of acquisition trials, then it would be expected that the number of correctly recalled tasks for the TI condition would approximate that for the NT condition and exceed that for the T condition.

Methods

The subjects (N=18,n=6) for this experiment were right-handed students at the Pennsylvania State University, University Park. The tasks and apparatus for this experiment were the same as those used in Experiment 1. The design and procedure were similar to those used in Experiment 1. However, only a random sequencing of tasks over trials was used for acquisition. Since the Contextual Interference x Recognition Training interaction was not significant in Experiment 1, the use of both random and blocked acquisition conditions was considered unnecessary for the purposes of this experiment. A new group (TI) was added who received the same recognition training as the T group, but was instructed just prior to acquisition practice that the tasks they would be performing were the same as those on which they had received recognition training. In addition, no TNT group was used in this experiment because it was thought that the effect of the verification process on performance time and recall could be investigated adequately through the use of T and TI groups only. Furthermore, only three trials per task were given during acquisition. This was because the primary focus of this experiment was on the effect elimination of the verification process would have on recall performance. Finally, only a random sequencing of tasks was used for the retention performance test.

In summary, this experiment consisted of three groups (T, TI, and NT) receiving three acquisition trials on each of the three tasks used in Experiment 1 in a random sequence. Following a 10 min filled retention interval subjects were given cued, uncued, recognition, and performance retention tests. In all other respects the design and procedure for this experiment was identical to Experiment 1.

Results and Discussion

The same dependent measures were analysed for this experiment as for Experiment 1. Mean performance times were computed for individual trials and were collapsed across tasks for the acquisition analysis. In all other respects, the analysis of data was the same as for Experiment 1.

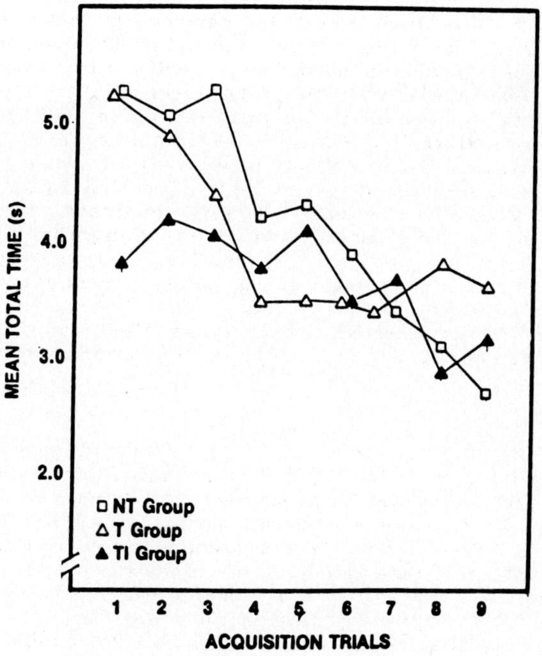

Figure 5. Group mean total time measures for acquisition trials in Experiment 2.

Figure 5 shows acquisition trial mean TT measures collapsed across tasks for the T, TI and NT groups. This analysis showed that instructing subjects that the tasks they would perform during acquisition were the same as those for which they received recognition training (TI group), substantially reduced the TT time on the first trial of practice below that of subjects who did not receive these instructions (T group) or subjects who were not given recognition training (NT group). It should be noted, however, that the results of Experiment 1 were not replicated concerning the faster performance of the T than the NT group on Trial 1. We feel that these findings did not occur due to a lack of statistical power. In Experiment 1, the reliability of TT means was increased by averaging trials into blocks of three. Also, the effect of the recognition test given before each practice phase elevated the TT of the T groups for the first trial of each practice phase. TT for the NT groups continued to get faster over practice phases and this accentuated these differences.

Table 1 shows the group mean percentage of correct recall measures for the cued and uncued recall tests. The analysis conducted on these measures showed no significant group differences for cued recall. However, the TI group recalled significantly fewer tasks than the T and NT groups for the uncued recall test. Additionally, the T group recalled significantly fewer tasks than the NT group for this test. The discrepancy in findings between the cued (no group difference) and uncued (differences among all groups) can be attributed to the cued test being more difficult than the uncued test, and the small number of acquisition trials given. Evidently, none of the groups had developed a detailed enough memory representation to support cued recall performance.

Table 1

Recognition Training group cued and uncued percentage correct recall means, $\underline{F}$, and $\underline{MS}_e$ error terms in Experiment 2

TEST	GROUP MEANS (% recall)			GROUP	
	NT	T	TI	F	MS_e
Cued	11%	11%	22%	.83	.07
Uncued	38%	22%	5%	4.50*	.50

*$\underline{p}$<.05

The analysis of retention performance measures showed that TT for the NT group ($\underline{M}$=2.97s) was faster than for the TI ($\underline{M}$=3.20s) and T ($\underline{M}$=3.10s), but that these differences were not significant. It is notable that these findings paralleled those for uncued recall with the NT group recalling a greater number of tasks and performing faster than the T and TI groups.

The findings for this experiment were consistent with the proposed model in Experiment 1 whereby verification process was performed by recognition training subjects on the first acquisition trial to determine if the acquisition tasks were the same as those for which they had received recognition training. The finding that the TI group performed faster on the first acquisition trial than either the T or NT groups demonstrates that the provision of instructions regarding the identity of the recognition and acquisition tasks eliminated the need for subjects to perform verification processing. The finding that the TI group recalled fewer tasks than either the T or NT groups provides convincing evidence that the verification process was not responsible for the T group recalling fewer tasks than either the TNT or NT conditions in Experiment 1. Notably, the finding that the TI group recalled fewer tasks than even the T group suggests that verification processing can contribute to improved rather than poorer recall performance. It must be concluded that recall performance is dependent on the type and amount of processing performed by subjects across all acquisition trials.

General Discussion

We wish to highlight three important points from the experiments we have presented which have implications for current approaches to motor skills research. First, these experiments provided evidence in support of Shea and Zimny's (1983) assumption concerning the separability of recognition and recall test performance. This was accomplished in Experiment 1 by demonstrating that recognition could be established at 100 per cent correct prior to and during acquisition but not change the usual pattern of blocked—random recall findings. We view this interpretation as differing from current theories which view recognition and recall as separate memory systems (Adams, 1971; Schmidt, 1975). Rather, recognition and recall are seen as tests which index different types (as well as amounts) of knowledge present in the memorial representation of the task. Recognition is more dependent on matching processes upon the presentation of a task/non-task at test, while recall can be characterized as being more controlled and dependent upon the use of retrieval structures.

Second, the finding that recognition training with the same tasks practiced during acquisition (T condition) resulted in depressed recall in comparison to recognition training with tasks different from those practiced during acquisition (TNT condition), or no recognition training (NT condition), provides support for the hypothesis that matching processes are important for learning (Neves & Anderson, 1981). The match obtained by the comparison of the acquisition tasks with those currently active in working memory from recognition training allowed T condition subjects to use identification processes during acquisition task performance. While this operation was sufficient to support performance during acquisition and retention, as well as recognition, it was deficient in terms of providing the retrieval routes necessary for recall purposes. The mismatch obtained by the TNT condition, however, when the recognition training tasks present in working memory were compared to acquisition tasks, caused these subjects to engage in a more analytical type of processing (Brooks, 1978; Elio & Anderson, 1984) that was sufficient for recall, in addition to performance during acquisition and retention, as well as recognition. The analytical processing described above was more consistent with that performed under the nonrecognition training conditions.

Our interpretation of the deficient processing phenomenon in terms of matching processes has important implications for a comprehensive understanding of other research areas in learning and performance. The cross trial use of matching processes in terms of available feedback from prior performance, including knowledge of results, determines the type as well as the amount of processing undertaken by the learner. From this perspective, motor learning is an error-correction based process (McClelland & Rumelhart, 1985), where the modification of memory representations is dependent upon error detection and subsequent correction of past performances.

Finally, the total pattern of recognition training findings from these experiments can best be viewed in terms of parallel-distributed models that emphasize learning and performance through the interplay of multiple sources of knowledge. The processing performed across acquisition trials lead to differential retention test performance among the recognition training groups that, importantly, did not interact with contextual interference. Thus, at one level, we have performance which is affected by blocked/random practice schedules during acquisition, which facilitates qualitative types of processing and which leads to superior recall performance for the random subject who has formed distinctions between tasks. However, we see at another level, differential quantitative processing by subjects as a result of recognition training, which leads to, for subjects with same-task pattern training, a deficiency in their ability to both elaborate and distinguish among tasks, thus causing a deficit in recall performance across both levels of contextual interference. Interestingly, knowledge was sufficient to maintain performance of tasks with patterns present during both acquisition and retention. Thus, it is this concurrent presence of both qualitative and quantitative processing during acquisition leading to differential recognition, recall, and performance retention findings which provides support for a parallel-distributed view of learning and performance.

References

Adams, J.A. (1971). A closed-loop theory of motor learning. Journal of Motor Behavior, 3, 111-149.

Anderson, J.R. (1983). The architecture of cognition. Cambridge, M.A.: Harvard University Press.

Baddeley, A. (1986). Editorial: Modularity, mass-action and memory. The Quarterly Journal of Experimental Psychology, 38A, 527-533.

Battig, W.P. (1979). The flexibility of human memory. In C.S. Cermak and F.I.M. Craik (Eds.), Levels of processing in human memory. Hillsdale, N.J.: Erlbaum.

Brooks, L. (1978). Nonanalytic concept formation and memory for instances. In E. Rosch and B.B. Lloyd (Eds.), Cognition and categorization. Hillsdale, N.J.: Erlbaum.

Dellarosa, D. & Bourne, L.E.Jr. (1985). Surface form and the spacing effect. Memory and Cognition, 13, 529-537.

Elio, R. & Anderson, J.R. (1984). The effects of information order and learning mode on schema abstraction. Memory and Cognition, 12, 20-30.

Lee, T.D. (1987). Testing for motor learning: A focus on transfer-appropriate practice. In O.G. Meijer and K. Roth (Eds.), Movement behavior: The motor-action controversy. Amsterdam: North-Holland, in press.

Lee, T.D. & Magill, R.A. (1983). The locus of contextual interference in motor skill acquisition. Journal of Experimental Psychology : Learning Memory and Cognition, 9, 730-746.

McClelland, J.L. & Rumelhart, D.E. (1985). Distributed memory and the representation of general and specific information. Journal of Experimental Psychology: General, 114, 159-188.

Meijer, O.G. & Roth, K. (Eds.) (1988). Movement behavior: The motor-action controversy. Amsterdam: North-Holland.

Morris, C.D., Bransford, J.D., & Franks, J.J. (1977). Levels of processing versus transfer appropriate processing. Journal of Verbal Learning and Verbal Behavior, 16, 519-533.

Neves, D.M. & Anderson, J.R. (1981). Knowledge compilation: Mechanisms for the automatization of cognitive skills. In J.R. Anderson (Ed.), Cognitive skills and their acquisition. Hillsdale, N.J.: Erlbaum.

Pew, R.W. (1984). A distributed processing view of human motor control. In W. Prinz and A.F. Sanders (Eds.) Cognition and motor processes. Berlin: Springer-Verlag.

Reder, L.M., Charney, D.H., & Morgan, K.I. (1986). The role of elaboration in learning a skill from an instructional text. Memory and Cognition, 14, 64-78.

Rosenbaum, D.A., Kenney, S.B., & Derr, M.A. (1983). Hierarchical control of rapid movement sequences. Journal of Experimental Psychology: Human Perception and Performance, 9, 86-102.

Schmidt, R.A. (1975). A schema theory of discrete motor skill learning. Psychological Review, 82, 225-260.

Shea, J.B. & Morgan, R.L. (1979). Contextual interference effects on the acquisition, retention, and transfer of a motor skill. Journal of Experimental Psychology: Human Learning and Memory, 5 (2), 179-187.

Shea, J.B. & Zimny, S.T. (1983). Context effects in memory and learning movement information. In R.A. Magill (Eds.), Memory and control of action. Amsterdam: North-Holland.

Shea, J.B. & Zimny, S.T. (1987). Knowledge incorporation in motor representation. In O.G. Meijer and K. Roth (Eds.) Movement Behavior: The motor-action controversy. Amsterdam: North-Holland.

Cognition and Action in Skilled Behaviour
A.M. Colley and J.R. Beech (Editors)

LEVELS OF INTERFERENCE BY IRRELEVANT SPEECH: ONE, SOME OR MANY?

Christopher Miles, Clare Madden and Dylan M. Jones
University of Wales Institute of Science and Technology

Several theoretical possibilities proposed to account for the effects of irrelevant speech on performance are outlined. They suggest the effect to be perceptual, memory-based, or attentional. By way of testing these possibilities, a number of experiments, using different tasks, are reported. No evidence for an effect of irrelevant speech at the level of perception was obtained. Irrelevant speech was shown to disrupt short-term memory by acting at rehearsal, rather than input or output, of the information. This effect was apparent when the irrelevant speech was both familiar and foreign to the listener. Effects of irrelevant speech on a proof-reading task were present only when the speech had meaning for the listener, and were confined to perceptual analysis rather than semantic analysis of the text. The results suggest that irrelevant speech exerts an effect on short-term memory which is separate from, and additional to, that found for proof-reading. Possibilities for further research are outlined.

During the last ten years there has been an increased research effort concerned with the effects of irrelevant speech on human function. In particular, there has been interest in the effects of irrelevant speech upon those tasks requiring language. The present chapter is consistent with this approach, and reports experiments involving both short-term memory for visual material, and also proof-reading. In the present context the term "irrelevant speech" does not necessarily preclude that speech from having meaning for the listener; it is irrelevant only to the performance of the task at hand. Thus typically, the reported experiments compare forward speech with that same speech played backwards. By such means, the spectral properties of the auditory signals are the same, but one (the reversed) is devoid of meaning. This allows an examination of the effect of meaningful with non-meaningful irrelevant speech.

Before turning to the empirical bases of the investigations, a brief account of the theoretical possibilities proposed to account for the effects of irrelevant speech will follow. The first theory, known as "phonological interference theory", is perhaps the strongest to be discussed, and suggests that interference between the written word and spoken word is post-perceptual. That is, it is due to the phonological codes of each interfering in that part of memory concerned with phonological codes. It assumes further that the spoken word has direct and privileged access to that particular part of the memory. Thus, any auditory signal containing phonology for the listener should interfere with visual items being committed to memory.

The second possibility, the arousal theory, posits that the effects of speech are due to increased arousal levels in the listener. Increased arousal has consequences for the individual in that it restricts the range of cue utilization in complex tasks (Easterbrook, 1959). It is not the intensity of the speech that produces the arousal, but rather, it is the speech itself.

A final possibility, the attentional theory, suggests that the attentional system is responsible for the effects of irrelevant speech. Here, two possible attentional mechanisms exist, concerned with either "early" or "late" selection.

An "early" selection mechanism is favoured by Broadbent (1971, 1983) who argues that irrelevant speech causes interference in the attentional system at the level of perception. Those visual tasks with no memory component should therefore be susceptible to the disruptive properties of speech. In contrast, the "late" selection theory suggests that interference is due to competition for meaning between the spoken and written word. Here, only that speech with meaning for the listener should disrupt performance.

We now turn to some experiments performed in our laboratory which attempt to distinguish between these theoretical possibilities.

Effects of Irrelevant Speech at Perception

The perceptual interference theory states that speech interferes with the ability to register the visual image, and it is not dependent upon either the phonology or meaning of the speech. Further, tasks which do not require memorization of visual stimuli should be susceptible. One series of studies (Baddeley & Salame, in press) required subjects to classify visually presented pairs of consonants on the basis of either case or rhyme. No effect of continuous spoken Arabic (speech condition) compared to quiet was observed. A further experiment in the series required subjects to decide whether visually presented non-words were or were not homophonous with real words. Again, no effect of speech was observed.

Clearly, these data do not support the perceptual interference model of irrelevant speech favoured by Broadbent (1983). This conclusion is given further support by findings in our own laboratory which examined the effect of irrelevant speech on the Stroop task (Stroop, 1935). Subjects were required to read overtly each of the colour, word, and interference cards comprising the Stroop task, whilst listening to a continuous stream of the four colour names red, green, yellow and blue uttered monotonically in a random order, at the rate of one word per 2 secs. The auditory material was presented over headphones and comprised three conditions: forward speech, reversed speech (both at 75 dB (c)), and quiet. A comparison of reading speeds between the three conditions produced no differences for any of the cards.

In order to exclude the possibility that the subject's overt articulation of the visual material masked the incoming auditory stimuli, a further experiment required subjects to whisper their responses. Again, no effect of irrelevant speech upon speed of processing was observed. In order to remove altogether the requirement to articulate a response, a computer-based version of the Stroop task was developed. This was a self-paced task and required subjects to press a "same" or "different" key in response to the simultaneous presentation of pairs of stimuli. Three blocks of 50 trials each represented the word, colour and interference conditions of the Stroop test. No effects of irrelevant speech were apparent for either speed of reading, or number of errors, for any of the three Stroop conditions.

Taken together, therefore, our own results and those of Baddeley and Salame (in press) provide strong evidence that speech does not act by interfering with the perceptual coding of visual material. One further experiment, however, investigated the possibility that the introduction of a single-item memory load to the Stroop task would render it susceptible to the effects of irrelevant speech. In this instance, <u>single</u> stimuli were presented consecutively in a self-paced task, requiring subjects to make a "same" or "different" response with respect to the present and previous stimulus. Three blocks of trials represented each of the three Stroop conditions. However, once again no effect of speech upon either speed or accuracy of processing was apparent.

As argued earlier, the phonological interference explanation of the irrelevant speech effect suggests that it is the phonological properties of the speech which cause the disruption. In the above experiments, spoken colour names constituted the speech. Consequently, the phonological content of the speech was low, comprising five distinct phonemes; red, green, yell, low and blue. One possibility is that the absence of an effect of irrelevant speech was due to its relatively impoverished phonetic content. To check this, subjects listened to a 1985 Reith Lecture by J.R. Searle (1985, BBC Publications) whilst performing the computer-based version of the interference condition of the Stroop task. For both the conventional Stroop test used previously and the single-item memory load versions, no effects of irrelevant speech were observed.

Effects of Irrelevant Speech on STM

The above data strongly suggest, therefore, that irrelevant speech does not interfere at the level of perceptual analysis of the visual stimuli. In addition, it does not interfere with a single-item memory loaded task. The most likely candidate to explain the irrelevant speech effect does however appear to be associated with short-term memory. Specifically, the interfering effect of speech may be explained by reference to the articulatory loop component of working memory (Salame and Baddeley, 1982). They argue that working memory comprises at least two components; the phonological store and the articulatory control process. Whilst the spoken word has direct and privileged access to the phonological store, visual items require registration in this store via the articulatory control process. Simply put, the irrelevant speech impairs short-term memory by corrupting those items held in the phonological store. An effect of irrelevant speech is not apparent when only a single item is held in memory, possibly because the store has the capacity to hold both the visually and auditorily presented items simultaneously.

Experiments in our own laboratories have reliably shown that immediate ordered recall of a visually presented string of items is impaired by irrelevant speech. This effect occurs both when the language of the irrelevant speech is foreign to the listener, for example Welsh, or when English speech is played backwards (Jones, Miles & Page, submitted), see Figure 1.

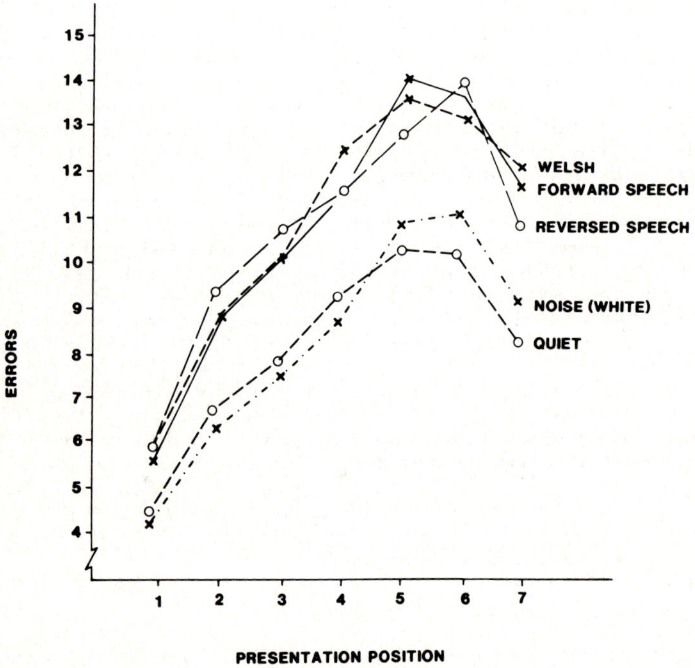

Figure 1. The serial position curves show the effects of five types of sound on serial recall in short-term memory. Three types of speech sound were presented: English, reversed English, and Welsh. White noise (at 70 dB(C)) and silence (approximately 37 dB(C)) acted as control conditions.

Two points of clarification should be made at this juncture. First, the irrelevant speech does not interact with serial position. That is, an impairment in recall is apparent across all serial positions. Second, the effect of irrelevant speech occurs for ordered recall only. Free recall appears to remain immune to any interference (Salame, personal communication). The first point, therefore, argues against any explanation which suggests that the phonological properties of the irrelevant speech act by a "knock-down" mechanism:- they do not simply displace the codes of the visual items. Rather, the memory trace of the visual items is in some way overwritten. The second point is difficult to explain; it may be that ordered recall is more difficult for the individual than free recall, and therefore the individual's capacity to ignore the irrelevant speech is reduced. A problem here of course is to define precisely what is meant by "difficult".

Stages of Interference

The short-term memory paradigm used in our laboratory typically comprises three stages; presentation of the visual stimuli, rehearsal of the stimuli for a period of 10 s, and ordered recall of the stimuli. It is possible that the irrelevant speech exerts its disruptive effect at one or more of these task stages. In order to investigate this possibility more fully, the following experiment was conducted. In a repeated measures design, subjects were presented with irrelevant speech at perception only, rehearsal only (a period of 10 s), or output only. A control condition consisted of silence for the duration of the task. Precise control over the onset and offset of the speech was achieved by software which "gated" the speech at the appropriate task points. Subjects performed 20 trials in each of the four conditions, and mean error performance for blocks of 10 trials for each condition can be seen in Table 1.

Table 1

The effects of irrelevant speech and quiet at each of three stages of the short-term memory paradigm on mean errors per task half

	Presentation	Rehearsal	Output	Quiet
1st half	3.14	3.75	2.39	2.33
2nd half	3.10	3.07	2.23	1.99

Analysis of Variance shows the mean error scores across the four conditions to differ significantly ($F(6,35) = 36.9$, $p < .0001$). However, the effect does not interact with task half ($F < 1$). The implication of the data is that irrelevant speech acts at both input and rehearsal of visually presented items. Further, for each half of the task the degree of disruption remains consistent, suggesting a genuine impairment of function, which the subject cannot ameliorate over time via a change of strategy. That an effect is apparent at input requires some explanation. Subjects will normally covertly articulate the visually presented items for rehearsal purposes before the presentation of the visual items has ceased. Thus, the irrelevant speech effect in this instance is not incompatible with the phonological disruption theory. Phonological codes for the visual items are being formed before the subject formally commences the rehearsal stage of the task.

In conclusion, it appears that irrelevant speech does impair short-term memory by interfering with rehearsal of the to-be-remembered information. However, the explanation is not one of simple masking, because the effect is only apparent for ordered recall. This suggests the possibility that a mechanism responsible for imposing order upon the stored material is disrupted, rather than the material itself. Second, the "phonological interference" argument seems to run into difficulties when faced with the fact that a language unknown to the subject disrupts short-term memory. If the language is not known, then the phonology will also be "foreign". This issue will be returned to in the final section of this chapter.

Effects of Irrelevant Speech on Proof-reading

A further set of experiments has examined directly the effect of irrelevant speech on proof-reading. Given that short-term memory is important in the reading process (Mitchell, 1982), one might predict an impairment in this type of function whilst speech is present in the environment. Particularly, children learning to read may be especially susceptible if speech interferes with the translation of the visual image to its corresponding phonetic code. To examine these possibilities a proof-reading task was developed which required subjects to identify two different classes of error: contextual errors and non-contextual errors. The former class required meaning to be extracted from the text and comprised two types: grammatical errors which involved violations of the rules of grammar, such as tense changes, and inappropriate word errors which involved the substitution of legitimate words which were acoustically simlar to the correct word. The second class of error also contained two types: these were incorrectly spelt words, which preserved the shape of the original word but became a non-word, and omission errors, which involved the removal of single letters from words. Each subject proof-read for 15 minutes and was instructed to identify an error by drawing a ring around it.

Using this task, we have manipulated the irrelevant speech in a number of ways in an attempt to identify which particular features of the speech are responsible for the disruption. Previous work (Weinstein, 1974; 1977) has shown that both bursts of teletype sound, and bursts of speech exert similar effects on a proof-reading task. That is, the detection of contextual errors (of grammar, and missing words) was impaired, whilst the detection of non-contextual errors (mis-spellings and typographical errors) remained unimpaired. The precise interpretation of these effects, particularly the role of meaning, remains ambiguous due to the complicating action of bursts of sound. It is unclear whether the impairment may be attributed to the meaning of the speech, the bursts *per se*, or a combination of each. Our initial experiments therefore examined directly the effect of meaning on proof-reading by comparing forwards speech with reversed. In addition, we examined the role of intensity of the speech by playing each tape at two intensities, (50 dB(C) and 70 dB(C)). The results of this experiment are shown in Table 2.

Table 2

The effects of type of irrelevant speech (normal and reversed) and its intensity (50 dB(C) and 70 dB(C)) on an index of reading speed (lines read) and the four error types (per cent errors detected)

	NORMAL SPEECH		REVERSED SPEECH	
	50 dB	70 dB	50 dB	70 dB
Grammatical	38.7	43.6	39.1	41.4
Inappropriate	74.7	71.9	68.7	72.0
Mis-spelling	64.0	58.8	68.7	73.1
Omission	51.7	51.4	60.8	63.4
Speed	195	220.3	212.3	209.7

Separate analyses for each of the five measures revealed no effects of intensity of the speech. However, detection rate was impaired in the forward speech condition compared to the reversed speech condition for both mis-spellings ($\underline{F}(1,30) = 4.03$, $p < .05$) and omissions ($\underline{F}(1,30) = 6.42$, $\underline{p} < .01$). There was no interaction effect between type of, and intensity of, speech for any of the measures.

Clearly, such a result is consistent with explanations proposing meaning as the distracting factor, and is therefore in line with the "late" selection model of attention. There is no evidence here that changes in arousal, due to the intensity of the speech are responsible for the disruption. In addition, this type of result differs to that shown for short-term memory which supports the phonological interference explanation. A somewhat curious result here is that the meaning of the speech did not impair the ability to extract meaning from the text, it impaired detection only of those errors requiring a more superficial level of processing. Further, the intensity of the speech was not important in determining the degree of disruption. Such a finding has obvious implications for the design of open-plan classrooms and offices where tasks involving language are frequently undertaken. Dampening of irrelevant speech may be inadequate for maximum performance.

In summary, the present results cannot be understood by supposing that the irrelevant speech impairs reading via a short-term memory store. Contemporary models of reading propose a short-term store used for assembling the grammatical structure of the material being read (Mitchell, 1982). Thus, disruption of this store by speech should produce impairment in detection of grammatical errors. Such a finding was not produced here. One possibility, therefore, is that the effect on short-term memory is separate from, and additional to, that found for proof-reading.

The role of physical features of the speech

A further set of experiments in our laboratory has manipulated physical features of the speech, and examined their effect upon the proof-reading task. In particular, we have examined the effect of a moving voice against a stationary voice, and the effect of several streams of speech. In the first instance, a single voice moving left to right in a sinusoidal fashion was compared to a control condition of a stationary voice positioned roughly at the median plane. In the second instance, three streams of speech were used and the main comparison of interest was the physical separation of the speech. The three streams of speech were presented in either (i) separate planes, one at each ear and the third in the centre of the head, or (ii) the same plane at the centre of the head. A positive result for either of these manipulations would lend support to an "early" selection attentional model, which classically proposes physical characteristics of the speech to be attention-catching (Treisman, 1969).

However, neither manipulation produced impairment on any of the five measures of the proof-reading task. Thus, it appears that meaning is the important feature of the disrupting nature of speech for proof-reading tasks.

Manipulation of the proof-reading text

The final experiment to be reported in this chapter manipulated the text rather than speech parameters. Such a manipulation is based on the rationale that whilst reading, analysis of the written word may proceed at several partially interacting levels. For instance, analysis at the semantic level does not necessarily succeed complete analysis at the phonemic level. Reading may encompass units of analysis larger than the letter or word.

From the finding that meaningful speech impaired analysis of non-contextual errors, it is suggested that irrelevant speech interferes by restricting lower levels of analysis. This is the case only when the prevailing level of unitization is high, such as when reading prose. It is not the irrelevant speech itself that alters the level of unitization, rather it restricts analysis of the products of reading.

To examine the idea that a high level of unitization is required for irrelevant speech to exert an effect, the level of unitization was manipulated in the following way. The proof-reading text was displayed on a computer screen. In one condition subjects could view only one line of text at a time, in another, five lines of text were available. In the one-line condition, only parts of sentences are available for analysis, and this will necessarily restrict the level of unitization. However, in the five-line version full sentences would be available for analysis, thus facilitating a larger level of unitization.

Such a paradigm allows for the prediction that size of the display will determine both the number and type of errors detected. Specifically, the five-line display should facilitate detection of errors of the contextual type, whilst exerting no influence on detection of errors of the non-contextual type. The effect of irrelevant speech should be apparent only when the level of unitization is high (the five-line condition) and should result in impairment of detection of contextual-errors. Note that an alternative approach might suggest short-term memory as the candidate most vulnerable to the effects of irrelevant speech, and therefore impairment of error detection should be most apparent in the one-line condition where reliance upon short-term memory is greatest. The results of this experiment can be seen in Table 3.

Table 3

The effects of irrelevant speech (at 70 dB(C)) and dispıay size (one line versus five lines) on five measures of proof-reading efficiency. Accuracy scores are per cent errors, and speed of reading is number of lines read.

	NORMAL SPEECH		REVERSED SPEECH	
	One line	Five line	One line	Five line
Grammatical	48.9	56.7	41.0	66.6
Inappropriate	75.3	75.0	77.0	76.6
Mis-spelling	72.0	67.8	70.4	85.1
Omission	46.5	53.0	50.5	60.4
Speed	92.8	110.2	95.0	92.4

Separate analyses of each of the five measures were performed. As predicted the larger display size facilitated detection of contextual errors, although this was limited to the grammatical errors. Irrelevant speech and display size interacted for the mis-spellings measure. With the larger display, irrelevant speech impaired detection of these error types. This finding supports the prediction that the higher level of unitization renders the lower levels of analysis more susceptible to the disruptive effects of irrelevant speech.

Future Research

In conclusion, our experiments have produced two general results, the first is that immediate, ordered recall for visually presented items is impaired by speech-like sounds. Contemporary literature suggests that interference between competing phonological codes is responsible for the effect. Proof-reading, in contrast, appears to be sensitive to the meaning of speech, suggesting that irrelevant speech does not impair reading by supplanting phonological codes of the written word within short-term memory.

Our concern now is to identify more precisely those properties of irrelevant speech responsible for the short-term memory impairment. A direct test of the "phonological interference" explanation is underway, and is being attacked in two ways. The first involves the comparison of the repeated presentation of a single phoneme "Ah" with the same phoneme presented continuously, in this case "Aaaa...h". The second involves a comparison of the effect of the repeated presentation of a group of digitized phonemes, each acoustically dissimilar, with the presentation of a single, repeated digitized phoneme. Thus, no meaning is apparent to the listener, but one sound is phonetically complex in comparison to the other. If the phonological interference theory of irrelevant speech and short-term memory is correct, then both manipulations should prove disruptive.

Conclusion

At a practical level, the most important finding to date is that regarding intensity of the irrelevant speech. A quiet voice would appear to disrupt reading to the same degree as a loud voice. The implications for the design of libraries, offices and classrooms are obvious. At a theoretical level, we do not yet have a satisfactory explanation for why the ordered recall of events is more sensitive to irrelevant speech than free recall. The presently termed "phonological interference" explanation for the effects of irrelevant speech on short-term memory may prove to be overly simple. A more precise definition of those properties of speech that are responsible for the disruptive effect is required.

References

Baddeley, A.D., & Salame, P. (in press). The unattended speech effect: Perception or memory? Journal of Experimental Psychology: Learning, Memory and Cognition.

Broadbent, D.E. (1971). Decision and stress. London: Academic Press.

Broadbent, D.E. (1983). Recent advances in understanding performance in noise. In G. Rossi (Ed.), Proceedings of the Fourth International Congress on Noise as a Public Health Problem, Volume 2. Milano: Centro Ricerche E Studi Amplifon.

Easterbrook, J.A. (1959). The effect of emotion on cue utilization and the organization of behaviour. Psychological Review, 66, 183-201.

Jones, D.M., Miles, C., & Page, J. Disruption of reading by irrelevant speech: Effects of attention, arousal or memory? Submitted for publication.

Mitchell, D.C. (1982). The process of reading: A cognitive analysis of fluent reading and learning to read. Chichester: Wiley.

Salame, P., & Baddeley, A.D. (1982). Disruption of short-term memory by unattended speech: Implications for the structure

of working memory. Journal of Verbal Learning and Verbal Behaviour, 21, 150-164.
Stroop, J.R. (1935). Studies of interference in serial verbal reactions. Journal of Experimental Psychology, 18, 643-662.
Treisman, A. (1969). Strategies and models of selective attention. Psychological Review, 76, 282-299.
Weinstein, N.D. (1974). Effects of noise on intellectual performance. Journal of Applied Psychology, 59, 548-554.
Weinstein, N.D. (1977). Noise and intellectual performance: A confirmation and extension. Journal of Applied Psychology, 62, 104-107.

Cognition and Action in Skilled Behaviour
A.M. Colley and J.R. Beech (Editors)

WORKING MEMORY IN THE ACQUISITION OF COMPLEX COGNITIVE SKILLS

Robert Logie
University of Aberdeen

Alan Baddeley
MRC Applied Psychology Unit, Cambridge

Amir Mane, Emanuel Donchin and Russell Sheptak
University of Illinois at Urbana-Champaign

Three experiments are reported which used secondary task methodology to study the acquisition of complex cognitive skills. Unlike earlier studies of working memory, the primary task relied on perceptuo-motor skills and accurate timing of responses as well as short and long term strategic decisions. Expert performance was found to be affected by generation of concurrent, paced responses and by concurrent working memory load, but not by production of a response to a secondary stimulus. Effects of working memory load were not contingent upon the nature (verbal or visuo-spatial) of the processing requirement. Early in training paced generation of responses had little effect on performance. Novice performance was affected by working memory load, but a wider range and different aspects of performance were disrupted by a visuo-spatial rather than by a secondary verbal load. With further training the differential nature of the disruption by a secondary visuo-spatial task was much reduced. However there was disruption by paced generation of responses. Subjective ratings of task difficulty were found to be poor predictors of performance. These results suggest that response timing and general working memory load are important aspects of expert performance. They also suggest that tracking control is an important and demanding aspect of novice performance but that it is a highly automated skill in the performance of experts. The implications of this methodology for the study of cognitive workload, of skill acquisition and the potential implications for the theoretical development of working memory are discussed.

The concept of working memory (Baddeley & Hitch, 1974) refers to the functional analysis of temporary storage and manipulation during information processing, incorporating a central executive for complex decision and control processes, and a number of subsidiary slave systems, thought to be involved in specific processing. A major contribution of this approach has been in providing a coherent, functional description of short-term verbal storage and manipulation, within the context of an articulatory loop; a slave system thought to act as a subvocal rehearsal buffer (e.g. Salame & Baddeley, 1982; Vallar & Baddeley, 1982). A second slave system, the Visuo-Spatial Sketch Pad, is thought to provide similar functions for visuo-spatial material (Baddeley & Lieberman, 1980; Logie, 1986).

The potential scope of this concept is, in principle, sufficiently wide to provide insight into an enormous number of everyday tasks of widely varying complexity. Some studies have shown working memory to be useful in the study of reading (Baddeley, 1979; Baddeley, Logie, Nimmo-Smith, & Brereton, 1985), and counting (Logie & Baddeley, 1987). However, most of the tasks so far chosen for study have been relatively simple or have had strong cognitive components, with relatively little perceptual motor or speed content.

This study investigated the changes in performance with training on a complex computer game, Space Fortress. In contrast to earlier studies of working memory, the primary task relied on both perceptuo-motor skills and more cognitive skills such as those involved in both moment to moment decisions and in more long-term strategies. The experiments described had two aims; first to provide an analysis of a fairly complex task in terms of subcomponent skills, and second, to investigate the use of a complex task environment as a test of the generality of the working memory framework and secondary task methodology. These experiments were part of an extensive project on learning strategies which involved a number of subcontractors worldwide. All subcontractors studied learning strategies and training in Space Fortress to allow comparability between projects.

The secondary task procedure rests on the assumption that where mutual interference occurs in performing two tasks simultaneously when compared to performing each task alone, that the tasks share some cognitive resource. The secondary tasks are chosen to involve specific resources and therefore, any mutual disruption of the game and a particular secondary task might suggest that the cognitive functions thought to be important for the secondary task are also involved in the game. This assumption is not entirely without polemic (e.g. Allport, 1980; Navon & Gopher, 1979). Nonetheless it has been particularly fruitful in providing coherent sets of converging evidence for the various components of working memory (Baddeley, 1986).

The experiments were concerned with four questions, first the role of response competition in performance, second the importance of general working memory load and third, the relationship between visuo-spatial processing and perceptuo-motor control in the game. Finally, the experiments studied the role of these factors at various levels of expertise.

Space Fortress

The computer game Space Fortress involves controlling the movement on a screen of a spaceship by means of a joystick control. A diagram of the layout of the computer screen is shown in Figure 1. The spaceship moves in a frictionless environment, and the joystick controls the forward direction only. A button inset into the top of the joystick controls the firing of missiles from the spaceship. In the centre of the screen is a space fortress. This pivots around a central point, attempting to track the spaceship and destroy it with missiles. The spaceship in its turn attempts to destroy the fortress.

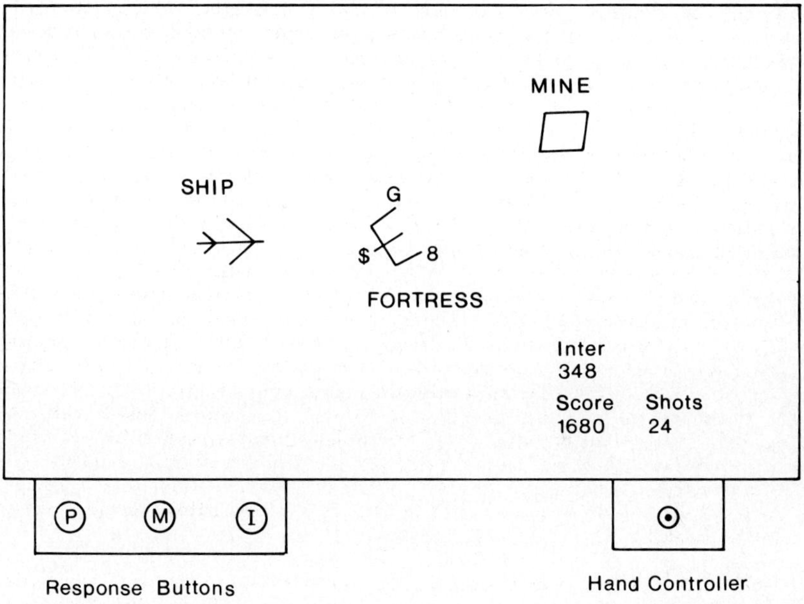

Figure 1. Display and layout of controls for Space Fortress.

From time to time a space mine appears from a random position at the edge of the screen. This tracks the spaceship, and can cause damage if they meet. The mines are of two types; a friend mine or a foe mine. If the mine is a friend, a successful hit by a missile from the ship causes the mine to crash into and damage the fortress. If the mine is a foe, the subject must change the status of the weapon system on the ship and destroy the mine with a successful shot. The weapon system is changed by pressing a button on a separate control with the left hand. The mine is identified as a friend or a foe by letters which appear above the fortress.

One further complication is that from time to time, a variety of non-alphabetic symbols appear below the fortress. The appearance of two consecutive dollar signs ($) signifies the availability of bonus points or a new supply of missiles for the ship. The subject may choose which is the most appropriate at that stage of the game.

An overall measure is given by a points total. Points are gained by successful hits or destructions of the fortress or mines, as well as choice of bonus points when these are available. Points are lost when the ship is hit or destroyed either by a mine or by the fortress. Points are also lost if the ship fires missiles "in the red". The ship has an initial supply of 100 missiles. Once this supply is exhausted, the ship may continue to fire missiles, but at a cost of points being deducted from the score. The selection of a missile bonus when this is available helps avoid this problem. Given the possibility of points being subtracted as well as added, it is common for a novice player to have a very large negative score.

In addition to this rather arbitrary measure of performance, a large number of individual measures of aspects of game performance were recorded. Over fifty parameters were measured, including efficiency of firing the missiles, the time taken to destroy a fortress or mine, the general movement of the ship around the screen, the choice of missiles or bonus points when the dollar sign appears.

The task is obviously complex with a number of component perceptuo-motor and cognitive tasks involved. Our main approach was to provide a fairly complete analysis of the components of working memory which might be involved in learning and performing this task. However, a complete analysis of this sort is beyond the scope of the present paper and a more complete account of these data will be reported in Logie, Baddeley, Mane, Donchin and Sheptak (in preparation).

Experiment 1

Method

Secondary Task Procedures.

The secondary tasks for Experiment 1 were chosen to cover a wide range of cognitive and perceptuo-motor functions that might be involved in the game, including response factors, timing, and memory load.

The first secondary task investigated the effects of a secondary response on the organisation of responses appropriate to events in the game. This involved auditory presentation of a random sequence of days of the week, presented at a rate of one day every three seconds. The subject's task was to repeat as quickly as possible the day presented. The next set of tasks involved the generation of a response at a pre-set rate, but with no stimulus present. The intention with these tasks was to study the effect on those aspects of the game that require timing of responses. In the first of these conditions, subjects were to alternate taps between two foot pedals at a two per second rate. In a second condition subjects were to repeat a single word ("GO") at a rate of two per second. The last set of tasks involved an investigation of the working memory load required by the game.

The first of these conditions was identical to "repeat GO", or articulatory suppression, considered in the context of its effect on memory performance. Numerous previous studies have shown repeated articulation of an irrelevant word to be associated with specific impairment of short-term verbal memory (e.g. Baddeley, 1986).

In a second (word span) condition, the experimenter read to the subject, lists of single syllable, high frequency words for immediate ordered recall. In the final condition for this experiment (sentence span) subjects were given sets of simple sentences, such as "The butcher ate the apple; the artist cut the grass". The experimenter then read either "the objects" or "the subjects". The task was to recall the objects or the subjects of the sentences as appropriate, in the order in which they were presented. In the example given, if "the objects" were required, the subject should respond "apple, grass" (Daneman & Carpenter, 1980).

General Procedure.

Subjects were tested over three sessions, with a gap of at least one day between sessions. The first session was to provide practice and to collect control data on the game and on each of the secondary tasks alone. In the two subsequent sessions, subjects' control data were collected for each task, followed by the appropriate dual task condition with the game.

After each game, the subjects were asked to recall the letters that had been assigned to foe mines for that game, and after every condition to rate the difficulty of the task just completed. They were given a ten point scale, where a rating of one indicated that the task was extremely easy and a rating of ten indicated that the task was virtually impossible.

Subjects.

Experiment 1 involved expert performance in six subjects who were given a minimum of twenty hours' practice on the game, prior to the introduction of any secondary tasks. Other investigators who have used Space Fortress, have found that ten hours' practice is sufficient to gain relatively skilled performance on the task. Subjects were all right-handed males, aged 18-20 years, and who were students at the University of Illinois at Urbana-Champaign.

Results.

The intention at the first stage of analysis, was to look for general indications as to patterns of impairment in game performance. As such, the data were first examined in terms of the overall, relative effects on the gross measure of game score and the effects of game playing on secondary task performance. The more detailed measures of performance were considered in a second set of analyses of effects on game microstructure.

Dual task performance was measured in terms of percentage changes from control, single task performance. Table 1 summarises the percentage decrements in mean game scores for all dual task conditions and decrements in secondary task performance, along with the mean rated difficulty of each task alone and with the game. Taken as a whole, it is clear that, with the exception of articulatory suppression, all of our secondary tasks resulted in some impairment in performance when combined with the game, although with repeat-a-day this impairment only appeared in the secondary task. However, the relative efforts differed with the particular secondary task chosen. Initial inspection suggests that the relative impairments shown could not be predicted simply on the basis of subjective levels of difficulty. On the basis of a model of cognition that suggested the use of general purpose resources, it would be reasonable to expect that the secondary tasks rated as most difficult when performed singly, should also result in the largest performance decrements in the dual task conditions. This is clearly not the case. For example, the task which appears to produce the greatest overall decrement in game score, rapid tapping, was rated as one of the easiest tasks when performed alone.

The picture is similar if we consider decrements in secondary task performance. Repeat-a-day was rated as being the easiest of any of the tasks when performed alone, but showed the largest percentage impairments when performed with the game.

Table 1

Percentage decrements in game score and secondary task performance, and mean rated difficulty in Experiment 1.

	Decrement in Game Score	Decrement in Secondary Task	Rated Difficulty
Game alone			3.72
Repeat day	0	37.3**	1.39
Articulation	10.41	10.2	3.33
Sentence span	13.62**	7.0	4.67
Word span	18.64**	14.5**	4.17
Tapping	23.54**	17.7	2.00

** $p < 0.01$

These results thus suggest that impairments due to a secondary task are not simply due to general cognitive load, and that the effects may be specific to particular aspects of the primary task. We examined this notion further in an analysis of game microstructure.

Effects on Game Components.

Table 2 summarises the results in terms of the groups of component measures affected by particular secondary tasks. From the Table, it appears that the overall effects on game score did not reflect a general load on processing resources, but rather that the secondary tasks affected different aspects of game performance. Tapping affected the number of times that the fortress was hit by a missile or by a mine (NFOHITS), the number of times the fortress was destroyed (NFODES), and the proportion of missiles fired by the ship that hit an appropriate target (SHTEFF). Repeated articulation

Table 2

Effects of secondary tasks on component measures in Experiments 1 and 2

Secondary Task (Experiments 1 and 2)	Components Affected
Repeat day	None
Tapping	NFOHITS, NFODES, SHTEFF
Articulation	NBDINT
Word span	NFODES, RTIFF
Sentence span	RTIFF, TOTSHOTS
(Experiment 2 only)	
Limerick	RTIFF, TOTSHOTS, TIMKLFO
Map	RTIFF, TOTSHOTS
Brooks Verbal	NBDINT, NFOHITS, NFODES, RTIFF, TIMKLFO, TOTSHOTS
Brooks Spatial	NSHDMG, NFOHITS, NFODES, RTIFF, TIMKLFO, TOTSHOTS

affected only one variable (NBDINT); a measure of timing of button presses. In contrast, word span and sentence span both affected the delay in responding to the appearance of a foe mine (RTIFF). In addition, word span affected the number of times the fortress was destroyed (NFODES), while sentence span affected the total number of shots fired by the ship (TOTSHOTS).

The number of fortress destructions (NFODES) can arise from a variety of factors. In this sense, it can be taken as a relatively gross measure of performance. However, shooting efficiency (SHTEFF) and number of hits on the fortress (NFOHITS) could both be thought of as measures of aiming and timing of responses to events in the game. These appeared largely unaffected by the requirements to respond to secondary stimuli, but were affected by the requirement to generate responses at a set rate. A further measure of timing, the number of bad time intervals (NBDINT) was also affected by one of these secondary tasks, namely repeated articulation. In this respect, concurrent articulation appears to produce impairment due to the timing and generation of responses, rather than any effect on short term verbal memory load. For example subjects could accurately recall the foe letters at the end of each game, regardless of whether or not there was a secondary task.

Therefore, it appears that two major aspects of game performance were identified by secondary task methodology, namely accuracy and timing of responses, and the more complex monitoring of several sources of information. However, none of the secondary tasks were chosen specifically to study the involvement of visuo-spatial processing, for example in control of ship movement, and a second experiment was carried out to investigate this issue.

Experiment 2

Method

The set of secondary tasks chosen for Experiment 2 were selected largely to study the relation between perceptuo-motor control in the game and visuo-spatial processing functions in contrast to general working memory load or verbal processing. Two sets of tasks were chosen for present purposes. While the verbal/visuo-spatial contrast was maintained in each set, the major difference between the sets was in terms of the relative general processing load required by each. These are described below.

Secondary tasks.

1. Brooks visuo-spatial task and verbal tasks. These were based on a task originally reported by Brooks (1967), that involved the subject retaining a sequence of movements through a 4x4 matrix pattern. Subjects were given a starting square which was always the square in the second row and second column. They were then presented through headphones with a sequence of eight sentences describing a path through the matrix, with consecutive numbers in adjacent squares. An example might be:

In the starting square put a 1
In the next square to the right put a 2
In the next square to the right put a 3
In the next square down put a 4
and so on.

At the end of this sequence, the subjects were required to repeat the sequence verbatim, and to use a visual image of the path through the matrix as the means for retention. Performance on this task is typically disrupted by visual tracking tasks such as a pursuit rotor, suggesting some overlap between perceptuo-motor control and the visuo-spatial content of the main task (e.g. Baddeley & Lieberman, 1980). Tracking tasks interfere much less, or not at all with a verbal version of this task where the subject again hears a sequence of sentences, but with the words "good", "bad", "slow" and "quick" substituted for directions in the visuo-spatial version. Here, subjects were encouraged to use verbal rehearsal in order to retain the sequence.

2. Map and Limerick tasks. These were based on a technique developed by Moar (1978), and involved presenting subjects with a map of an island, on which were marked six locations. On a given map, the names of the locations were chosen from a particular category. For example, one map contained the names of well known scientists such as "Darwin Gardens" or "Newton Monastery". The name and type of location (e.g. Monastery, Airport etc.) were unique to a particular map and location, and no location was directly north, south, east or west of any other location. Subjects were given one minute to study the map and were then asked questions concerned with the relative direction between pairs of locations,

for example:

Is Newton Monastery north of Darwin Gardens?
Is Einstein Hospital southwest of Curie Stables?

The Limerick task was designed as a verbal equivalent of the map task, and involved the subject learning a short poem in the form of a limerick. These were chosen from Green (1956), or devised by the first author. One example was:

There was a young thief of repute,
Whose ideas were surprisingly cute.
He built a balloon,
By the light of the moon,
And used it to gather his loot.

The subject was then given a number of questions concerned with the relative position of various words in the poem, for example:

Does thief come before surprisingly?
Does light come after gather?

In both tasks, subjects were given one minute to learn the poem or map and the questions were presented through headphones. Responses were timed with a voice key, and error responses were recorded by the experimenter.

In addition, two of the tasks from Experiment 1 were included, namely repeat-a-day and rapid tapping.

General procedure.

Subjects were tested over three sessions, with the procedure identical to that for Experiment 1, except with a new set of secondary tasks. Six expert subjects took part, five of whom also took part in Experiment 1. Experiment 2 took place approximately three months after Experiment 1.

Results

As with Experiment 1, effects on mean game score and secondary task performance are reported first, followed by an examination of effects on game component measures.

Table 3 summarises the effects on game score and secondary task performance in terms of percentage decrements, along with mean rated difficulty. Unlike Experiment 1, rated difficulty on the secondary tasks alone appeared to be associated with the largest decrements in game score. The major exception to this was rapid tapping, which appeared to produce a relatively large impairment in game performance but received a very low difficulty rating when performed alone.

The results on tapping and repeat-a-day were replicated in this study, supporting the view that generating a secondary response appears to require resources that overlap with some crucial aspects of game performance.

Table 3

Percentage decrements in game score and secondary task performance, and mean rated difficulty for all conditions in Experiment 2.

	Decrement in Game Score	Decrement in Secondary Task	Rated Difficulty
Game alone			2.42
Repeat day	6.36	41.10**	1.22
Limerick	19.68**	6.05	3.78
Tapping	20.13**	11.03	1.72
Map	25.08**	2.64	4.61
Brooks Verbal	33.05**	19.89**	5.67
Brooks Spatial	36.22**	34.99**	4.72

** $p < 0.01$

The results of the remaining secondary tasks provide a less clear picture. Although all of the tasks were associated with impairments in performance, there was no clear differential disruption by the spatial as opposed to the verbal tasks. The relatively larger disruption by the Brooks tasks can easily be accounted for in terms of general processing load, since both of these tasks were rated as the most difficult of the set. However, it is possible that this lack of differential impairment results from combining game component measures in a single score, and this is explored below.

Effects on game components.

Table 2 shows a summary of the effects of particular secondary tasks on groups of component measures. The results for repeat-a-day and tapping were identical to those for Experiment 1, and have not been repeated in the Table.

The limerick task affected the response time to the presence of a foe mine (RTIFF), and the time to destroy the fortress, or a foe mine (TIMKLFO), along with total number of shots fired (TOTSHOTS). The map task affected only RTIFF and total shots fired. The Brooks verbal task and spatial tasks affected broadly similar sets of factors, with two exceptions: The verbal task affected timing of button presses (NBDINT), while the spatial task affected ability to steer the ship away from damage (NSHDMG).

Discussion

One fairly striking observation from these data is that measures of tracking control (NWRAP, NMOVIN, MOVMNT) were unaffected by any of our secondary tasks, in particular the visuo-spatial memory tasks. The Brooks spatial task was affected by simultaneous game performance, but so too were other secondary tasks. In addition, the alternative visuo-spatial task (maps) was largely unaffected by dual task conditions. Indeed, what is most striking about both of the Brooks tasks is the range of game components which they affect. This further supports the view that the interference produced by these tasks results from general rather than specific processing.

However, this begs the question as to the processes that may underlie game performance. The specific disruption of visuo-spatial processing, including tracking a moving target, by the Brooks task is well established (Brooks, 1968; Baddeley & Lieberman, 1980). This suggests that the cognitive processes involved in tracking on a pursuit rotor or following a randomly moving target (e.g. Baddeley, Bressi, Della Sala, Logie, & Spinnler, 1986) are not involved in control of ship movement in Space Fortress. This seems incongruous as the tasks seem superficially very similar.

The most plausible explanation lies in the level of expertise involved. In earlier studies, the subjects are given sufficient practice to be familiar with the task. This is generally of the order of several minutes. The task in Space Fortress is somewhat more complex, however all of our subjects had a minimum of 20 hours' practice on the game prior to the introduction of our secondary tasks. Few studies have investigated the effects of secondary tasks where tracking has been practiced for extended periods, and this factor may well be crucial. One possibility is that the visuo-spatial tracking elements of the task are largely automatic (e.g. Shiffrin & Schneider, 1977) in experts on the game. In Experiment 3 we attempted to test this possibility by studying the effects of our secondary tasks on the performance of subjects who had relatively little practice on the game.

Experiment 3

Method and Procedure

The aim in Experiment 3 was to investigate the effects of our various secondary tasks on performance during the early stages of training. We chose those of our tasks which appeared to yield the most interesting results with experts, namely the tasks used in Experiment 2. In particular we were interested in whether visuo-spatial or verbal memory loads would have differential effects on game performance in novices, where this had not occurred in experts. The basic procedure for each task and its combination with the game was more or less identical to that adopted for Experiment 2.

The general procedure was designed to examine effects on performance at two different stages in training. Subjects were first given three hours of practice on the game. Next, they were given one session consisting of practice on each of the secondary tasks. There then followed two sessions where each secondary task was performed alone or with the game. Next, subjects were given a further five hours' practice on the game alone, followed by a further two sessions involving the secondary tasks.

Subjects were nine students at the University of Illinois at Urbana-Champaign. None had played Space Fortress prior to this experiment.

Results

Tables 4 and 5 show the percentage decrements in game score and secondary tasks, along with mean ratings of difficulty. From Table 4 it is clear that early in training, repeat-a-day and tapping had no effect on game performance, nor were they affected in turn. The two Brooks tasks produced roughly the same amount of disruption. However there was a striking contrast between the effects of the map and the limerick tasks. The map task disrupted game performance at about the same level as did the Brooks tasks. The limerick task produced much less of an impairment. This distinction is not reflected in secondary task performance, and therefore is unlikely to be due to a trade-off in allocation of resources, nor can it be explained in terms of the relative difficulty of the two tasks, as their ratings of difficulty did not differ significantly.

Table 4

Percentage decrements in game score and secondary task performance and mean rated difficulty for all conditions after three hours of training in Experiment 3

	Decrement in Game Score	Decrement in Secondary Task	Rated Difficulty
Game alone			1.89
Repeat day	3.54	6.43	1.33
Tapping	20.66	4.10	2.89
Limerick	42.85**	7.79	3.94
Brooks Spatial	71.06**	42.10**	4.33
Map	74.68**	11.8	4.28
Brooks Verbal	76.77**	30.90**	5.50

** $p < 0.01$

Table 5

Percentage decrements in game score and secondary task performance and mean rated difficulty for all conditions after eight hours of training in Experiment 3

	Decrement in Game Score	Decrement in Secondary Task	Rated Difficulty
Game alone			1.89
Repeat day	7.66	59.5**	1.28
Limerick	25.39**	7.7	3.00
Tapping	26.96**	4.8	1.89
Map	33.97**	4.5	3.83
Brooks Verbal	46.94**	31.8**	4.50
Brooks Spatial	50.34**	32.2**	3.39

** $p < 0.01$

Table 5 shows that the pattern is rather different after further training. Repeat-a-day now is affected by dual task conditions, although it does not affect game performance as with expert players. Tapping now shows a significant decrement in performance on the game. There is still no distinction between the two Brooks tasks, however, the differential effects of the map and limerick tasks have been considerably reduced. Both significantly impair game performance, but the difference in relative impairment is no longer significant.

The ratings of difficulty appear to be relatively good predictors of dual task performance early in training, but this relationship breaks down as training progresses.

Effects on game components.
Table 6 shows a summary of the effects of particular secondary tasks on groups of component measures. There is insufficient space to consider these in detail, and a brief summary will be given here.

As before, repeat-a-day had no effect on any of the game components that we examined. Unlike the results for experts, at an early stage of training tapping affected only one variable.

Table 6

Effects of secondary tasks on component measures in Experiment 3

Secondary Task	Components affected - Early in Training	Late in Training
Repeat day	None	None
Tapping	TOTSHOTS	TOTSHOTS, NFOHITS, NFODES, SHOTEFF
Limerick	PCNTBON	NFOHITS, NFODES, TOTSHOTS
Map	NSHDMG, NFODES, RTIFF, PCNTBON	NFODES, RTIFF, PCNTBON, NFOHITS, TOTSHOTS
Brooks Verbal	NFOHITS, NFODES, PCNTBON, TOTSHOTS	NFOHITS, NFODES, PCNTBON, TOTSHOTS, RTIFF
Brooks Spatial	NFOHITS, NFODES, TIMKLFR, PCNTBON, TOTSHOTS	NFOHITS, NFODES, TIMKLFR, PCNTBON, TOTSHOTS, RTIFF, TIMKLFO

The map task clearly affects a wider range of factors early in training than does the limerick task, and this distinction is less clear with further training. This supports the results for game score.

Unlike game score, there is also a distinction between the two Brooks tasks in the range and type of components affected at different levels of training.

Overall Discussion

The original aim of these studies was twofold: to provide an analysis of a complex task in terms of decomposition into component skills, and to act as a study of the use of secondary task methodology and the working memory framework in a relatively novel environment. Space Fortress provided a set of task demands which lent themselves fairly readily to this type of methodology, and on the whole, the results are encouraging. The results of Experiment 1 suggested that at least two different classes of skill were required; one involved in response timing and accuracy, and the other in monitoring of events and strategic control. Experiment 2 supported these conclusions. However, the lack of any differential disruption of the perceptual-motor control aspects of game performance by secondary visuo-spatial tasks was a little puzzling. A possible explanation lies in the extent of subject training. Since all of the subjects were highly practiced on the game, certain aspects of game performance may have been highly automated, and as a result much less prone to disruption.

Experiment 3 showed that the pattern of disruption in game performance associated with our range of secondary tasks changes as a result of training. Further, the changes were not wholly characterised by a general decrease in the disruptive effects of our secondary tasks. In particular, the effect of a secondary tapping task increased as our subjects became more expert. The role of visuo-spatial processing was not quite so clear cut. However, there were suggestions in the data that the importance of visuo-spatial processing as measured by the differential disruption by secondary visuo-spatial tasks, changed as subjects progressed from relatively novice status to a moderate level of expertise on the game. The role of this component appeared to be less crucial for those with many hours of training on the game. Finally, general working memory load appeared to be important at all levels of training.

These results underline the importance for training procedures of considering which skills are necessary at specific stages in training. That is, it may be crucial for efficient training on this game to concentrate on ship control during the early stages. As training progresses, it may be appropriate to concentrate more on timing of responses.

It is important at this point to consider whether the working memory approach has proved to be any more useful than alternative approaches in the study of the acquisition of complex cognitive skills. A traditional approach to the study of cognitive workload in complex tasks relies on subjective judgements from the trainee of the task or aspects of the task. This can provide useful insights for those involved in training design. However these judgements should be treated with caution for a number of reasons. For example, the requirement to make subjective judgements about a task may well change the way in which the task is carried out. The extent to which individuals have access to the relevant information about their own performance is also unclear. That is, many aspects of skilled performance may not be available to conscious inspection (e.g. Ericsson & Simon, 1980; Nisbett & Wilson, 1977). Our own data support this view, since the subjective ratings of difficulty were, on the whole, poor predictors of performance, particularly with expert players.

A more theoretical approach is to adopt the view that different components of the task compete for general purpose resources. As expertise is gained, some of the processes become relatively automatic and therefore demand less of the available resources (e.g. Shiffrin & Schneider, 1977). Our own data suggest that this approach may miss crucial aspects of skilled performance. It is true that general working memory load appeared to have pervasive effects on a number of game components. However, one prediction from the general resources view would suggest that those secondary tasks which were, in some sense, most difficult, should produce the greatest degree of performance decrement when combined with the game. It should also be true that tasks which were, by some criteria, relatively simple, should produce very little impairment in game performance. In so far as the ratings of difficulty can be used as measures of difficulty, it is clear that these predictions were not supported by our data.

A second difficulty for the general resources view comes from the pattern of disruption shown by different secondary tasks. Our different classes of secondary tasks appeared to affect different clusters of game components. This suggests the involvement of separate specialised resources rather than general resources. This in turn supports the view that the working memory approach to the acquisition of complex skills is indeed fruitful.

What then do these studies contribute to the development of the concept of working memory? There are strong hints in our data that a working memory in the sense of a set of mechanisms that are involved in monitoring and acting upon several near-simultaneous events is indeed useful. This application of the Baddeley and Hitch (1974) working memory model is largely unexplored. There is also evidence that is consistent with the notion of mechanisms that specialise in visuo-spatial processing (Baddeley & Lieberman, 1980; Logie, 1986), and in the timing of responses. Further, this importance of these mechanisms changes with an increase in expertise on the game. However, the structure and more detailed characteristics of the mechanisms involved remain somewhat unclear in this context.

The results of the three experiments reported here have important implications for the framework of working memory in terms of its applicability to rather more complex tasks than hitherto. Thus an important area for exploration lies in the generality of this methodology and its applicability to other complex tasks with rather different characteristics, such as greater memory load or more complex and long-term strategic content.

The advantage of this course would be threefold. It would provide insight into the rather more general question as to the processes which underlie skill acquisition. It would offer a possible new methodology for the measurement of cognitive workload. Finally, it would act as a basis for theoretical advances in the development of an increasingly influential and fruitful explanatory framework.

Acknowledgements

This work was funded by the Defense Advanced Research Projects Agency (DARPA), under contract MDA903-84-K-0065, and subcontracted through the University of Illinois to the Medical Research Council (UK). We are grateful to DARPA for its support. We are also grateful to the technical staff at the University of Illinois at Urbana-Champaign.

References

Allport, A. (1980). Attention and performance. In G. Claxton (Ed.), Cognitive psychology: New directions. London : Routledge and Kegan Paul.

Baddeley, A.D. (1979). Working memory and reading. In P.A. Kolers, M.E. Wrolstad & H. Bouma (Eds.), Processing of visible language 1. New York : Plenum.

Baddeley, A.D. (1986). Working memory. Oxford : Oxford University Press.

Baddeley, A.D., Bressi, S., Della Sala, S., Logie, R., & Spinnler, H. (1986). Dementia and working memory. Quarterly Journal of Experimental Psychology, 38A, 603-618.

Baddeley, A.D., & Hitch, G. (1974). Working memory. In G.H. Bower (Ed.), The psychology of learning and motivation, 8, 47-90.

Baddeley, A.D., & Lieberman, K. (1980). Spatial working memory. In R. Nickerson (Ed.), Attention and performance VIII. Hillsdale, N.J. : Erlbaum.

Baddeley, A.D., Logie, R.H., Nimmo-Smith, I., & Brereton, N. (1985). Components of fluent reading. Journal of Memory and Language, 24, 119-131.

Brooks, L.F. (1967). The suppression of visualization by reading. Quarterly Journal of Experimental Psychology, 19, 289-299.

Daneman, M., & Carpenter, P.A. (1980). Individual differences in working memory and reading. Journal of Verbal Learning and Verbal Behavior, 19, 450-466.

Ericsson, K.A., & Simon, H.A. (1980). Verbal reports as data. Psychological Review, 87, 215-251.

Green, R.L. (1956). The book of nonsense. London : J.M. Dent & Sons.

Logie, R.H. (1986). Visuo-spatial processing in working memory. Quarterly Journal of Experimental Psychology, 38A, 229-247.

Logie, R.H., & Baddeley, A.D. (1987). Cognitive processes in counting. Journal of Experimental Psychology: Learning, Memory and Cognition, 13, 310-326.

Logie, R.H., Baddeley, A.D., Mane, A., Donchin, E., & Sheptak, R. (in preparation). Working memory and the analysis of a complex skill by secondary task methodology.

Moar, I.T. (1978). Mental triangulation and the nature of internal representations of space. Unpublished Ph.D.thesis, University of Cambridge.

Navon, D., & Gopher, D. (1979). On the economy of the human-processing system. Psychological Review, 86, 214-255.

Nisbett, R.E., & Wilson, T.D. (1977). Telling more than you know: Verbal reports on mental processes. Psychological Review, 84, 231-259.

Salame, P., & Baddeley, A.D. (1982). Disruption of short-term memory by unattended speech: implications for the structure of working memory. Journal of Verbal Learning and Verbal Behavior, 21, 150-164.

Shiffrin, R.M., & Schneider, W. (1977). Controlled and automatic human information processing: II. Perceptual learning, automatic attending and a general theory. Psychological Review, 84, 127-190.

Vallar, G., & Baddeley, A.D. (1982). Short-term forgetting and the articulatory loop. Quarterly Journal of Experimental Psychology, 34A, 53-60.

Cognition and Action in Skilled Behaviour
A.M. Colley and J.R. Beech (Editors)

THE USE OF MEMORY BY EXPERTS AND NOVICES

K.J. Gilhooly and A.J.K. Green
University of Aberdeen

This chapter concerns symbolic problem-solving skills and discusses differences in memory use by experts and novices in a number of problem domains, including chess, physics, mathematics, computer programming, map reading and political science. Early studies of chess skill supported a pattern-recognition model of chess expertise. This model accounted for the observed superiority in recall for realistic chess position by experts and the lack of difference in recall for randomised positions between experts and novices. Further, the model suggested that move-choosing skill reflected superior pattern recognition coupled with appropriate actions in a production-system type of organisation. More recent studies of chess skill, however, suggest strongly that the pattern recognition model is over-simple; players at the same skill level can vary in efficiency of pattern encoding and more skilled players choose better moves even when no familiar patterns are present. Current research on chess skill stresses the role of mental search, position-evaluation and general knowledge of chess strategy and tactics. Chess inspired pattern-recognition models have been developed for many of the other fields reviewed here and have been successful in the analyses so far reported. However, given the re-examination of the role of search in chess skill, we argue that studies of expertise in non-adversary domains might benefit from a similar re-evaluation of search-based explanations. It is surmised that more complex models than those currently in use will ultimately be required for all areas of expertise.

This chapter concerns symbolic problem-solving skills and discusses differences in memory use by experts and novices in a number of problem domains. Expertise we define as the possession of a large body of knowledge and procedural skill. The novice we conceive of as a beginner, an individual whose performance lacks the speed, accuracy and efficiency of the expert. It is generally agreed that experts and novices do not differ in their "cognitive architectures". Both experts and novices are much the same in terms of basic working memory and long term memory capacities. To anticipate a little, it may be said that what experts know and how they utilise that knowledge are the key differences between experts and novices. Thus, the major differences are located in long term memory contents, their organisation and utilisation. Since working memory may be usefully conceived of as activated portions of long term memory, it is clear that changes in long term memory contents will also affect working memory content.

Our main objective is to contrast explanations of expertise in adversary and non-adversary domains. In this way, we employ chess as the "case study" for adversary domains. Search based explanations of chess skill gave way to an account of skill in terms of a superior memory for patterns of chess pieces. This proved influential in developing models of expertise in non-adversary domains, as we later show. However, the question arises as to whether researchers have over-emphasized knowledge-based interpretations of expertise.

We will be focussing mainly on cross-sectional comparisons between experts and novices in our attempt to develop the foregoing sketch. The important question of the mechanisms that transform the novice into an expert is not dealt with extensively here. For a fuller treatment of issues in the acquisition of problem solving skill, see Gilhooly and Green (in press).

The general task areas to be considered are those of (a) adversary problem solving, and (b) semantically rich, non-adversary, problems. Historically, adversary problems were the first to be studied in terms of expertise, e.g. De Groot's work in the 1930's (published in English in 1965). More recently, semantically rich problems in which no adversary is present, have also received considerable attention, both as intrinsic challenges to cognitive psychology and as targets for automation, e.g. as computerised "expert systems". (See Alty, in press, for a discussion of expert systems).

Adversary Problems

In tackling adversary problems, solvers must consider not only their own possible actions but also those of an opponent. Games such as chess, GO, bridge and poker provide good examples of adversary problems and have been studied from psychological, artificial intelligence and normative points of view. (The normative approach is concerned with how best to play the game concerned.) Psychologists have found it helpful to use some of the terminology and concepts that have been developed in the normative Theory of Games (Von Neumann & Morgenstern, 1944) and in studies of machine game playing (Clark, in press). Accordingly, we will first outline the basic notions of "game tree", "look-ahead" and "minimax" before considering empirical studies of human game playing. The focus will be on chess play, since this has been by far the most frequently studied adversary task.

Game Trees, lookahead and the Minimax Principle

In board games the possible sequences of moves and counter-moves from a given position can be represented by diagrams known as "game trees". If it is possible to look ahead from the start to all the possible endings of the game then the best starting move can be chosen by application of the "minimax" strategy. The idea of a game tree and of minimax may be illustrated by the artificially simple game shown in Figure 1. The first player determines his or her best move by looking ahead to the possible endings and then works backwards, applying the minimax strategy to assess the worth of intermediate states. This strategy assumes that the opponent will do his or her worst to you and that you will always choose the best alternative available. Working backwards, minimaxing would label W3 as a win (+), W2 as a loss (-) and W1 as a draw (0), and recommend W3 as the best starting move, since it is bound to lead to a win whereas the other moves lead to a loss or a draw.

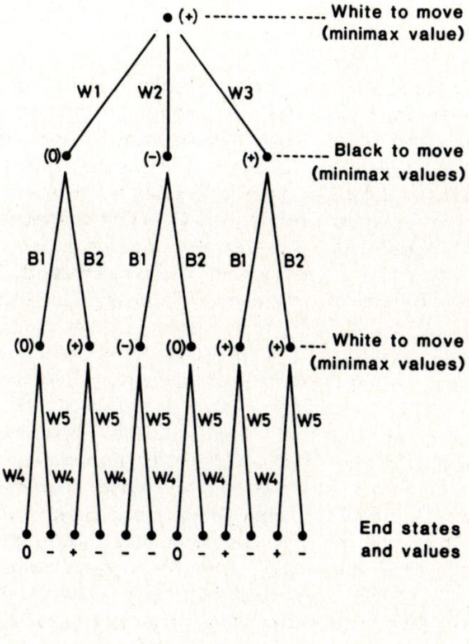

Figure 1. An example game tree.

The problem with a simple application of this approach to many games, including chess, is that in order to determine the consequences of a move the player must consider the opponent's possible replies and then his or her own replies to each of the opponent's replies to those, and so on. In theory, a "brute force" computer program could generate such information and always select the best move. However, the tree of possibilities is just too big -

approximately 10^{120} possible sequences of moves in chess and only 10^{16} micro seconds per century to explore them all.

The cognitive effort required to explore all the possible chess games is just too much for any human, or for any present or likely future machine. Computers and humans can only investigate and keep track of the consequences of relatively few moves, and then only to a limited extent. So, in order for humans or computers to play reasonable chess some strategies must be available to restrict search to plausible moves and to evaluate lines of development in the absence of complete information about their remote consequences, (i.e. with a limited degree of lookahead).

The main thrust of development in computer chess programs has been to look ahead in the game tree as far as possible within time and memory constraints, evaluate positions at the limits of look-ahead and to back-up, using minimax to choose the best starting move. This approach leads to vast, but rapid, searches and has yielded high levels of performance (see Holding, 1985, Chapter 6). However, the magnitude and speed of such a search is outside human capabilities. How then do humans achieve high levels of performance, which are still, at the top level, better than those of existing chess programs? This question is addressed in the following sections.

Search in chess : early studies.

Perhaps the most direct way to try to find out about thought processes during chess play is to present subjects with a chess problem and ask them to think aloud as they decide which move should be made next by one of the players (usually white). This method was followed by De Groot (1965), Wagner and Scurrah (1971), Newell and Simon (1972) and Charness (1981b), among others.

De Groot was particularly interested in possible differences between players of differing degrees of expertise. Five Grand Masters and five expert players were given the same chess position and thought aloud while choosing a move. The search trees that they developed could be abstracted from their protocols. A number of points emerged from these data. First, there was little or no difference in the quantitative aspects of the search patterns of the Grand Masters and the experts. The only major difference was in the quality of the move finally chosen. (Move quality was rated by independent experts.) Whilst De Groot obtained differences in the expected direction for depth of search, number of branches, total moves and speed of processing, none of these reached significance. Although, as Hearst (1977) suggested, the Grand Masters might be able to search deeper and broader if they were sufficiently motivated (e.g. in competition), it is still noteworthy that they consistently reached a better conclusion without significantly more search than the weaker players. Also, of course, the amount of sheer search is very small compared to that of the best computer chess programs.

How is it that expert human chess players can be so selective to such good effect when they search for a next move? According to a much investigated hypothesis, known as the pattern recognition hypothesis, the answer may lie in the extensive repertoire of chess patterns and schemata built up by experts over many years' study of the game. These patterns may help the expert players structure their perceptions of the board appropriately and could be attached to recommendations for possible actions, in a production system organization. Evidence suggesting this possible explanation was obtained from the chess memory task described in the next section.

Chess memory task

De Groot (1965) put chess positions involving 20/24 pieces and taken from actual games, in front of subjects for five seconds; then, he removed the positions and asked subjects to reconstruct them. Chess masters could reconstruct the positions almost without error (91% correct), while poor players made many errors (41% correct). A clue to understanding the chess masters' performance is given by another of De Groot's findings. When good and poor players were shown boards with the pieces arranged at random, both groups did equally poorly.

Chase and Simon (1973a, b) argued that the chess memory data are consistent with the view that perceivers of the chess board store about seven familiar units or "chunks" (Miller, 1956) in short term memory during the inspection period irrespective of their skill level. However the chess masters' seven chunks of information are much richer than the novices', i.e. they are larger units.

Chase and Simon (1973a, b) sought to demonstrate quite directly the proposed superiority of master players' chunks compared to those of weaker players. In their study, three players varying in skill were given chess perception and memory tasks. The perception task required the subjects to reconstruct on one board a chess position which remained in view on another board. The main variables of interest were the numbers of pieces placed following each glance at the stimulus board, the times between piece placements and the nature of the relationships between the pieces placed between one glance and the next. For all players the average number of pieces placed after a glance was similar (between two or three). However the master's glances were significantly shorter, indicating more rapid encoding. The chess recall tasks were similar to those of De Groot and involved five seconds' presentation followed by board reconstruction. Times between placements of pieces were recorded and intervals of two seconds or more were taken to correspond to boundaries between chunks in recall. On this basis, the number of pieces per chunk varied systematically (if not dramatically) with skill level from 2.5 to 1.9 pieces per chunk from strongest to weakest player. Pieces within a single chunk tended to have relations of defence and attack, be close together and be of common colour and type. Thus, Chase and Simon's studies indicated that, compared to weaker players, the stronger player encodes chess information more rapidly when perceiving the board and encodes a given position in larger chunks when recall is required.

The Memory-Aided Pattern Perceiver (MAPP) Model

Simon and Gilmartin (1973) converted the general notion of the pattern recognition hypothesis into a working computer model for the chess memory task. This model, known as the Memory-Aided Pattern Perceiver (MAPP), assumes that a position is encoded as a set of chunks (pattern labels) that occupy a limited-capacity short term memory. The pattern labels are then decoded during the position reconstruction phase. The chunks or pattern labels are produced by a pattern recognizer that seeks to match board configuration to known patterns permanently stored in a long-term memory. The pattern recognizing component consists of a discrimination net that is organized around salient pieces. It is assumed that the skilled player has a large discrimination net that incorporates a great many different patterns while the weaker player has fewer patterns available with which to describe any given position. The program can thus simulate different levels of expertise by varying the number of patterns in its long term store.

Two versions of MAPP were explored. One had available 894 patterns and the other 1144 patterns. Given the same board positions, the more "knowledgeable" version was able to encode the positions more efficiently into its short term memory and thus scored better on position reconstruction than the less knowledgeable version.

Simon and Gilmartin estimated that a MAPP-like system could replicate master level performance on the chess memory task with somewhere between 10,000 and 100,000 patterns in long-term memory. However, the estimated number of patterns required may be reduced if, as Holding (1985, p.109) points out, it is assumed that the patterns are not simply arrangements of particular pieces on particular squares. If the chunks remain recognizable when shifted a few squares or when they are changed from black to white, then the estimated number of patterns needed for master level performance can be reduced to the more manageable levels of 500 to 5,000 patterns. Acquisition of this many patterns is clearly possible with extended study.

Tests of MAPP assumptions

Some of MAPP's assumptions have been tested independently by Frey and Adlesman (1976) and Charness (1976). Frey and Adlesman examined the assumption that chess chunks are stored in a limited capacity short term memory. In their study subjects were presented with chess positions for eight seconds and then required to count backwards from a three-digit number for either three seconds or 30 seconds before attempting to reconstruct the position. The counting backward procedure is usually assumed to "clear" short term memory by preventing rehearsal and/or displacing the contents of short term memory (Brown, 1958; Peterson & Peterson, 1959). However, this manipulation had only a very slight effect. Correct recall after three seconds' interpolated activity was 13.1 pieces and after 30 seconds was 11.6 pieces. These data cast doubt on the assumption that chunks are held in short term memory. Further strong evidence against the short term memory assumption was reported by Charness (1976). He carried out a number of studies using five second presentation and Brown-Peterson interference paradigms. The 30 second interpolated tasks varied in complexity and modality (shadowing digits, summing digits, copying symbols, rotating and then copying symbols, studying other chess problems, naming pieces on a chess board). Recall of chess positions was only reduced by about 6-8% by the most effective of these manipulations. (Control conditions indicated that recall of trigrams was markedly affected by some of the interpolated tasks.) As usual, the skilled players performed better across all the memory task conditions than the weak players.

The degree to which memory for briefly presented chess positions resists interference, strongly suggests that the information is stored in long term memory rather than short term memory. The results reviewed in this section support a "depth of processing" interpretation whereby the skilled player can encode to a deeper level, more rapidly, than the less skilled player.

Age and skill in chess

Charness (1981a, b) investigated possible player-age effects additional to skill effects. Ageing is generally thought to affect memory operations, particularly those of retrieval, and so Charness hypothesised that players of equivalent skill, but widely differing ages, might differ in the underlying processes that yielded similar molar results (i.e. similar skill ratings).

Charness (1981a) assembled a sample of 34 chess players who varied independently in age (16-64 years) and skill level (Chess Federation of Canada skill ratings ranged from 1283 to 2004). The players were presented with four positions in which they had to choose a move while thinking aloud. Next, they were asked to rapidly evaluate end-game positions as being wins, draws or losses for White. After this task, the players were asked unexpectedly to recall the four initial positions by reconstructing them. Finally, a recognition task was administered in which the subjects attempted to identify the first four problem conditions among a set of 26. Only skill level was predictive of performance in the move-choosing task and in the end-game evaluation task. Skill level was positively, while age was negatively, related to chess recall scores. Measures of chunk size in recall were obtained using a procedure similar to that of Chase and Simon (1973a, b) described above. This indicated that chunk size was positively related to skill and negatively related to age. That is to say, the older subjects made use of more but smaller chunks in recall than did younger subjects of similar skill levels. These results then suggest that differences in encoding efficiency may not be sufficient to explain differences in skill levels. It should be noted however that Charness's (1981a) memory task involved delayed testing while the usual chess memory study has involved immediate memory. A follow-up study (Charness, 1981c), however, confirmed the result by showing age effects on immediate recall of chess positions, independent of skill levels.

Direct counter-evidence to the pattern recognition theory of chess skill

The results of Charness described in the previous section may have raised doubts in the reader's mind about the explanation of chess skill in terms of pattern storage and recognition. In its strongest form, the pattern recognition hypothesis, as proposed by Chase and Simon, stated that chess skill is explained by superior memory storage and recognition of familiar patterns. Holding (1985) points out that the reverse is in many ways more plausible, i.e. that superior storage and recognition of chess patterns is explained by greater skill. Charness's results show that the same skill level can be achieved even when chess memory performance varies. At the least, this implies that chess memory cannot be the sole determinant of chess skill.

Holding and Reynolds (1982) tested the further possibility that skill differences could be shown even when no memory differences were present. They did this by having high and low rated players attempt (a) to recall random positions after eight seconds' exposure and (b) to decide on the best move when they were shown the correctly reconstructed random positions. As usual, there was no skill effect on memory for the random positions. However, there was a marked linear increase in the quality of the moves chosen by the players as their skill ratings increased. Such a trend cannot be explained by the pattern recognition theory of chess skill.

These results have thus led to a re-evaluation of the pattern recognition theory and have made other difficulties with the theory appear more salient. For instance, the sizes of the chunks reported by Chase and Simon (1973a, b) are rather small (two-four pieces) to represent important chess patterns and the exact mechanisms for linking pattern recognition to choice of moves is unclear. Indeed, Holding (1985) lists some 40 objections to the pattern recognition hypothesis of chess skill! Rather than chess skill being determined by chess memory it seems that chess memory is an incidental side-effect of chess skill. Consistent with this view, Pfau and Murphy (in press) found that ratings of chess skill in 60 players were better predicted by a tactical skill test, a positional judgement test and a 75-item chess knowledge test ($r = .70$ with the criterion) than by memory scores following five second exposures of chess positions ($r = .44$ with criterion). General chess knowledge, rather than chess memory for specific patterns, appears to be critical to chess skill.

Re-examination of human search in chess

The results of De Groot (1965) which showed few differences between highly skilled and less skilled players in their search patterns helped motivate the concentration of research on the pattern recognition hypothesis. In view of the difficulties with that hypothesis, research attention has begun to switch back to search in chess; this is particularly evident in the work of Holding (1985) and Charness (1981b).

From analyses of thinking-aloud records obtained from 34 players in a move choosing task, Charness (1981b) found steady increases in the depth, breadth and speed of search as skill increased from ratings of 1283 to 2004; similar findings were also reported by Holding and Reynolds (1982). Thus, it appears that De Groot's early results were somewhat misleading and probably reflected the small sample sizes and the relatively small range of skill levels in his study.

Accepting then that forward mental search increases in scope and speed with increasing skill, are any other changes in search patterns detectable with changes in skill? One important aspect of search is evaluation. If poor evaluations are made at the limits of search, then the choices made at the top level of the search tree are likely to be in error. Indeed, it has been shown in computer studies that when evaluation procedures are poor, deeper look-aheads can lead to worse decisions than shallower look-aheads (Pearl, 1983).

Holding (1979) investigated the relationship between overall skill level and quality of evaluation. He asked 50 players to assess the relative advantages of whichever side they thought was winning. The assessments were made on a 10 point scale over 10 board positions. The results indicated clearly that judgements of which side was winning were much better in the more skilled players and that the different classes of player differed in the degree of discrimination they showed among the game positions. Thus, skilled players used a wider range of the scale than weaker players.

Holding also compared the subjects' judgements with evaluations of the positions delivered by Seale and Atkin's (1977) highly rated program, Chess 4.5. This programme assigns overall scores to positions on the basis of features such as king defence, pawn structure, rook connection, file control, and queen mobility and attack. The program's evaluations correlated very highly with those of the top half of Holding's players ($r = .91$). The correlation with the lower half of Holding's sample was lower, but still striking ($r = .80$). These results suggest a reasonable measure of analogy between the factors entering into expert human chess evaluation and those incorporated into the evaluation function used in the Chess 4.5 program.

An important difference between more and less skilled players then is in procedural knowledge of how to evaluate the promise of board positions accurately.

Non-Adversary Problems

This section focuses on skill-related differences in non-adversary problem-solving, in semantically rich knowledge domains, such as physics, mathematics, computer programming, map reading and political science. A common theme of investigations of expertise in such domains is the role of the structure of knowledge in high-level cognitive performance. Studies typically show that experts, in contrast with novices, know more and what they know is better organised. In addition, the superior performance of experts is highly domain specific and disappears with tasks outwith the area of expertise. Furthermore, instead of perceiving and remembering individual pieces of information, experts process meaningful groups of information, making their perception more efficient and recall performance much higher than that of novices.

Physics

Consider the domain of physics problem-solving. To solve a textbook physics problem, a solver must first apply certain principles to produce several equations, which are then combined to yield the desired expression. Firstly, then, a problem representation must be constructed in the context of knowledge available for a certain type of problem. If knowledge useful for a problem is accessed when the problem is categorised, Chi, Feltovich and Glaser (1981) hypothesized that expert-novice differences may be related to the nature of problem categories. To test this hypothesis, expert and novice physicists were asked to sort problems on the basis of similar solution methods. No quantitative differences emerged between the two groups, suggesting that capacity differences were not at the root of the difference. The categories were, however, qualitatively dissimilar. Experts sorted problems on the basis of major physics principles, such as Newton's Second Law, while novices sorted problems according to similarities in surface structure, such as objects or key words specified in the problem statement. The results support the notion that problem categories corresponding to problem schemata exist. Thus, the experiment provides evidence of a link, albeit indirect, between expertise and perception.

In many ways, the model of the physics expert is similar to the pattern recognition model of the chess expert discussed previously. The physics expert and the chess master are hypothesized to have large amounts of highly structured knowledge, subsets of which are triggered by meaningful aspects of the situation. These subsets of knowledge, whether they are physics principles or chess patterns, make available a response to the situation - generation of equations or chess moves, respectively.

Mathematics

Schoenfeld and Herrmann (1982), in a study of problem perception and knowledge structure in expert and novice mathematical problem solvers, provide direct support for the perception/expertise hypothesis. Theories of problem solving typically hold that problem schemata influence the way problems are perceived and that with experience, the quality of a problem representation is expected to improve with a corresponding improvement in problem perception. Schoenfeld and Herrmann controlled for age and ability, two factors possibly confounded with expertise in other contrasting-group designs, and found that after a period of training in the solving of mathematical problems, novices showed sorting different to that of the control (no training) and more like that of experts. Specifically, the experimental group perceived problem relatedness more like the experts - according to methods governing problem solution - than did the control group, although the experimental group's performance could not truly be called expert-like. This experiment provides direct support for the hypothesis that criteria for problem perception shift as a person's knowledge base becomes more richly structured.

Computer Programming

What of models of experts and novices in the domain of computer programming? Adelson (1981) addresses the question of how novice and expert programmers represent and use programming concepts. Fundamental to this study is the notion of "chunking". Whilst long-term memory is a limitless repository of permanent knowledge and skills, any information active at a given time is held in a limited capacity working memory. Chunking increases capacity and allows a single concept to represent a collection of related items, which in time enables much more information to be processed automatically and efficiently. In Adelson's study novice and expert programmers were shown randomly ordered lines of PPL code which could be organised syntactically or on the basis of principles of program function. Experts recalled more lines of code than novices. In addition, chunk size for experts (i.e. lines of code recalled with inter-response times of 10 sec or less) was larger than that for novices. Scaling solutions showed that novices cluster terms from the same syntactic category whereas experts cluster items belonging to the same program. This suggests that both experts and novices have conceptual categories for elements of a programming language, the novices' being syntactically and the experts' being semantically based. The results do not, however, indicate whether the programmers' skill was due to encoding or retrieval.

A rather similar study was carried out by McKeithen, Reitman, Rueter and Hirtle (1981), again looking at expert and novice computer programmers. Subjects of three skill levels were shown a 31-line ALGOL W program in either normal or scrambled version for five two-minute study trials. Skill level was found to differentiate recall performance for the normal version but not the scrambled version, replicating the Chase and Simon (1973a, b) results for random chess patterns. Their next step was to examine differences in the way subjects organise their recall. Using the measure PRO (possible recall orders) it was apparent that experts were not more organised than novices, and that their organisations were not deeper than either intermediates or beginners. What of the content of organisations? The homogeneity of organisations within skill levels was examined and a connection found between expertise and particular mental organisations of concepts in the field of expertise. The data do not prove that this organisation produces expertise. They do show that experts know more or less the same things, and know them in the same way, as indicated by the fact that several chunks are shared.

A certain anomaly in the Adelson study was a failure to demonstrate superior recall and changes in the nature of conceptual categories between long-term and short-term novices. Long-term novices were those individuals who had completed more than two programming courses plus the expert with the least experience. The short-term novices were those currently enrolled in their first programming class. This seems to conflict with McKeithen's results which suggest a gradual acquisition of knowledge, as indicated by the fact that, at the end of their first programming course, novices had begun to acquire some of the experts' chunks. A study by Ehrlich and Soloway (1982) supports the gradual transition hypothesis. Their study examined the use of tacit plan knowledge by expert programmers. Ehrlich and Soloway adhere to the theory that expert programmers use their higher level knowledge to code programs for ease of recall, but depart from Adelson and McKeithen in that they hypothesise that experts encode this higher level knowledge in the form of script-like plans which represent certain stereotypical actions in a program. Since experts may be unaware of using a structure such as the "Running Total Loop Plan", the focus of the study is on procedural as opposed to declarative knowledge. The technique used was essentially a "fill-in-the-blank" task, and the programming language, PASCAL. Problems concerned the initialisation of variables and context effects. Results are consistent with the hypothesis that experts use tacit knowledge enabling them to react appropriately to constraints operating on initialisation and update of variables, and to contextual constraints implicit in a program. One advantage of the study is that it captures something of the stereotypical nature of programming skill, which is absent in the Adelson and McKeithen studies. Skilled programmers seem to engage in a process of selecting from memory an appropriate plan and adapting this to meet the needs of the current situation. That novices were able to initialise counter variables would suggest that they share with non-novices a piece of tacit knowledge, but of course this does not mean that they share a particular plan. Their solutions may be based on entirely different knowledge bases.

Map Reading

We turn now to consider research on expert/novice differences in map memory. Preceding research might lead one to predict better memory for map information amongst skilled as opposed to unskilled users of maps. However, the study by Thorndyke and Stasz (1980) presents something of an anomaly, since their expert users failed to perform consistently better than novice map users in a map memory task, leading the authors to conclude that domain knowledge did not contribute to performance differences. A study carried out by Gilhooly, Wood, Kinnear and Green (in press) resolves the issue. Thorndyke and Stasz employed schematic maps rather than contour maps. Thus, the maps used may not have allowed the experts' advantage to show; schematic maps are mainly used for tourist purposes and were probably equally familiar to both expert and novice subjects. Gilhooly et al. employed both contour maps and schematic maps. They report two experiments which found that better memory by experts held for the contour maps, but not for schematic maps, thus suggesting that the possession of specialised schemata facilitates map memory in experts. This interpretation was supported by an analysis of thinking-aloud protocols in the second experiment.

Political Science

Political science problems are usually regarded as non-adversary, and ill-structured, in that there is seldom an agreed-upon solution. Voss, Greene, Post and Penner (1983) carried out an interesting study employing thinking-aloud protocols. Subjects were asked how to increase crop productivity in the Soviet Union. Voss et al. found that all subjects attempted to isolate one or more factors producing the problem, but experts also carried out an extensive problem analysis. The solution was accompanied with an examination of the implications of the proposed solution. Such an examination is similar to search in chess, in that the ramifications of candidate moves or solutions are considered. In contrast with experts, novices were not effective in using their knowledge, and spent little time on developing arguments to support their solution. Voss et al. suggest that it is the knowledge of the inter-dependencies that exist within a domain that enables the individual to develop argumentation. In addition, the development of hierarchical structures, where a set of subproblems are seen as subordinate to a more abstract concept, such as "lack of capital investment", is held to enhance the ability to retrieve information. They concluded that the experts' superior performance was due to the organisation of knowledge, gained as a result of experience in the domain, into effective patterns. These patterns are then accessed during the application of domain-specific strategies. The explanation is very similar to the model of chess expertise in its focus on patterns, although a second factor contributing to the expert's performance was the level of support backing up a candidate solution. Here, "search" or considering the implications of a proposal may play a key role.

Problem solving procedures

What of the problem-solving procedures adopted by novice and non-novice solvers? Experts seem to represent a problem in terms of schemata containing factual knowledge and procedural knowledge of appropriate solution methods. In addition, experts in the domain of physics, for example, are able to minimise working memory load by adopting a "working forwards" strategy. Larkin, McDermott, Simon and Simon (1980) describe experts as generating equations forward from the givens toward the goal, whereas novices solve problems using means-end analysis, working backward toward the givens by choosing new equations that might solve for unknowns in preceding equations. Once equations allowing a solution are obtained, novices reverse the process and work towards the goal. An interesting paper by Sweller, Mawer and Ward (1983) suggests that means-end analysis retards the acquisition of appropriate schemata characteristic of expert problem solvers, because control of moves is vested heavily in the goal, leaving little attention to be directed at essential aspects of problem structure, thus reducing learning. Experts, on the other hand, employ a knowledge-based strategy which is dominated by previous experience. Their results indicated that presenting problems with non-specific as opposed to specific goals facilitated the acquisition of expertise in mathematical problem solving. So, it seems that the strategy typically employed by novices is also the one most likely to inhibit the processing of aspects of problem structure required for expert problem solving. During problem solving then, the nature of the goals and subgoals held in working memory are perhaps equally as important as the structure of knowledge in long-term memory.

Discussion and Conclusions

Research on adversary problem solving, and chess in particular, has led to the development of the chess expert model which is based on the pattern recognition hypothesis. Specifically, the chess expert's skill is proposed by Chase and Simon (1973a, b) to be explained by superior memory storage and recognition of familiar patterns. Thus, chess memory is held to determine chess skill. To a large extent, this model of the chess expert has been borrowed by researchers studying non-adversary problem solving in the domains of physics, computer programming, mathematics, political science and map reading. Overall, the adoption has been a success. The model has provided a framework in which to examine differences in the structure and organisation of knowledge in experts and novices.

However, it is now apparent that the chess expert model requires, at the least, some modification. Recent research on chess skill, as we noted earlier, has raised questions about the adequacy of the pattern recognition theory. The work of Charness (1981a, c) on age and skill in chess has shown that individuals of equivalent skill differed in performance on a chess memory task. Chess memory, then, cannot be the sole determinant of chess skill. In addition, Holding and Reynolds (1982) found that skilled players selected better moves than unskilled players when confronted with random positions. Again, this is not consistent with the pattern recognition theory.

As we saw earlier, these findings led to a re-evaluation of the pattern recognition theory and a return to an examination of the role of search and evaluation in chess. No such parallel exists in the adjoining field of non-adversary problem solving. Research on non-adversary problem solving suggests that expertise is associated with better memory for items within the field of expertise. In addition, a central role is assigned to old knowledge in the acquisition of new knowledge, although researchers vary in the extent to which "knowledge" is defined as domain specific information, general world knowledge or knowledge about strategies for knowledge acquisition and application. Clearly, research in the domain of physics by Chi et al. (1982) places much emphasis on the structure and organisation of knowledge, arguing that the problem-solving difficulties of novices can be attributed mainly to inadequacies of their knowledge bases. Such an emphasis ignores the fact that the nature of goals and sub-goals in working memory can influence skill acquisition (Sweller et al., 1983).

In addition, although Voss et al. (1983) interpret their results in terms of the pattern recognition theory, it is clear that search and evaluation are important aspects of skill in social science problem solving. Indeed, Voss et al. state that "whereas the first time that the expert was confronted with the problem it was necessary to conduct an 'organised search', this becomes less necessary with repetition". In other words, as knowledge is acquired in a particular domain, problem solving becomes more schema driven as opposed to search driven. Gick (1986) raises an interesting point with regard to this. Researchers employing the expert-novice paradigm must use tasks that are sufficiently familiar for a novice to be able to solve them. For an expert, however, such problems may range from transparently easy to only moderately difficult. Thus, it is hardly surprising to find that experts solving physics problems work forward from a schema. The nature of the problems precludes the use of search based strategies by experts. This suggests that studies of expertise may well have failed to capture the essence of expert performance in their disregard of the role of search and in their focus on knowledge organisation and structure.

Accounts that play down the role of information processing in experts seem vulnerable to questions about how expertise developed in the first place, and why it is that two individuals with equivalent experience differ in level of skill development? Brooks (1977) in a study of cognitive processes in computer programming stated that differences between novice and non-novice subjects are to be expected, but what <u>is</u> surprising are the "large differences among subjects of the same general background, intelligence levels and experience", and the fact that a programmer good at writing one kind of program is not necessarily good at writing other, similar programs. What are the factors that preclude the use of relevant knowledge?

Clearly, knowledge and process must work interactively in a complex and as yet not understood manner.

It seems that future research must aim to redress the discrepancy between approaches to adversary and non-adversary problem solving. This means examining search-based strategies as well as schema-driven strategies in experts. Only then will we be able to construct a picture of expertise that is both accurate and useful to researchers and educationalists alike.

References

Adelson, B. (1981). Problem solving and the development of abstract categories in programming languages. Memory and Cognition, 9, 422-433.

Alty, J. (in press). Machine expertise. In K.J. Gilhooly (Ed.), Human and machine problem-solving. London and New York: Plenum Press.

Brooks, R. (1977). Towards a theory of the cognitive processes in computer programming. International Journal of Man-Machine Studies, 9, 737-751.

Brown, J. (1958). Some tests of the decay theory of immediate memory. Quarterly Journal of Experimental Psychology, 10, 12-21.

Charness, N. (1976). Memory for chess positions : resistance to interference. Journal of Experimental Psychology : Human Learning and Memory, 2, 641-653.

Charness, N. (1981a). Aging and skilled problem-solving. Journal of Experimental Psychology : General, 110, 21-38.

Charness, N. (1981b). Search in chess : age and skill differences. Journal of Experimental Psychology : Human Perception and Performance, 7, 467-476.

Charness, N. (1981c). Visual short-term memory and aging in chess players. Journal of Gerontology, 36, 615-619.

Chase, W.G.,& Simon, H.A. (1973a). Perception in chess. Cognitive Psychology, 4, 55-81.

Chase, W.G., & Simon, H.A. (1973b). The mind's eye in chess. In W.G. Chase (Ed.), Visual information processing (pp.215-282). New York : Academic Press.

Chi, M.T.H., Feltovich, P.J., & Glaser, R. (1981). Categorisation and representation of physics problems by experts and novices Cognitive Science, 5, 121-152.

Clark, M. (in press). Adversary problem-solving by machine. In K.J. Gilhooly (Ed.), Human and machine problem-solving. London and New York : Plenum Press.

De Groot, A.D. (1965). Thought and choice in chess. The Hague : Mouton.

Ehrlich, K., & Soloway, E. (1984). An empirical investigation of tacit plan knowledge in programming. In J.C. Thomas & M.L. Schneider (Eds.), Human factors in computer systems. Norwood, N.J. : Ablex.

Frey, P.W., & Adlesman, P. (1976). Recall memory for visually presented chess positions. Memory and Cognition, 4, 541-547.

Gick, M.L. (1986). Problem solving strategies. Educational Psychologist, 21, 99-120.

Gilhooly, K.J., & Green, A.J.K. (in press). Learning problem-solving skills. In A.M. Colley & J.K. Beech (Eds.), The acquisition and performance of cognitive skills. Chichester : John Wiley & Sons.

Gilhooly, K.J., Wood, M., Kinnear, P.R., & Green, C. (in press). Skill in map reading and memory for maps. Quarterly Journal of Experimental Psychology.

Hearst, E. (1977). Man and machine : chess achievements and chess thinking. In P.W. Frey (Ed.), Chess skill in man and machine. New York : Springer-Verlag.

Holding, D.H. (1979). The evaluation of chess positions. Simulation and Games, 10, 207-221.

Holding, D.H. (1985). The psychology of chess skill. Hillsdale, N.J. : Lawrence Erlbaum Associates.

Holding, D.H. & Reynolds, J.R. (1982). Recall or evaluation of chess positions as determinants of chess skill. Memory and Cognition, 10, 237-242.

Larkin, J.H., McDermott, J., Simon, D.P., & Simon, H.A. (1980). Models of competence in solving physics problems. Cognitive Science, 4, 317-345.

McKeithen, K.B., Reitman, J.S., Rueter, H.H., & Hirtle, S.C. (1981). Knowledge organisation and skill differences in computer programmers. Cognitive Psychology, 13, 307-325.

Miller, G.A. (1956). The magical number seven, plus or minus two; some limits on our capacity for processing information. Psychological Review, 63, 81-97.

Newell, A., & Simon, H.A. (1972). Human problem-solving. Englewood Cliffs, N.J. : Prentice-Hall.

Pearl, J. (1983). On the nature of pathology in game searching. Artificial Intelligence, 20, 427-453.

Peterson, L.R., & Peterson, M.J. (1959). Short-term retention of individual verbal items. Journal of Experimental Psychology, 58, 193-198.

Pfau, H.D., & Murphy, M.D. (in press). The role of verbal knowledge in chess skill. American Journal of Psychology.

Schoenfeld, A.H., & Herrmann, D.J. (1982). Problem perception and knowledge structure in expert and novice mathematical problem solvers. Journal of Experimental Psychology : Learning, Memory and Cognition, 8, 484-494.

Simon, H.A., & Gilmartin, K. (1973). A simulation of memory for chess positions. Cognitive Psychology, 8, 165-190.

Seale, D.J., & Atkin, L.R. (1977). Chess 4.5 - the Northwestern University chess program. In P.W. Frey (Ed.), Chess skill in man and machine. New York : Springer-Verlag.

Sweller, J., Mawer, R.F., & Ward, M.R. (1983). Development of expertise in mathematical problem solving. Journal of Experimental Psychology : General, 112, 639-661.

Thorndyke, P.W., & Stasz, C. (1980). Individual differences in procedures for knowledge acquisition from maps. Cognitive Psychology, 12, 137-175.

Von Neumann, J., & Morgenstern, O. (1944). Theory of games and economic behavior. Princeton, N.J. : Princeton University Press.

Voss, J.F., Greene, T.R., Post, T.A., & Penner, B.C. (1983). Problem solving skill in the social sciences. In G. Bower (Ed.), The psychology of learning and motivation, Vol.17, pp.165-213. New York : Academic Press.

Wagner, D.A., & Scurrah, M.J. (1971). Some characteristics of human problem-solving in chess. Cognitive Psychology, 2, 451-478.

Cognition and Action in Skilled Behaviour
A.M. Colley and J.R. Beech (Editors)

DISCUSSION: CHANGING REPRESENTATIONS OF SKILL

Ann M. Colley and John R. Beech
University of Leicester

One of the most obvious ways in which performance changes during the acquisition of a skill is in the use of processing resources by the performer. Early in acquisition of both cognitive and motor tasks the learner is able to attend to only a small portion of the task, at the expense of the rest. Although this observation is hardly novel, we are still some way from producing a coherent and comprehensive explanation of it.

Three of the papers in this section focus on topics which are relevant to this issue. Logie, Baddeley, Mane, Donchin, and Sheptak look at changes in the way in which working memory is used during the acquisition of a complex cognitive skill. The ACT* theory of Anderson (1982) suggests a major role for working memory early in skill acquisition when facts about performance, given by instruction or retrieved from declarative memory, are being assembled and proceduralised. These facts are assembled in working memory for proceduralisation into task-specific productions. Later in acquisition, when procedures (Productions) are well-established, working memory is used to initiate sequences of mental operations or to shift strategy during performance. The model of working memory first produced by Baddeley and Hitch (1974) is still under development, and part of the aim of the Logie et al. paper is to further our knowledge of the way in which different subsystems, i.e. the articulatory loop and the visuo-spatial sketchpad are used in the different components of a complex computer game.

They achieved this by examining the effects of a secondary task on the performance of a game requiring complex cognitive and motor skills. In the first experiment on well-practised subjects, they found that a number of secondary tasks (such as word repetition and the syntactic analysis of sentences) impeded game performance or were themselves impaired. A more detailed analysis of over 50 parameters of performance on the game revealed that secondary tasks had different effects on these parameters. The effects were quite reliable, for instance, when two of the secondary tasks (continuous articulation and tapping) were used in the next experiment with most of the previously tested subjects, exactly the same components manifested interference. This time the visuo-spatial sketchpad was tested as well as equivalent conditions requiring verbal processing. All of the secondary tasks produced interference. Thus a task such as the Brooks spatial task, intended to have specific effects in the game-playing environment, had a more general or pervasive effect on several components of game performance, in this case on aspects of game playing requiring spatial processing. The final experiment, on relative newcomers to the game, revealed that after three hours, repetition and tapping tasks showed no interference effect and there was a marked difference between a visualisation and equivalent verbal task with the former showing relatively more impairment. Further training resulted in interference effects in the repetition and tapping tasks. The computer game studied here required a much greater diversity of demands than is usually the case. This makes interpretation of the results rather difficult. One might conclude that secondary tasks that require concurrent verbal, semantic or visual processing will interfere with overall game performance. Given that so many parameters in the game were monitored, it is not entirely clear why particular parameters were impaired by the secondary tasks. It would be fair to say that it would be difficult to predict which game components would be affected for each secondary task, except in a few minor cases; for instance, the Brooks spatial task actually impaired steering. However, given that a particular secondary task specifically interfered with a particular configuration of game components in certain cases, the existence of specialised areas of resources is implied, as suggested by Logie and Baddeley.

A popular methodology in the study of the changes in performance which occur during skill acquisition is the comparison of expert and novice performance on a given task. Gilhooly and Green review literature on the use of memory by experts and novices in problem-solving tasks from both adversarial and non-adversarial domains.

One suggested distinction between experts and novices known as the pattern recognition hypothesis (e.g. Chase & Simon, 1973), derived from work on chess, is that experts have an extensive repertoire of patterns and schemata which have developed over a number of years. This repertoire is used to encode and structure new information relevant to their area of expertise. Computer simulation of this model by Simon and Gilmartin (1973) demonstrated that a richer repertoire of patterns in long term memory leads to more efficient encoding of board positions in short term memory. Gilhooly and Green cite experimental evidence against the pattern recognition hypothesis, which suggests instead that chess memory is associated with chess skill but does not determine it (Holding, 1985). What appears to be more important is procedural knowledge of the way in which board positions lead to various game states. In non-adversarial problem-solving, such as in physics, explanations of differences between experts and novices borrow heavily from the pattern recognition hypothesis. There has been, as yet, little attempt to look at differences between experts and novices in procedural knowledge, although some investigators have traced the acquisition of procedural knowledge in cognitive skills, for example the study by Anderson, Farrell and Sauers (1984) on learning LISP. The way forward seems to lie in what Gilhooly and Green describe as the interaction between "knowledge and process".

In the attention literature, a major focus of debate in recent years has been the concept of automaticity. It has long been observed that after many hours of practice at certain tasks, performance has the appearance of being "wired in" or automatic. Such changes in performance have been problematic for theories of attention and information processing, for example Single Channel Theory partly owes its demise to reaction time experiments which found that after a large amount of practice the Hick-Hyman Law breaks down (Siebel, 1963), and to our ability to perform two resource-demanding activities at once (Shaffer, 1975).

Although performance may appear to be automatic, providing an adequate definition of automaticity has proved to be a major problem as Phillips and Hughes point out. A number of characteristics have been used to distinguish between automatic and controlled processing (Shiffrin & Dumais, 1981). Those referred to most frequently in the literature are that: automatic processing is activated without conscious awareness, usually without intention and may be activated in parallel with other processing. Controlled processing requires attention, usually involves awareness and intention and uses up processing resources which cannot then be applied elsewhere.

Some investigators (e.g. Cheng, 1985) have taken issue with such hypothesised properties. She argues against the necessity for assuming capacity-free processes and makes the analogy between resource limitations in processing and hardware limitations in a computer. Automaticity overcomes hardware limitations, but resource limitations can also be overcome by modifications to the software or "restructuring" of the task components. Phillips and Hughes also tackle the problem of defining automaticity and examine the internal consistency of the definitions used by two-process theorists such as Posner and Snyder (1975) and Schneider and Shiffrin (1977).

Phillips and Hughes have examined the effects of manipulation of awareness on controlled and automatic processes. Their task was an auditory two-choice reaction time, requiring a movement lasting less than 250 ms. Phillips and Hughes argue that the reaction time prior to the response requires controlled processing, whereas the subsequent fast movement time is automatic. Since two-process theories assume that awareness is involved in controlled but not automatic processing, any manipulation of awareness should affect reaction time but not movement time. Awareness was manipulated by requiring subjects to rate the duration of the reaction time or movement time of their response. They found greater effects of this manipulation on movement time than on reaction time. This, they argue, suggests that awareness is coordinated with automatic processing, and is evidence against a simple two-process view. Their study therefore adds to the steadily-mounting evidence against the simple automatic-controlled distinction. Part of the problem with this distinction is, as Shiffrin and Dumais (1981) point out, that most tasks require a mixture of controlled and automatic processing so it is difficult to find exemplars of either type. This problem, in itself, suggests that the distinction in its present form may not be a particularly useful one. It may well be that a number of different mechanisms underlie the apparent decrease in processing resources used as a particular skill becomes established, and that we should be looking at changes in the way mechanisms are used during skill acquisition, rather than assuming that a qualitatively different form of processing becomes established. For example, Anderson (1982) has demonstrated that ACT* can account for speed-up by its processes of composition, generalisation and discrimination of productions (algorithmic improvement which reduces the number of productions used in a given task), and by strengthening of productions. As learning progresses, processing is reduced in terms of the number of procedural steps, and becomes more task-specific. The use of working memory is therefore reduced. According to Hunt and Lansman (1986) it may be absent altogether. In their production activation model automatic processing occurs through spreading activation between productions and is independent of working memory. Controlled processing requires the manipulation of the contents of working memory by productions. This kind of model focuses on changes in the way in which processing mechanisms are used. It therefore does not rest solely on definitions drawn from the behaviour to be explained, which, as Phillips and Hughes suggest, is a feature of two-process theories which has been criticized for its circularity. If automaticity is defined according to this model, then it does not involve awareness in the sense that working memory is not used. Some processing may be initiated by productions rather than via working memory or via an external cue and therefore does not require an explicit intention. The role of intention and awareness varies with the task or task component in question, and disparate findings in the automaticity literature can potentially be reconciled. Dual task performance may be explained by the lack of data-specific or function-specific interference between tasks, which either require the use of different mechanisms or which are structured over learning to involve different mechanisms (Allport, 1980).

One of many factors which can potentially affect the performance of a cognitive or motor task is interference from other task components, or from sources extrinsic to the task. Such interference, while impairing performance, is of potential use for the researcher since it allows inferences to be made concerning the source of the interference, and hence underlying mechanisms.

The literature on motor short term memory is rife with results which are contaminated by interference effects from the experimental tasks used which have affected the encoding of movement information (Colley & Kitchen, 1983; Gentile & Nemetz, 1978; Kerr, 1978). Problems of interpretation pervade many studies in this area which has now ceased to attract the attention of researchers. Interference effects on the encoding of movements have re-emerged in the growing literature on contextual interference (Lee & Magill, 1983; Shea & Morgan, 1979; Shea & Zimny, 1983). Contextual interference results from the way in which movement patterns are presented during task acquisition. Blocked practice and random practice have different effects on acquisition and retention, with random practice resulting in poorer acquisition performance but better retention. The Shea and Zimny (1983) explanation is in terms of the intraitem processing which occurs for both practice conditions and the interitem processing which occurs only for the random condition. Interitem processing is more elaborative and distinctive and aids recall by providing multiple retrieval routes. The contextual interference effect can be consistently demonstrated. What is proving more difficult is the provision of an adequate theoretical explanation of the effect.

The original aim of the study by Limons and Shea was to follow up a conclusion drawn by Shea and Zimny concerning the separability of recall and recognition of movement patterns. Random practice results in good recognition and recall performance, whereas blocked practice results in good recognition performance only. This led Shea and Zimny to suggest that intraitem processing is necessary for recognition, while intra- and interitem processing is necessary for recall. Limons and Shea used a standard contextual interference paradigm, which compares blocked practice with random practice, but added recognition training prior to acquisition trials in order to examine its effect on subsequent recall. Three types of recognition training were used: no training, training with the acquisition task patterns, or training with task patterns not used in the acquisition trials. This training had no effect on the contextual interference effect. Recognition performance was good for both blocked and random subjects. Random practice resulted in better recall regardless of recognition training. A more surprising result was that recall of subjects who had received recognition training with the task patterns was worse than that of subjects who had trained with patterns not used in the task or those who had received no training. Limons and Shea interpret this finding in terms of deficient processing. Subjects who saw the movement patterns used in acquisition trials during recognition training were able to retain these in working memory and use them during acquisition, rather than processing them completely as other groups who saw them only during acquisition trials were obliged to. Their intraitem processing (and interitem processing for the random subjects) was therefore deficient.

A different explanation of contextual interference effects from that of Shea and Zimny (1983) has been offered by Lee and Magill (1985). The "spacing effect" was first found in experiments in short-term retention of verbal materials using a modified version of the Brown-Peterson paradigm (Peterson, Wampler, Kirkpatrick, & Saltzman, 1963). In these experiments an item is presented twice before a filled retention interval and recall. The inter-presentation interval between the two presentations of the item is also filled to prevent rehearsal. For a given retention interval, recall was found paradoxically to improve as the inter-presentation interval got longer, so that the greater the forgetting of an item between its two presentations, the better was its subsequent recall. Forgetting therefore appears, in some circumstances, to facilitate retention. As an explanation of this effect Lee and Magill turn to Jacoby (1978) who suggested that if an event is repeated, the processing of that event is not necessarily also repeated. The previous solution, if still available, is used without the processing necessary to find it being repeated. This "short-cutting" of the processing required to encode an item in memory may impair long-term retention. Forgetting of an item between presentations can therefore facilitate retention. The explanation offered by Lee and Magill is easily-reconcilable with the deficient processing explanation used by Limons and Shea to explain their recognition training findings. By deficient processing, Limons and Shea are referring to the use of previously encoded material to reduce the amount of processing undertaken on subsequent similar material.

Whichever explanation of contextual interference eventually finds favour, the effect itself has important implications for motor skill learning. The way in which practice is administered can have a clear effect on the retention of movement-related information, and it appears that at least early in learning it may be important to ensure that the learner undertakes all of the processing required for a given task.

In cognition there has been much recent debate on the effects of irrelevant speech on performance. Quite apart from the practical implication of being distracted by irrelevant speech, this work also has important theoretical implications. Miles, Madden and Jones examine the theoretical issues and present their own experimental evidence from short-term visual memory tasks and proofreading. Three types of explanation have been offered to explain the disruptive effects of irrelevant speech. These are first, phonological interference, which occurs when memory for phonological codes is dealing with two simultaneous inputs; second, that speech increases arousal which restricts cue utilization; third, various attentional theories propose interference due to competing verbal messages. In the last case, the locus of the interference depends on whether a given theory proposes early or late selection. Miles et al. review studies from other investigators, and from their own laboratory which support the phonological explanation for the disruptive effect of irrelevant speech on visual memory. Their results on proofreading, however, suggest a separate disruptive effect of irrelevant speech on the early stages of processing by meaningful speech.

One of their findings is particularly interesting in the context of the previous discussion of contextual interference. In experiments examining the effects of backwards or forwards English speech or Welsh on visual short-term memory, they found a general impairment across all positions for serial recall but not for free recall. As Miles et al. point out, serial recall is more "difficult". It requires the maintenance of information concerning the ordinal positions of items in short-term memory, as well as the items themselves. This requirement may place extra importance on the role of rehearsal, which will presumably allow these ordinal relationships to be retained. Irrelevant speech may interfere with rehearsal sufficiently to prevent ordinal information from being encoded, but the interference may not be sufficient to prevent encoding of the items themselves. Parallels can be drawn between this effect and the "deficient" encoding found by Limons and Shea. It is necessary for full processing to take place in the case of movement patterns or for full rehearsal to take place in the case of visually-coded items in order for necessary task-related information to be retained.

The papers in this section point to two major areas in which our knowledge of the mechanisms underlying skilled performance is currently expanding. Firstly, further investigations of the roles of working memory, domain-related knowledge and procedural knowledge in performance will help to clarify the way in which they are used at different levels of expertise. The way in which the use of these mechanisms interacts with skill level may account for findings attributed to two different processes of attention. Secondly, the studies reported by Miles et al. and by Limons and Shea remind us that we must not neglect to examine how task-related information is encoded. There are strong practical implications of this work, not only in the design of laboratory tasks, but in training and skilled performance outside of the laboratory.

References

Allport, D.A. (1980). Attention and performance. In G. Claxton (Ed.), Cognitive psychology: New directions. London: Routledge & Kegan Paul.

Anderson, J.R. (1982). Acquisition of cognitive skill. Psychological Review, 89, 369-406.

Anderson, J.R., Farrell, R., & Sauers, R. (1984). Learning to program in LISP. Cognitive Science, 8, 87-129.

Baddeley, A.D. & Hitch, G.J. (1974). Working memory. In G. Bower (Ed.), Recent advances in learning and motivation. Vol.8. New York: Academic Press.

Chase, W.G. & Simon, H.A. (1973). Perception in chess. Cognitive Psychology, 4, 55-81.

Cheng, P.W. (1985). Restructuring versus automaticity: Alternative accounts of skill acquisition. Psychological Review, 92, 414-423.

Colley, A. & Kitchen, S. (1983). Criterion movements in motor short-term memory experiments. Acta Psychologica, 53, 119-128.

Gentile, A.M. & Nemetz, K. (1978). Repetition effects: A methodological issue in motor short-term memory. Journal of Motor Behavior, 10, 37-44.

Holding, D.H. (1985). The psychology of chess skill. Hillsdale, N.J.: Erlbaum.

Hunt, E. & Lansman, M. (1986). Unified model of attention and problem solving. Psychological Review, 93, 446-461.

Jacoby, L.L. (1978). On interpreting the effects of repetition: Solving a problem versus remembering a solution. Journal of Verbal Learning and Verbal Behavior, 17, 649-667.

Kerr, B. (1978). The effect of invalid task parameters on short-term motor memory. Journal of Motor Behavior, 10, 261-273.

Lee, T.D. & Magill, R.A. (1985). Can forgetting facilitate skill acquisition? In D. Goodman, R.B. Wilberg, & I.M. Franks (Eds.), Differing perspectives in motor learning, memory and control. Amsterdam: North-Holland.

Peterson, L.R., Wampler, R., Kirkpatrick, M., & Saltzman, D. (1963). Effect of spacing presentations on retention of a paired-associate over short intervals. Journal of Experimental Psychology, 66, 206-209.

Posner, M.I. & Snyder, C.R.R. (1975). Attention and cognitive control. In R.L. Solso (Ed.), Information processing and cognition: The Loyola symposium. Hillsdale, N.J.: Erlbaum.

Schneider, W. & Shiffrin, R.M. (1977). Controlled and automatic human information processing: I. Detection, search and attention. Psychological Review, 84, 1-66.

Shaffer, L.H. (1975). Multiple attention in continuous verbal tasks. In P.M.A. Rabbitt & S. Dornic (Eds.), Attention and Performance V. London: Academic Press.

Shea, J.B. & Morgan, R.L. (1979). Contextual interference effects on the acquisition, retention and transfer of a motor skill. Journal of Experimental Psychology: Human Learning and Memory, 5, 179-187.

Shea, J.B. & Zimny, S.T. (1983). Context effects in memory and learning movement information. In R.A. Magill (Ed.), Memory and control of action. Amsterdam: North-Holland.

Shiffrin, R.M. & Dumais, S.T. (1981). The development of automatism. In J.R. Anderson (Ed.), Cognitive skills and their acquisition.

Hillsdale, N.J.: Erlbaum.

Siebel, R. (1963). Discrimination reaction time for 1023-alternative task. Journal of Experimental Psychology, 66, 215-226.

Simon, H.A. & Gilmartin, K. (1973). A simulation of memory for chess positions. Cognitive Psychology, 8, 165-190.

AUTHOR INDEX

SUBJECT INDEX